Did You Know Your Diagnosis Is Bullshit?

(a how-to guide to diagnosing with kindness)

Steven Paglierani
(with Maria Kirsch)

Published by
The Emergence Alliance Inc / Emergence University Press
55 Old Nyack Tpke., Ste 608
Nanuet, NY 10954

SAN 859-5380

https://stevenpaglierani.com (The author site for this book)

https://theEmergenceSite.com (This site contains many of the early discoveries which led to the ideas in this book. And while I've since refined a lot of my terms and ideas, some readers may find it of interest.)

Paglierani, Steven. T., 1946-

Did You Know Your Diagnosis Is Bullshit
(a how-to guide to diagnosing human suffering with kindness)

Book V in the Finding Personal Truth series

Includes bibliographical references.

ISBN 978-1-948911-02-3 (soft cover, color interior)
ISBN 978-1-948911-03-0 (ebook, fixed pages, color interior)

1. Psychopathology / Assessment, Testing & Measurement 1. Mental Health Diagnosis 2. Emergence Personality Theory
1. title

302 pages. 103,318 words. 133 color illustrations.

PSY042000 PSYCHOLOGY / Assessment, Testing & Measurement
MED018000 MEDICAL / Diagnosis
PSY022000 PSYCHOLOGY / Psychopathology / General
PSY029000 PSYCHOLOGY / Reference

Library of Congress Control Number: 2024937153

Printed in The United States of America

Printing Number
29 28 27 26 25 24 10 9 8 7 6 5 4 3 2 1

Dedication

To my life partner and closest friend, Hanna. Thank you for convincing me to believe in my dreams again. And for silently sitting with me when I so often have wanted to quit.

Other Books by Steven Paglierani

Solving the Mind Body Mystery (Why Do Some People Lose Their Words)
[978-0-9844895-3-4 Soft Cover 2010]

Unraveling Human Nature (How Well Do You Know Yourself?)
[978-0-9844895-4-1 Soft Cover 2011]

The Science of Discovery (Why Do Scientists So Rarely Make Breakthroughs)
[978-0-9844895-5-8 Soft Cover 2016]

Therapy For Therapists (a guide to changing lives)
[978-0-9844895-9-6 Soft Cover 2020]

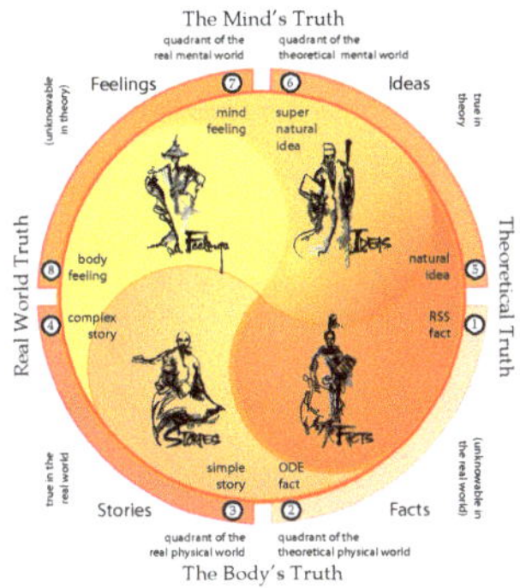

Table of Contents

Reader's Guide

An Unvarnished Book 1569

A Few Words From a "Still Becoming Human" Author 1569
Everyone Diagnoses—Some of Us Do It Professionally 1569
My Early Career as a Diagnostician 1570
What Is This Book About? 1571
What Were The Four Prior Books About? 1572
A Few Things To Keep In Mind As You Read 1576
Finally, Few Words of Encouragement 1577

Introduction

The Art of Diagnosis 1579

Can Diagnosis Become a Science? 1579
Could (and Should) You Explain "Diagnosis" to a Patient? 1582
Why Are Diagnostic Manuals Called "Manuals?" 1586
Aren't These Manuals Supposed to Teach You How To Diagnose? 1587

What's Wrong With Dictionaries (Mere Lists of Single Points)? 1588
Why Haven't I Felt Unsure When I've Diagnosed? 1590
So How Do I Diagnose? 1592
A First Look At The Diagnostician's Funnel 1593
Could You Visually Teach Bipolar Mania to a Patient? 1595
What Will We Address In This Book? 1596

Chapter 1

The Invisible Mind 1599

Can We Make What's In The Mind Visible? 1599
How Many Variables Do You See In This Drawing? 1602
How Many Variables Will You Need To Learn? 1603
What Does Any of This Have To Do With The Depression Line? 1604
What Part Does The Information Variable Play In All This? 1606
A Single Moment Square with Multiple Dots 1607
Contrasting and Comparing The Rectangle and The Square 1608
What's the Big Deal About the Space in Between Corner Dots? 1611
Introducing the "Three Information Sinks" 1611
How Does A Series of Single Moments Become An Event? 1613
A Blank Event-Line Rectangle 1614
The "Normal State of Mind" Event Line 1615
How Does Depression Differ From a Normal State of Mind? 1616
How Does Mania Differ From the Normal State of Mind? 1617
How Does Mania Differ From Depression? 1618
How Does Dysthymia Differ From Depression? 1619
How Does Dysthymia Differ From the Normal State of Mind? 1620
Can You Possibly Have Trouble Telling These Four Lines Apart? 1621
Should You Believe This Stuff Without It Being Peer Reviewed? 1621
What Will We Look At Next? 1623

Chapter 2

Wounds or Symptoms? 1625

What Should Diagnosticians Be Looking For? 1625
What Will We Talk About In This Chapter? 1626
Change Type One: Getting Overwhelmed 1630
Change Type Two: Getting Wounded 1633
Change Type Three: Reliving a Wound 1636
What's the Most Painful Change? A Hint. It's Not Getting Wounded 1638
Change Type Four: Healing a Wound 1640
Regression and Transference: the Symptom Making Machine 1642
So Where Do Symptoms Come From? 1644

Where's My Proof That The Mind Does This? 1645
How Much of What Patients Remember is a Reconstruction? 1646
Are All Wounds, "Context Independent?" 1647
What Does It Mean to Say Wounds Are "Context Independent?" 1648
How Does Healing Alter Regression Transference Loops? 1648
How Do You Diagnostically Discern Clinical Significance? 1651
The First Kind of Meta-Symptoms: Wincing and Flinching 1652
Have You Ever Noticed A Client Wincing? 1652
To Diagnose, You Must Learn to See Winces 1653
The Second Meta-Symptoms: Sudden-Onset Mental Blankness 1654
The Third Kind of Meta-Symptoms: Being Unable to Picture Things 1654
Lastly, a Brief Look At The Word "Disorder" 1656

Chapter 3

Measuring Personality 1657

How Many Drawings Should It Take To Define Personality? 1657
How Many Qualities Will It Take To Define Personality? 1658
Can Human Beings Ever Become Fully Conscious? 1660
A Brief Look at Those Five "Fractal" Filters 1667
Have You Ever Opened a Russian Nesting Doll? 1667
The Core Personality as The Four Nested Sublayers of Layer 7 1670
Character State / Type Urges: the 1st Sublayer of Layer 7 1671
Character Type - The Primary and Secondary States 1672
Social Priorities Urges: the 2nd Sublayer of Layer 7 1674
Identifying Regressions Based on Social Priorities 1675
Decision Tree Urges: the 3rd Sublayer of Layer 7 1680
How Can Ralph and I Have the Same Decision Tree? 1682
Decision Trees as a Factor in Majority vs Minority Personalities 1682
Majority vs Minority Personalities: Part 1 - the Social Priorities 1684
Majority vs Minority Personalities: part 2 -the 4 Decision Trees 1686
The KA Social Priority Grouping (1 - 6) 1688
Determining a Person's Diagnostic Baseline 1688
The OCD Social Priority Grouping (7 - 12) 1689
The AS Social Priority Grouping (13 - 18) 1690
The ADD Social Priority Grouping (19 - 24) 1690
Rant Warning: Unprofessional Words Ahead 1692
What Makes Minority Personalities Measurably Different? 1693
Finally, Here Comes the Rant 1694
Can We Scientifically Define "Autism?" 1694
What Does the Word "Autism" Actually Refer To? 1696
Autism, OCD, Asperger's, and ADD as Normal Responses to Life 1697

What is Autism? 1697
We All Suffer From Some Degree of Autism 1698
Personality is Not *Behavior*. It's What Does Not Get Filtered Out. 1702

Chapter 4

Classifying "Disorders" 1703

Can We Stop Treating People Like They're Broken? 1703
The Diagnostic Sequence (the Next Three Chapter's Topics) 1705
There Are Two Kinds of Disorder—One Kind Is *Not* Diagnosable 1706
Diagnosable Disorders Come in Two Sizes—Event & Personality 1708
Primary Causes of the "Disorder" in Event-Sized Disorders 1710
Secondary Causes of the "Disorder" in Event-Sized Disorders 1711
How Do Personality-sized Disorders Differ? 1713
The Two Kinds of Event-sized Disorders: Simple and Complex 1715
There Are Two Kinds of Personality-sized Disorders 1716
The Two Kinds of Personality-sized Disorders: Fixed and Transitional 1716
The Two Kinds of Bipolar Information (affective vs schizophrenic) 1718
Picturing the Diagnostic Lines in Three-Dimensional Space 1720
What About All The Other Kinds of "Personality" Disorders? 1729
The First Year of Life - Undifferentiated Information 1729
Differentiation: the Key to Diagnosing Personality-sized Disorders 1731
Information-Based Differentiation in The First Year of Life 1732
Personality-Based Differentiation in The First Year of Life 1736
What Happens to Babies in the Second Six Months? 1738
What Develops in Most Babies During The Second Year? 1739
Seeing a Baby Tip From First to Second Year of Life Development 1739
What Then Is A "Personality Disorder"? 1740
What Must A Personality-sized Disorder Diagnosis Include? 1742
Finally, A Few Thoughts On The Scientific Method I'm Using 1743

Chapter 5

Evidence Gathering (a guide) 1745

How To Diagnose: Part One | Evidence Gathering 1745
What Do I Mean By "Evidence?" 1746
What About Using Scientific Inferences (Hypotheses) As Evidence? 1747
What's Wrong With Hypotheses? (The Drunk Who Lost His Keys) 1748
How Is The Diagnostic Process Like A Journey? 1749
A Few Things You'll Need To Do During The Diagnostic Process 1750
Why Divide The Diagnostic Process Into Two Parts? 1751
Can You Recall The Five Things You Need to Keep In Mind? 1751
Can Math Ever Accurately Measure People? 1752

What's Wrong With Using Existing Maths To Measure People? 1752
How Accurate Is Math In General? 1755
What's Wrong With Using Counting Math to Diagnose People? 1756
What's Wrong With Using Scale-Based Math to Diagnose? 1758
What's Wrong With Using Statistics to Diagnose People? 1760
What About Tipping-point Based Math? Any Flaws There? 1762
Evidence Gathering: Introducing The Four Steps 1762
Evidence Gathering's Four Steps: The Importance of This Sequence 1763
Step One - Use Initial Data to Begin to Set The Diagnostic Baseline 1763
Bonus Points - Have the Patient Write Down Their Problems 1764
Step Two - Have the Patient *Slowly* Elaborate the Presenting Problem 1764
Bonus Points - Physically Document and Separate the Gathered Evidence 1764
Step Three - Construct a Detailed Mental Image of the Disorder Present 1765
Bonus Points - Bookending & Complex Event-sized Disorders 1765
Step Four - Note The Direction of The Patient's "Internal Tide" 1765
Bonus Points - Spend Time Learning Measurable Personality Measures 1765
Four Things *to Keep in Mind* As You Begin to Gather Evidence 1766
Four Things *to Not Do* As You Begin to Gather Evidence 1767
The Flashlight Metaphor (Is All Evidence Developmental?) 1768
The Idea That Evidence Exists on Two Experiential Time Lines 1770
Composite Triggers | A Kind of Falsely Reported Evidence 1770
Composite Triggers | An Example: Rich and Leeanne 1773
Do These Few Details Tell Us Anything Useful? 1773
An Exception To The Warning Against Inferring Evidence 1774
A Second Example of Composite Triggers: Derrick and Nicolette 1775
Correcting "Assumed to Be False" Evidence | A Diagnostician's Error 1778
The Case of The Piece of Shit Boyfriend 1779
Does Determining The Truth of What Patients Tell You Matter? 1781
How The Novelty of An Event Affects A Patient's Sense of Truth 1782
The Patient's Truth: The Takeaway 1785
The Idea That "Evidence Gathering" Is "Pre-Learning" 1786
Why Do Babies Love Pre-learning? 1787
The Two Ways to Learn Who The Patient Is: Questions and Guesses 1788
Avoiding the Logic Trap: Why Logical Diagnoses Fail 1789
A Few Final Hints About What to Watch For 1790
Does Diagnostic, Evidence Gathering Ever Get Done? 1790
When Do We Get To The Diagnosis? 1792

Chapter 6

Letting The Diagnosis Emerge 1793

Diagnosis | Part Two - Allowing the Evidence to Speak For Itself 1793

Identifying "Birth to Six Months," Using Developmental Qualities 1797
Why Am I Calling These Cards, "Bingo Cards?" 1797
Identifying "Six Months to Age One," Using Developmental Qualities 1799
Identifying "Age One to Age Two," Using Developmental Qualities 1801
Identifying "Age Two to Age Four" Using Developmental Qualities 1803
Grand Rounds Case #1 - Introduction 1803
Linda's Case – A 13-Year-Old Girl Named Alyssa (pre-case intro) 1804
Linda's Case | A 13 Year Old Girl Named Alyssa - Intake (part 1) 1811
Evidence Gathering - Alyssa's Intake | First Thoughts 1824
My Apologies For What I've Just Put You Through: The Old Way 1827
Linda's Case | A 13-Year-Old Girl Named Alyssa - Linda (part 2) 1829
Evidence Gathered in Therapy Sessions | Do You Know Alyssa? 1834
Symptoms vs Personality | Which Kind of Evidence Matters More? 1834
My Short List of Diagnostic Baseline Elements 1836
Diagnosis & Treatment | Beginning the Differential Assessment 1837
The Overarching Clinical Concern: How Is Stress Affecting Patient Reporting? 1837
The 1st Differential: Sort Evidence to Determine Features of Personality 1837
The 2nd Differential: Determine Major vs Minor Personality 1839
The 3rd Differential: Diagnosable or Not? 1841
The 4th Differential: Creating the Diagnostic Hierarchy 1842
1st Hierarchical Differential | Level One vs Level Two 1844
2nd Hierarchical Differential | Natural vs Unnatural Subtype 1847
3rd Hierarchical Differential | Healthy vs Unhealthy 1847
4th Hierarchical Differential | Single Points vs A Constellation 1848
A Nine-Month Journey To A Provisional Diagnosis 1849
One Final Reminder: The Goal Here—Let The Diagnosis Emerge Naturally 1850

Epilogue

Questions & Comments **1851**

Diagnosis | What Have I Learned From Writing This Book? 1851
My Diagnostic Takeaways | A Short List 1852
A Few of My Takeaways 1854
My Most Surprising Personal Takeaway: ***Compatibility*** ***1855***
One—We Almost Exclusively Infer About Avoiding Bad Things 1856
Two—The Mind Treats Inferences As Facts; as Something That Has Happened 1856
A Few Places To Look When Trying To Find Inferences 1856
Using Context Independence to Determine Minority Personalities 1857
What Do We Do With The Existing Diagnostic Manual? 1859
Closing Comments And Thoughts on Future Books 1860

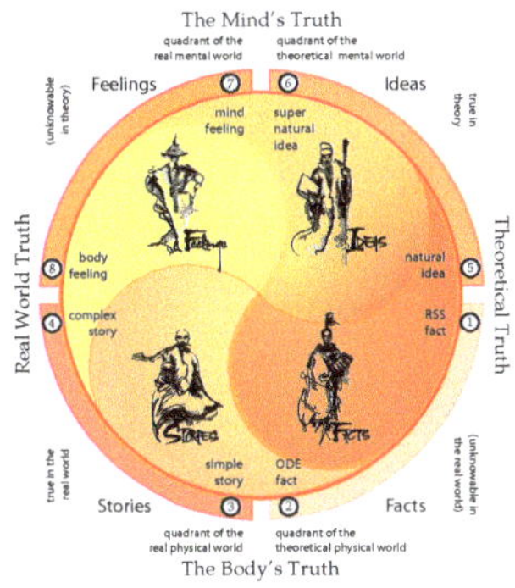

Reader's Guide

An Unvarnished Book
(what's in it for you . . . ?)

A Few Words From a "Still Becoming Human" Author

Based on this book's title, I imagine, many professionals will pass on it. When I think about them doing this, I feel surprised by my near-total lack of concern. I've purposely chosen this title in hopes I'll pique the interests of people who value being human more than being professional. No coincidence, this includes me and my many colleagues, most of whom have spent whole lives helping people.

Know I count among my colleagues warm-hearted grandmas and new mothers, many of whom function as the family diagnostician. If any of this fits you, then you are definitely in the right place—especially if you've wanted to call "bullshit" on the things many so-called professionals claim to know about you and those you love. In truth, if you've made it this far, I'm quite sure you've felt this way many times. Please (mad author shouting to the heavens), how about some chicken soup for the soul, rather than more chicken shit for the mind. This said, I would not expect you to read much further without me giving you the five-cent tour. What will this book do for you? What's in it for your patients? This is what I'm about to tell you.

Everyone Diagnoses—Some of Us Do It Professionally

Let's begin with this book's main point—that almost everyone alive diagnoses. Sadly, despite the word "manual" in the titles of existing diagnostic manuals, as of today, we have no manual to guide us.

No previous diagnostic manual offers anything even close to the warm, caring guidance we deserve. In truth, no existing diagnostic manual has even treated us like human beings. Not a one.

Am I angry about this? Yes. I admit, I am. But I'm feeling less angry than I felt a moment ago. Perhaps this is happening because I already feel so personally connected to you, the reader? As I think about it, I can see that I do feel this way.

How can this be? You and I have barely met and already, I've cursed a lot.

How?

Because somehow I know that you and your loved ones have suffered a lot. And maybe, just maybe, at times, you feel as angry about this as I do.

I also suspect that like me, you (or someone you love) may have, at some time, been diagnosed. I have. More than once.

If so, have you ever had your diagnosis properly explained to you, in a way that made sense? Or were you, like me, treated like a fragile moron, too dumb to understand or too weak to hear it?

Clearly, being treated like this is just plain wrong. This said, know I don't believe in bitching about the faults of others if I don't have something better to offer. In fact, in this book, I'm going to claim that part of making this better is up to all of us.

What will we need to do?

I'm going to claim that we all need to learn at least the basics of how to diagnose.

Why would we need to do this?

Because we all suffer. So we all should be able to know for ourselves the gist of what is wrong. Also, my career as a diagnostician began just after I turned seven. I suspect, yours may have begun at an early age too.

Me, I've waited most of my life for someone to teach me how to do this.

So who am I writing this book for? Can you guess? For one thing, I'm writing this book for seven-year-old me. Of course, I'm writing it for seven-year-old you as well. I'm also writing it for all the unborn children who will come into our world.

My Early Career as a Diagnostician

As I just told you, my career as a diagnostician began when I was seven years old. At seven, I began trying to diagnose my mom. She suffered from *undiagnosed* schizophrenia her whole life—and died at age 48 of *undiagnosed* anorexia.

Undiagnosed. Did this mean she was better off than her brother?

Not by much.

My Uncle, Constantine, who did get diagnosed, lived behind state hospital bars from age nineteen until his late fifties. Then, in the 1980's, medications which could adequately imprison him in his mind arrived. So they finally released his body. He then lived out the rest of his life in some sort of home for over-medicated schizophrenics. I saw him only a few times in my life. He never spoke one word.

Nineteen years as a human. Sixty plus years as a prisoner. I've always felt my uncle deserved better.

I've also always felt guilty that I couldn't be the one to help him, even a little. I still wish I could have. But of course, these wishes were just the dreams of an over-sensitive boy. And knowing I was as over-sensitive as he was only made me worry I'd break inside, just like he did.

Then there was my mother's mother. I've never been told her name. She too was a prisoner in that same state hospital. We'd drive there on Sundays to visit her and on the way in, we'd pass building after stone-cold looking building. I can still hear the screams and tortured cries coming from the faceless souls staring out at me from behind those iron-barred windows.

I recall, at age seven, desperately wishing I could in some way help them too. Now here I am, seventy plus years old, and I'm still trying. I've often wondered if my grandmother ever stood, howling and sobbing from behind those bars. I never knew. My family refused to talk about her, no matter how many times I asked.

Know that when I say, "we'd visit," I wasn't talking about me. Per doctor's orders, I was never allowed to see my grandmother, not even once in my life. My mother would go in. My father would stay with me. And on rare occasions, I'd be left to play on the lawn. And occasionally, I'd play with some other little boy whom I assumed had a similarly imprisoned uncle or grandma.

Know this book will not at all focus on my childhood struggles or on me. But I figured I should at least offer you a few of my qualifications as a fellow human.

Now, having done that, let me tell you about this book.

What Is This Book About?

This is my fifth book.

The previous four are more textbooks than easy reading.

Know this book is largely a practical composite derived from the previous four books. This one does have some textbook shit in it. But it's also filled with easy-to-read pages.

There are also dozens of interesting drawings—the kind young children love. My hope this time? That I can reach the five or six-year-old child in you.

The curious, wide-eyed, aspiring child diagnostician who loves looking at the pictures.

The seven-year-old who desperately wants to be taught how to help.

Know I had similar hopes each time I released one of my previous books. I hoped they would make a difference in at least a few people's lives. What I now know is that words alone, no matter how eloquently expressed, can never adequately describe the human mind.

The only way to reach the mind, in a lasting way, is with pictures.

This then is the first thing this book will offer you—a way to understand, and teach yourself to speak about—the mind, in fine detail. Not mainly with words, mind you. Rather, with a visual alphabet. This alphabet is comprised entirely of easily recalled drawings of colored shaped lines.

What are these lines like?

A flat one will teach you to know the state of mind we call "depression."

A jagged one will teach you what "mania" is like.

A curvy one will show you what a "normal" state of mind looks like.

A less-curvy one will teach you what "dysthymia" (low normal) is.

Then there are two, strangely shaped lines which reveal the nature of getting wounded and healing. How does getting wounded, and healing, change the mind? Imagine being able to teach your patients what these two things are, along with the nature of their diagnosis? Imagine giving this to them in ten minutes or less?

Know that each time you do this, that person will be able to effortlessly retain a sense of who he or she are for the rest of his or her lives. How can any of this be possible? It is. I promise. To do this though you'll need to learn to harness the visual power of fractal drawings. "Fractal?" You'll hear this word a lot in this book.

Like ocean waves and candle flames and cumulus clouds, fractal shapes are easily learned, recognizable patterns. Children learn these fractal patterns in minutes. They then effortlessly retain this knowledge for the rest of their lives.

The fractal drawings you'll be exposed to in this book will do the same for you. What you won't be required to do in this book, though, is to suffer through endlessly boring technical words. Rather, this book will mainly be a "look at the pictures" book. That's how I'll teach you to do this—to diagnose in such a human way that diagnosing someone can and will change this suffering person's life.

Imagine that.

Imagine teaching someone what their diagnosis means in a kind caring way.

Imagine doing this with such warmth and clarity that it changes their life, for the rest of their life.

This is what you'll learn how to do in this book. And yes, it will take work and a good amount of patience. But I believe in you. You **can** do this.

What Were The Four Prior Books About?

Something you'll hear over and over in this book is the idea that diagnosis begins and ends with understanding interpersonal relationships. In other words, you cannot hope to diagnose any person without first gaining evidence about how they interact with others. In a very real way then, the model this book uses for diagnosis parallels physicist Carlo Rovelli's physical model of the world.

Rovelli calls his model, "Relational Quantum Mechanics."

The essential idea behind RQM is that different observers may give different, but accurate accounts of the same system. The model I use in this book is similar. All things begin with understanding how human beings can give different, but accurate (from their point of view) accounts of their relationships. So a good way to understand this perspective is to see it as part of "The Relational Model of the Mind."

Know this model begins with, and is largely based on, what is contained in my prior four books. All these books function as parts of this Relational Model of the Mind. And the main ideas here are simple. We human beings cannot know ourselves in isolation. Ever. Rather, we can know ourselves only in relation to other human beings. As for the prior four books, here's the five-cent tour.

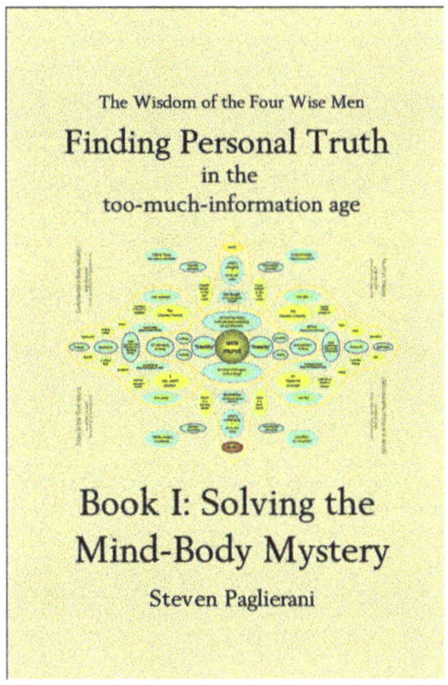

Book One—*Solving the Mind-Body Mystery (2010, Emergence Alliance Publishing, New York)*—is the foundation on which all the other books are built. Know the title of this book is somewhat misleading. The title mentions but one small part of this book. The main subject? That all of the changes we humans experience between birth and death begin with, and end with, how our minds do and don't ***differentiate*** what we experience—the Four Kinds of Information.

Oops. Difficult sentence. I'm likely talking about things you have yet to learn. If I confused you, I apologize. Even I sometimes lapse into unreferenced shit and technically difficult language. Forgive me. Let me try again. This time, we'll use a picture. So I'll need to ask you to use your mind. Try to imagine what it feels like to be one day old. What would your mind be like? What kinds of thoughts would you be thinking?

Here, a difficult word—but one you'll hear over and over in this book—is the only succinct way I know to describe what this experience is like.

The word?

Undifferentiated. Beyond "totally mixed up."

"Totally mixed up" infers there are separate, but unsorted, parts. But here, the word ***undifferentiated*** means something like "mentally driving in fog at night without lights on." Even this description misses the mark. It refers to the baby's mind as if it contains parts. A newborn baby's mind has no parts.

Rather, a newborn baby's mind is completely filled with raw data. Moreover the baby has yet to assign meanings to this data. This data has no meaning. Then, from day one on, babies continue to take in this kind of data. So at first, all they're doing is what I call, "pre-learning."

Pre-learning is the process by which babies gather data, ***without assigning meanings***. They then gather more data, then more data, and on and on. This is what pre-learning is. It's not understanding. It's just gathering data.

When does the learning occur?

To begin with, learning isn't a process.

What is learning then?

Learning refers to what happens whenever a fractal pattern emerges in a baby's mind. Realize, what actually emerges isn't like what your adult mind constantly fills with. Babies fill their minds with visual differences between two related patterns.

A square versus a circle. Mommy versus grandma. Doggie versus birdie. Me versus you.

Here again, we see that word—***relational.***

Learning is "seeing how similar visual things ***relate***."

This process is how babies ***differentiate*** the data they take in.

No coincidence, the fundamental skill in diagnosis is referred to as "finding the differential." The ***differential*** refers to the visual differences between two similar but different kinds of suffering people.

Where does my first book fit in with learning to diagnose?

It's the first book to differentiate the four ways the baby's minds sort information. This is one of the main things you'll learn to recognize and use in this book. You'll also learn how babies acquire these four abilities developmentally.

Why learn this? Because this can tell you a lot about who a person is and why they're suffering. Definitely a plus whenever you need to diagnose.

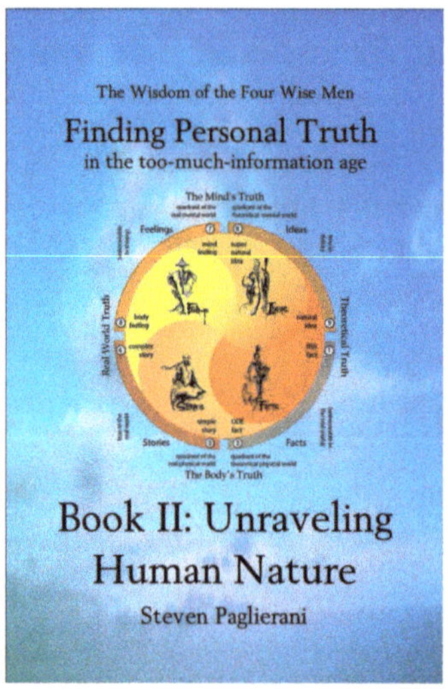

The second book? Book Two—***Unraveling Human Nature*** *(2011, Emergence Alliance Publishing, New York)*. The diagnostic skills in the present book draw a lot from the descriptions of personality in that 2nd book. That book describes an entirely new way of defining and measuring the differences between human beings. In it is the first personality theory to be based entirely on fractal patterns—as opposed to all previous efforts, all of which are based on statistical reductionist bullshit.

This said, the present book repeatedly references things from that earlier book. So anytime you need more explanation for things in this book, know, you can always find detailed descriptions of these things in that 2nd book.

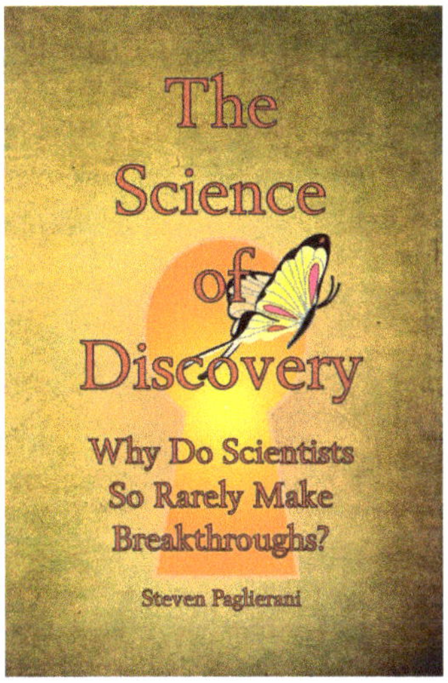

Book Three? *The Science of Discovery (Why Do Scientists So Rarely Make Breakthroughs?) (2016, Emergence Alliance Publishing, New York)*. All the science I base the present book on is described in depth, in that book.

What's different about the new science? For one thing, it's based entirely on two new maths—the two maths I use in this book. The first new math measures real world things about human beings—as they are, out in the world. It also does this with 100% accuracy. Then the second math marries logic and geometry in order to perfectly define the things the first math measures.

Together, these two new maths—for the first time—create theoretical concepts which then translate perfectly to the real world. This alone should tell you, something is special here. Current attempts to measure people rarely translate well to the real world. All the things you'll learn in this book do.

Know that in four of the chapters in that third book, I used this new science to make discoveries. I did this in four areas of life—sleep, weight change, deafness, and cancer. In all four cases, I had no idea how well the new method would work. Can you imagine the faith I needed to attempt to do this?

I was trying to make discoveries in areas I'm not professionally trained in.

In the end though, it all worked out well. Indeed, many of my patients have benefited from the things I discovered there.

How then does the idea of "scientific discovery" relate to diagnosis?

The act of diagnosing IS you trying to discover things about a human being.

Of course, to do this, you need an extremely good method. That third book supplies this method. I'm confident this process can work for you too.

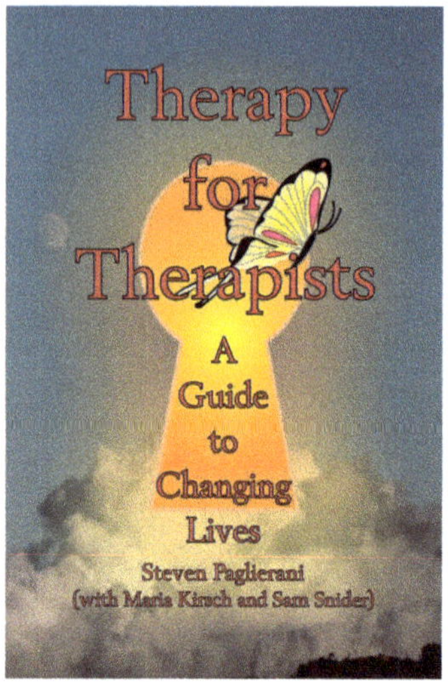

Finally there's Book Four—*Therapy for Therapists (A Guide to Changing Lives)* (2020, *Emergence Alliance Publishing, New York).* In this 4th book—and based on my thirty-plus years as a practicing therapist—I describe what a science-based therapy would look like. Here the science is Constellated Science, rather than the pathologically flawed old way.

Am I being too hard on the old science?

If you think so, consider this.

All existing diagnostic manuals base their claims and contents on the old science.

How's that been working out for you?

If you're still reading this book, I would guess, not so well.

A Few Things To Keep In Mind As You Read

Finally, a few things to keep in mind which will ensure you get everything you came to get out of this book.

One, and this is important, ***please do not try to memorize any of what's in this book.*** Rather, similar to how the best painters and sculptors create art, instead of a single read through, make many passes. This allows you to learn the same way young children do—by using ***pre-learning*** (unrestricted evidence gathering).

Pre-learning? What's that? Think about it.

No young child tries to memorize.

Rather they simply let their minds drive an "unrestricted, information gathering process." They then continue to do this until the learning naturally emerges in them.

Afterwards, they can effortlessly recall this thing (think waves, clouds, flames).

Know this book will claim, diagnosticians must use this same process in order to feel confident and be effective. So if at first, doing this feels unnatural and doesn't make sense to you, don't worry. You'll get a lot of hints along the way.

Two. ***Pay* more *attention to the subheads, than to the text in between the subheads.*** To do this, just stop each time you get lost, then reread that section's subhead. Then, try to connect this subhead to the content which has just confused you. The points I'm trying to make in that content will always be summarized in that subhead.

Three. ***Remember, I'm writing this book to the human being in you.*** This applies both to professionals and nonprofessionals alike. Know this is especially important for professionals to note. Be a human first. As for you nonprofessionals, know there will be times I choose to speak in technical terms. This is, after all, a technical topic. Just know these words will always be accompanied by what I hope will be my best attempt to translate these terms into everyday language. And if you find yourself struggling, use number two.

Four. This is the big one. ***Always spend time looking at the non-verbal parts of the drawings—before you read the text.*** Looking at diagrams in this order is the opposite of what most people do. Most people read the words first and only then look at the drawing.

Please do your best to not do this. It ruins your ability to learn. And for goodness sake, never try to memorize, let alone expect yourself to understand things completely, on the first pass. No one learns this way.

Five. This one is a small one. It involves ***this book's strange page numbering.*** This book starts way past page one. What's up with that? All five books share one and the same series of page numbers. So the only book that has a page one is Book One. From then on, each new book's page numbers begin from the previous book's last page.

Finally, Few Words of Encouragement

If someone was trying to convince me that I had to relearn much of what I thought I knew, I know I'd be biased towards looking for—and trying to find—flaws in what I was being told. If this is you, please realize, this is exactly what I myself went through as I wrote this book. Like you, everything I'd previously learned about diagnosis was either tainted with statistics or just plain wrong.

Also, as a therapist in private practice for some thirty years, I've hated giving suffering people more evidence they were broken. Most existing diagnoses do this to people. WTF. I also worried their diagnosis could be used against them at some time—the Internet gives people access to all manner of things which should remain private.

This book is not meant to make you doubt yourself.

It's meant to make you less accepting of things you already doubt.

In truth, I've never met a good therapist who doesn't see existing diagnostic manuals as flawed. As I think about it, I doubt I've ever met a therapist who doesn't know those books treat human beings like lab rats.

We humans deserve better.

We diagnosticians do too.

And yes, admittedly, this book's viewpoints radically depart from the norm.

Not once will you find a statistical claim based on artificially contrived lab results—such as those the old science creates. This said, everything in this book has, for years, been successfully used by me and my colleagues to help real people. And isn't this the whole point—to help suffering people to have better lives?

Realize I include you—the reader—in this group.

Wanting to help someone and not knowing how is a terrible burden.

With this book, I hope to lighten your load.

I also wish to reignite that drive and curiosity which first drew you to want to learn to diagnose.

Finally, keep in mind, getting these ideas to emerge in me took a long time. Three decades, to be precise. So please, please, please—do not expect yourself to get it all the first time through. I promise, though, that it will all make sense if you focus on pre-learning. You have it in you to become a world-class diagnostician. My hope is that this little book will be the "manual" you need to do that.

With warm regards,

Steven Paglierani

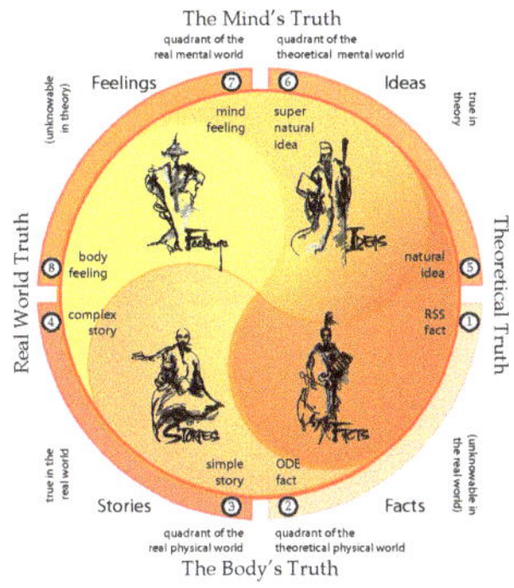

Introduction

The Art of Diagnosis
(what can we learn about . . . ?)

Can Diagnosis Become a Science?

Existing diagnostic manuals base their diagnoses primarily on how similar conditions differ. This idea, which therapists call, "differential diagnosis," should in theory have been one of the more useful aspects of these books. Unfortunately, none of these books define a scientifically sound set of universal diagnostic criteria. Overlaps and omissions, combined with poorly defined terms, make diagnosis more art than science.

Rectifying these errors and omissions will be the main goal of this book—to develop a universal set of diagnostic criteria such that diagnosis becomes more science than art. To do this, we'll need to find better ways to describe and define both existing, and future, diagnoses. Admittedly, this will be an ambitious goal.

We'll also need to address a second problem, something no prior diagnostic manual has offered—a way to distinguish between clinically significant features and what is normal. In part, this lack was due to a political problem. Prior books were created by consensus. To avoid conflicts between the various contributors, they omitted the component critical to defining "normal."

The component? A personality theory. No such theory, or even partial theory, is ever directly mentioned. Ironically, beneath each and every word in these manuals lie assumptions regarding the nature of personality. Strangely, nowhere do these authors enumerate the assumptions behind their claims. Again, a lack of science.

How did these authors think it possible to omit any mention of personality and still diagnose? They chose to focus on functioning—and the lack thereof, as the principal diagnostic criteria. To these authors, and based on the content of these books, who people are as persons matters little. All that matters is whether they function poorly or well.

In large part due to these books, eventually, functioning came to be the main measure for mental health. At which point, the diagnostician's primary task became assessing people for how well or poorly they function. No surprise then that all diagnostic manuals organize diagnoses into vaguely defined categories of poor functioning. Here differences in personality play no role in evaluations, and anything less than excellent functioning raises questions as to whether to diagnose.

This points to what may be the most significant omission in these manuals. Nowhere do they scientifically describe the actual mechanisms of injury or healing. The principal goal of diagnosis is to measure people's wounds—and to a true scientist, what you can't describe scientifically you can't possibly measure. So where are the scientific descriptions of the mechanism of wounding? They offer none.

To me, this particular omission is the most egregious of all. How could anyone claim to understand diagnosis if they can't describe the mechanism of wounding? And no, it's not enough to say injuries correlate to trauma. If this were true, how can the same traumas generate different symptoms in different people? Indeed, how can painful events which cripple some people and not even wound others?

Strangely, none of the eight diagnostic manuals acknowledge this omission. It seems we're just supposed to overlook the lack of actual science. And please, do not bore me with references to patently pseudo-scientific statistical data. Does no one see how these generalizations resemble the standard complaint against newspaper astrology—that by making claims broad enough, no one can say they are wrong?

Rather than seeking real science then, these authors spent their time arguing over words. How should we properly divide-up and name these "dys-functions?" What should we call them? Over time, they increasingly sorted human suffering into more and more vaguely defined categories. The six types of Schizophrenia. The eight paraphilias. The nine types of personality disorders. Or the ten, if you count the NOS category (not otherwise specified). And in case you don't know, NOS is pseudo-scientific code for "we have no freaking idea what to call this kind of suffering—let alone any science to back up what we're claiming."

Arguably, a clue to the source of this confusion lies in the never-mentioned elephant-in-the-room. The principal authors of these diagnostic manuals are American psychiatrists. Meaning what? Generally, American psychiatrists are good-hearted people whose main wish is to remedy suffering. Indeed, I've personally had two change my life, the two to whom I've dedicated this book.

In most cases though, unlike their European counterparts—whose educations require them to be trained as both MDs and psychotherapists, in America, the talk therapist's training part is either optional at worst—or minimal at best. This makes most, not all, American psychiatrists resemble carpenter-tool designers who have never hammered a nail—or plumbers who have never removed the tank cover from a toilet. Certainly, this is nothing like the European founders of their profession—Freud, Jung, Adler, and Janet. These men were both practicing MDs and practicing psychotherapists, as well as being published personality theorists who made significant contributions to that profession as well.

Does this sound like nonsense? Am I pissing you off? Then consider this. This same opinion was being expressed even in 1952, the year the first diagnostic manual came out. By whom? By a noted psychiatrist—and arguably the finest historian of the profession—a man whom I see as far more qualified than I to voice this opinion.

Consider what this man had to say, even back then.

> **A Comparison of European and American Psychiatry**
>
> After a three months trip in the United States in 1952, I was asked by some Swiss colleagues to tell them about my observations in America, and I tried to describe the difference between American and European psychiatry, seen from the point of a Swiss. Later, when I returned to the United States, a friend suggested that I translate the talk I gave in Switzerland into English. Thus, let us imagine that we are in Zurich, and that we are Swiss people interested in hearing about a very different kind of psychiatry.
>
> A European psychiatrist traveling in America is soon overwhelmed by such a wealth of new impressions, experiences, and human contacts, that he easily loses the general picture. Then a little incident will suddenly give him a clue. This happened to me a few weeks after my arrival, while attending a staff meeting where a case history was being discussed. A young psychiatrist was reporting on the life history and troubles of a patient and had begun to discuss the diagnosis, when the leader of the meeting gently interrupted him with this question: "What are his problems, and what can we do for him?"
>
> This meant that the nosologic discussion, interesting as it was for European psychiatrists, was considered idle talk and a waste of time by an American. The interruption meant "Let us go to the question," it was the voice of the principle of reality. It occurred to me then that American psychiatry differs from ours fundamentally in the way of approaching the subject. (Ellenberger, Henri MD. "A Comparison of European and American Psychiatry" Bulletin of the Menninger Clinic; Topeka, Kan. Vol. 19, Issue. 2, Mar 1, 1955)

"Life history?" "Troubles?" Not relevant? Get to the point?

"What are his problems and what can we do for him?"

Some would argue, psychiatrists today do discuss those "not relevant" questions and this is true—but only for the few psychiatrists professionally trained in personality and psychotherapy.

By those untrained in psychotherapy and personality, those for whom assessing functioning is all that matters? By them, not so much. The point is, would you trust a McDonald's cashier to advise you on managing your retirement account? Personally, I'd rather not. How then has it become acceptable for human beings to be judged as mentally well or broken, based mainly on a book authored by people untrained and unskilled in either psychotherapy or personality?

Could (and Should) You Explain "Diagnosis" to a Patient?

People who know me know I like to learn word meanings by taking words apart. I often do this in front of my clients and it awakens mutual curiosity in us both. It can also cause clients to have ahas, after which they can permanently recall what these words mean. This can be especially helpful when giving clients a diagnosis—where breaking words down can lead to important self discoveries.

I've chosen to include this excerpt from my 2020 book, *Therapy for Therapists (a guide to changing lives)* for a number of reasons. It's the opening paragraph to a chapter on "Visual Dialogue," Emergence Psychotherapy's main style of treatment. For one thing, in this paragraph, I admit to deliberately violating a professional tradition I myself personally eschew—the idea that therapists should not discuss with patients the nature of their diagnosis.

To begin with, I do believe there should be limits to doing this. Laypersons' interpretations of professional terms can at times be harmful. This said, much of the problem here can be traced back to how diagnostic manuals are written. Most words they employ more resemble Minoan Linear A than common everyday English.

Ironically, psychotherapy is supposed to improve people's ability to communicate with each other—not make it worse. All lasting personal human connections derive from some form of clear communication. Why write diagnostic manuals in ways which make it hard for us to connect with our patients? Shouldn't these words enable us to help them understand what is happening to them?

In addition, I especially hate (yes, hate) therapists of any kind who think they are above their patients. Based on the language used in existing diagnostic manuals, it seems, the authors of these books think doing this is fine.

I disagree. I see treating patients as beneath us as disrespectful and wrong.

Why do they think it's alright to do this then?

I have a few thoughts.

My best guess is, it's largely due to the overwhelming lack of science in these books. Most terms used in these manuals are either uselessly broad or patently pseudo-scientific. For instance, take the frequently referenced idea that people get "depressed." Have you ever tried to find a clear definition in these books for what they mean by this word?

Please allow me to save you the time. There isn't one. Nor do they scientifically contrast and compare this word to related states of mind like "mania," "dysthymia," or "normal."

In this book, I'll offer you a simple, visual tool with which to teach these states of mind to your patients. It's so simple, in fact, that you could use it to teach these four words to five-year olds—and do it in a single sitting. Yet once taught, patients (and five-year olds) will retain these differences for life.

This alone should make reading this book worthwhile.

Admittedly, some of what I've said so far makes it sound like I'm an insanely angry man. Cranky? Foul-mouthed? Ill-tempered? A resounding "yes" to all these things. Indeed, I suspect I may have already insulted you enough to make you want to hunt me down and professionally kill me.

If this is you, I want you to know, I do understand.

Many readers will have invested much of their lives learning to interpret these words—I do not wish to disregard these efforts. This said, in my career I have frequently had therapists admit to being thoroughly baffled by diagnostic manuals. They then turn to less-reputable sources for explanations, for instance, Dr. Google MD. This alone should tell you a lot about the nature of these manuals. Shouldn't the guidebooks which ground our profession be the ones we trust and turn to?

Finally, despite what it may sound like, know I am not one of those people who casually bash other people's life's work, even when I disagree. Thus for each criticism I make in this book, I intend to offer pragmatically better alternatives. I hope to infuse diagnosis with such kindness and clarity as to make it an inherent part of the healing process. Healing cannot occur when we sit in judgment, above our patients, or when they judge themselves. Rather it occurs only when we seek ways to better partner with our patients—heart to heart, human to human.

For example, consider how I—the cranky, foul-mouthed know-it-all—explain a patient's "diagnosis" to them. I do this looking to strengthen our human-to-human connection, in hopes this will set the stage for healing. The following excerpt also comes from that same chapter-opening in my 2020 book. Keep in mind, I'll be taking apart multiple but similar, and related, words—*dialogue* and *diagnosis* being the main two. Hopefully, this will give you a sense of what is to come in this book.

∞

What does any of this have to do with this chapter's topic, "Visual Dialogue"? Most people reading this phrase will assume they know what this phrase means. If this is you, let me ask you something. Do you know where the word "dialogue" comes from? If you noticed it begins with the same Greek prefix as "diagnosis," then you have a clue.

This prefix, "dia," refers to "going through" or "across" something. For example, take the word "diameter," which roughly means "a line which goes through or across a circle." Here the meaning of the "dia" prefix is obvious, largely because we can picture it. But like many languages, in English, words like "through" and "across" can have multiple meanings. And yes, going "through" or "across" a circle is one kind of meaning. But we psychotherapists often ask clients things like "what was it like to go through that?"

When therapists ask this question, they're using the word "through" to refer to the stuff clients are experiencing. And usually, this stuff is unpleasant, which brings us to the word "diagnosis." Here, the "dia" part I just explained, and the "gnosis" part is a Greek word which refers to personal knowledge. As opposed to intellectual knowledge, which refers to impersonal stuff.

This makes a diagnosis, "a line drawn through a constellation of the personal stuff we call symptoms and signs." Therapists get taught to draw these lines because the same symptoms and signs are often found in more than one diagnosis. Formally, therapists call the act of drawing these lines, "differential diagnosis." Here, clinicians try to place this line so it lands on the most symptoms.

This placement is then supposed to "differentiate" between similar diagnoses, telling clinicians which diagnosis fits best. Unfortunately, even on good days, this process is close to useless. It in no way resembles real science and is more like throwing shit at a wall to see what sticks. Which is why a lot of what therapists say is so incomprehensible to clients.

As for the other word, "dialogue," this word also has more than one meaning. To begin with, when we take this word apart, we again end up with two Greek word fragments. This time, we get "dia" and "logos." Here the "logos" part refers to "words" and "ideas"—in particular, reasonable (impersonal) ones. And the "dia" part refers to the path a conversation takes through these words or ideas.

In effect, "a path through words or ideas" is just another way to refer to what we do in conversations. The thing is, normally, the word dialogue refers to two or more people exchanging words. But when a therapist "visually dialogues" with a client, this conversation is a visual conversation.

Here both therapist and client visualize what's being explored—and words become secondary. By doing this, both therapist and client gain unfettered access to the client's mind, and this makes what's said far more memorable.

∞

Remember my claim a few pages back about teaching five-year olds the four states of mind? What you've just read about "visual dialogue" offers a clue as to how you can learn to do this. The single page I previously referred to uses very few words. Instead what it focuses on is the shapes of four distinctly-shaped lines.

Here each line represents one of the four states of mind—and the easily seen differences between the shapes of these lines is what teaches people how these states of mind differ. Know this idea—visual dialogue—will underpin everything I offer in this book. And in case this concept is still unclear, I've placed a version of that drawing on the following page. Obviously, it's far too soon for me to begin to explain how to use it. I suspect though, even without being told how to use it, it will immediately make sense to most people. The shapes carry the entire meaning.

The Four Life Intensities

(mania, normal, dysthymia, depression)

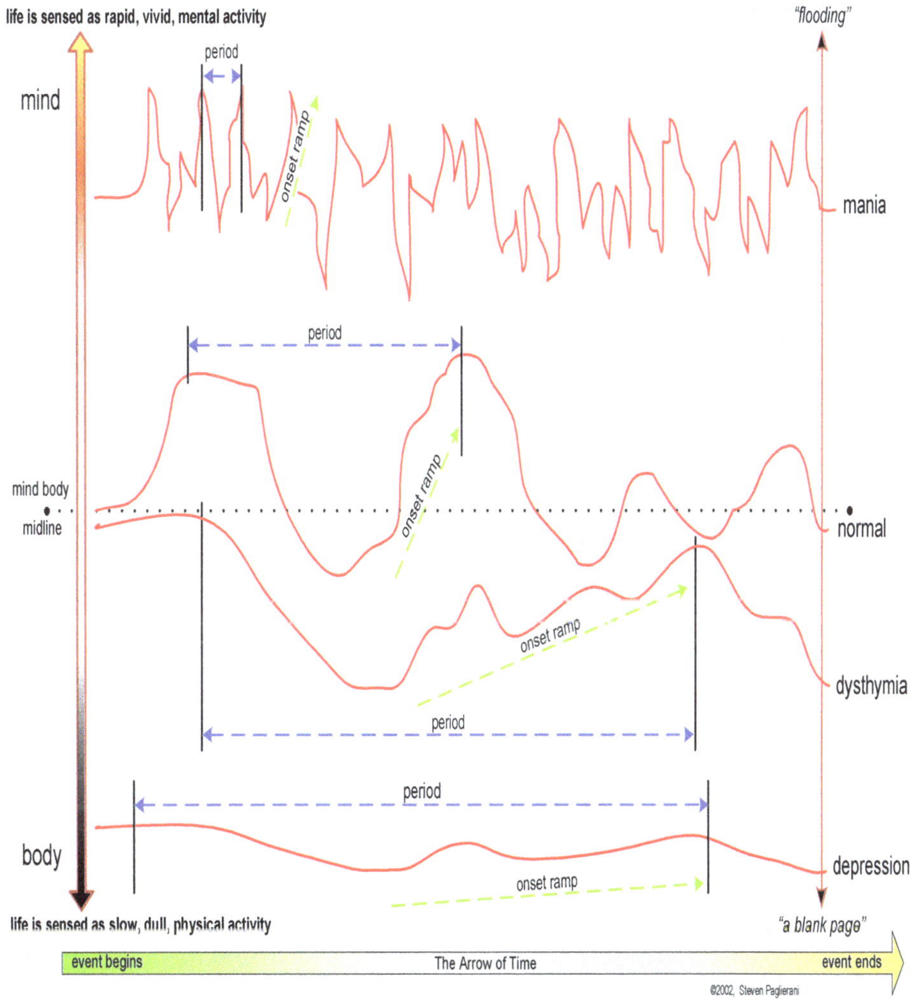

Visual Intensity	Period (peak to peak)	Onset Ramp
mania	very short	very abrupt
normal	medium	moderate
dysthymia	long	gradual
depression	very long	very gradual

At the end of this introduction, I'm going to offer a (hopefully) brief list of what we'll be looking at in this book. Obviously, re-imagining an entire diagnostic manual will require me to address quite a lot. Before I make this list though, I first need to ask you a simple question. Based on what you saw in that previous drawing, the one titled "The 4 Life Intensities," how many words would it take you to explain to someone what's in this drawing—but without showing them the drawing?

How about I make it simpler. The only thing you need to explain is the differences between the four "life-intensity" lines. How many words would you need to use to do just that? Curious? Then try it. Try writing out a description of what you see. Keep in mind, your words must enable a patient or colleague to recognize and understand the essential differences between those four lines—without effort—and for the rest of their lives.

Obviously, words could never accomplish what those four lines do in this drawing. Fortunately, you will have this drawing. So there's no need to worry about this. Of course, you'll need to know how to use it, which by the end of this book I promise, you will. Once you do, you'll be amazed by how helpful it can be.

Why Are Diagnostic Manuals Called "Manuals?"

Speaking of having to learn things, I now have a confession to make. This involves something I realized when I reached this point in writing the book. Up to now, I'd felt good about what I'd written. But each time I tried to write past this point, nothing felt right. Clearly, I was missing something. But what? I had no idea.

This made no sense. I love diagnosing and have been doing it for close to three decades. I've also spent almost five years planning how to organize and write this book. This includes making hundreds of drawings, creating several dozen outlines, and writing thousands of notes. Despite doing this—and despite several attempts to write what I thought should come next, everything I wrote felt flat.

Clearly authors of non-fiction books do not normally admit to such things, certainly not in the actual book. Then again, if you've ever written anything longer than a two-page email, you've likely felt this way yourself. Don't all writers feel stuck at times? Isn't this just part of being a writer? My answer? Yes. But this felt different. I was missing something big. But what?

What added to this confusion involved Marilyn, one of the people I supervise. Marilyn had recently begun a new job after previously working as a nurse for some years. Now, she was a Psychiatric Nurse Practitioner, her first job which included the choice to do psychotherapy. So Marilyn had asked me to do supervision with her to augment areas missing from her education—mainly psychotherapy.

No surprise then that she had been asking me loads of questions. Like most American Psychiatrists, she too had never been trained to do psychotherapy. Strangely though, most of her questions did not involve psychotherapy. Mostly, they were about diagnosis. This seemed odd. After all, wasn't the main focus of her education—and profession—giving and monitoring diagnoses. What was up?

The more I thought about this, the more I realized something that should have been obvious the whole time—everything Psychiatric Nurse Practitioners do centers on a diagnosis. They begin every case by deciding on a diagnosis. They prescribe medication based on what they decide. They also often do psychotherapy based on this diagnosis as well. Then they monitor the patient in both of these areas.

Obviously, Psychiatric Nurse Practitioners aren't the only ones who do this either. The same thing is true for most mental health based practitioners. Everything they do begins and ends with the patient's diagnosis. How was it possible then that Marilyn, a fully licensed Nurse Practitioner, felt insecure about having to diagnose?

Marilyn had also told me, on several occasions, that she loved our talks about diagnosing. If she loved this, shouldn't diagnosis have been a subject she excelled in back in school? This would have made more sense. Yet somehow, here she was, admitting that diagnosing made her feel insecure. Then it hit me. She and I had been feeling similarly lost. But Marilyn was feeling lost about *how to* diagnose. Whereas I'd been feeling lost because of something else.

In that moment, I realized that in all my years trying to re-imagine the diagnostic manual, I'd somehow missed the worst flaw of all. Despite the word "manual" being in the titles of these books, none of them actually explain *how to* diagnose. This then is why I'd been so stuck—all these books call themselves diagnostic "manuals." After all, the word "manual" is literally in the titles of all these books.

In truth though, not one of these books is an actual manual. A manual describes *how to* do things. No diagnostic manual has ever described how to diagnose. What do they do then? Mainly, they make lists of words and phrases which refer to vague categories of human suffering. So rather than how-to guides for diagnosis, these diagnostic manuals are just poorly written psychiatric dictionaries.

How is it possible that in all these years, I had never noticed this—not even once? And what of all the intelligent people in our profession? How is it none of them ever mention this either? To be honest, even now, when I think about this, it still surprises me. Holy shit. This was my stuckness? They're not manuals? They're just dictionaries? So what does this mean? We're about to find out.

Aren't These Manuals Supposed to Teach You How To Diagnose?

Ok. Now I'm going to claim we've just arrived at this book's most important question. Shouldn't the diagnostic manual be a guidebook—shouldn't it teach you *how to* diagnose? After all, despite obvious differences, all psychotherapy-related licenses begin and end in the same place; with a diagnosis. Psychologist. Social Worker. Licensed Mental Health Counselor. Marriage and Family Therapist. Regardless. We all base what we do around our patient's diagnosis.

What does it mean then that we've been basing diagnoses on a poorly written dictionary? As I think about this question, my mind is flooding with thoughts.

Is this why so many otherwise brilliant therapists, including Marilyn, feel insecure when they diagnose a new patient? Surely, this must be part of it.

And what about new therapists—is this why they so often can't think of their next question in sessions? And scientists—is this why they claim psychologies and psychotherapies are at best, soft-sciences? Argh. This one bothers me to no end.

As an aside, after finally writing these last few pages, to my surprise, I found several references to this same idea. For one thing, the American Psychological Association (APA)—the publishers of the DSM-V—on their website, call this book the "APA Dictionary of Psychology." More interesting though, in 2013, NIMH director, Thomas Insel, wrote the selection I've quoted below. It seems I was wrong. I am not the only one to have realized this.

> ***The DSM: A "Dictionary," Not a "Bible"***
>
> *(May 7, 2013) NIMH Director Thomas Insel set the mental health world abuzz last week when he blogged that the National Institute of Mental Health will be "re-orienting its research away from DSM categories." A new edition of the Diagnostic and Statistical Manual for Mental Disorders (DSM-5) is due to be released later this month.*
>
> *"While DSM has been described as a 'Bible' for the field, it is, at best, a dictionary, creating a set of labels and defining each (psychopathology)," said Insel in "Transforming diagnosis" (Director's Blog, April 29). He said that people "with mental disorders deserve better" than a menu of diagnoses that ensures clinicians use the same terms in the same ways but lacks scientific basis.*

What's Wrong With Dictionaries (Mere Lists of Single Points)?

It occurs to me that some readers may see nothing wrong with using dictionaries to diagnose. They may see what's in these books as obvious and self-evident to professionals. If this is you, then consider the way a proper science defines things—versus how dictionaries do it. Dictionaries use lists of vaguely related, single points. A proper science bookends its definitions with pairs of complementary opposites.

Does this difference confuse you? If so, I understand. Most people will never have heard of using pairs of complementary opposites to define things before. Know that once you're taught this difference, it's easy to see why it matters. Dictionaries define things by listing one or more broad references to "what a thing is." Whereas a proper science defines things by telling you not only "what a thing is," but also "what it is not."

The point is, lists of single points can never define things without leaving things out—whereas pairs of complementary opposites (the Tao symbol, for instance) can account for an entire topic. Want to see what this difference looks like? Then ask yourself this. How would an ordinary dictionary define the word "depression?" How much better is the close to useless list of symptoms in any diagnostic manual?

I'm claiming a proper scientific manual would define "depression" so clearly that five-year olds could learn it in minutes. They'd also understand what this word means for the rest of their lives. For example, consider the drawing on the next page. Does it look familiar? It should. It's a smaller version of the drawing from five pages back. Now look at the shape of the Depression line. Now contrast and compare it to the shape of the Dysthymia line. Given you'd learned to see the differences between these two lines, do you think you could mistake depression for dysthymia? Could the differences between these two states of mind be any easier to understand—let alone learn? Can you imagine teaching a patient you've just diagnosed with depression, what their diagnosis means—using just these two lines?

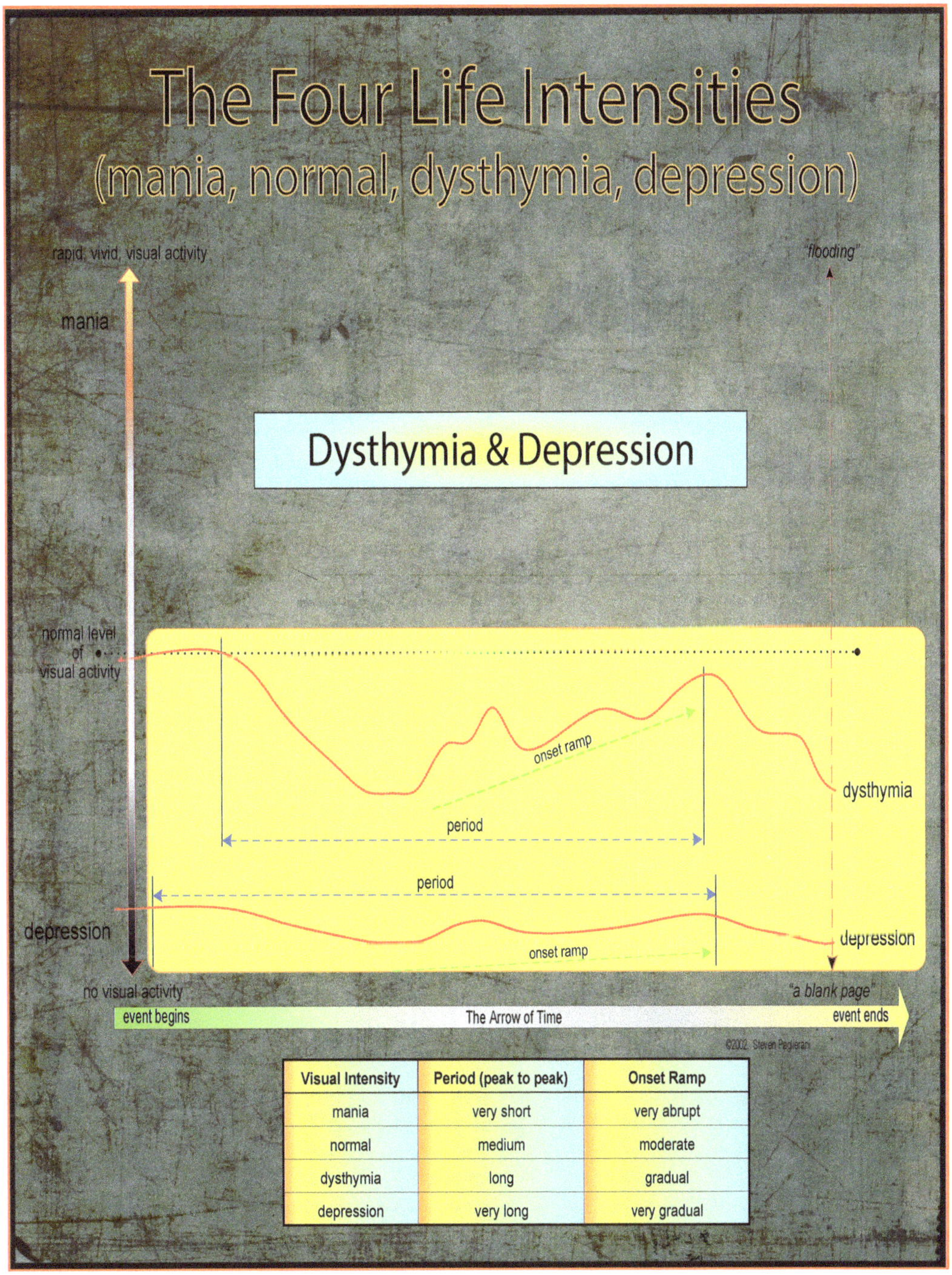

Visual Intensity	Period (peak to peak)	Onset Ramp
mania	very short	very abrupt
normal	medium	moderate
dysthymia	long	gradual
depression	very long	very gradual

Imagine how you could also use these lines to have patients self-evaluate—by drawing the prior week's line? This simplicity is the beauty of a **Visual First | Conceptual Second** diagnostic manual. Are you beginning to have glimpses of what a real diagnostic manual would be like? Visual definitions are the key.

Why Haven't I Felt Unsure When I've Diagnosed?

This led me to ask a question I'd never asked myself before. If diagnostic manuals are so flawed, where has my confidence been coming from? Please note, by "confidence," I am not saying I find diagnosing trivial or easy—nor do I ever do it casually, quickly, or in a fixed amount of time.

On the contrary, I often need two to four sessions before I even make a provisional diagnosis. I also occasionally adjust a diagnosis when previously unreported things emerge. Why? Because being open to adjusting a diagnosis is critical to a therapist's ability to offer proper care. These changes often improve outcomes. So the patient's diagnosis should be periodically revisited and reviewed.

The source of my confidence then? Clearly it can't have come from consulting a dictionary I don't believe in or trust. Re-imagining the "diagnostic manual?" How could I think I could do that? I also don't criticize other people's life's work without having at least some idea of better solutions. So where was my confidence coming from? Can you guess?

The more I considered this question, the more I realized, I never start with a diagnosis. Even in my early days as a therapist, I began with—and focused on—getting to know my patients. And lest you think this beginning was limited to doing a small number of hour sessions with a few dozen souls, consider this. In my first two years, I saw 700 teens with their families—each for seven to eleven, eight-hour Saturdays, as well as for a sequence of four more whole days during family week.

How was this possible? Because I began my career in the late 1980's. Back then, insurance companies would often pay for seven to eleven whole weeks of inpatient treatment for teens. I'd been hired as the family therapist in an inpatient JCAHO rehab for teens—all of whom had been diagnosed with substance abuse issues. And for them to get into treatment, family members had to agree to attend as well.

Today, I imagine, most therapists will have a hard time imagining getting this much time to help. What was it like? For new intakes, after detox, it would begin on a Saturday. They and their family members would join the already admitted patients and their families, usually some 100 to 200 people. They'd then spend six to ten more eight-hour Saturdays in multifamily groups.

Some of this was Psycho Education. Some was experiential. And some of this was me sitting with as many family members as I could find time to fit in, doing psycho-socials for every single family member. Then came family week, where four to eight teens and their family members attended four more straight days of groups. Four days of multifamily psychodramas. Four days of multifamily genograms. Four days of multifamily fish-bowl groups, art therapy groups, and play therapy groups.

Can you picture doing all this never having been trained as a therapist? I still can't explain how I was able to do it, let alone well. Odd as this seems, I cannot imagine getting a better education. Why mention this though? Because at the time, I was not licensed to diagnose. So my focus was never on making a diagnosis. All I cared about was helping these teens and their families to begin a better life.

Then in the early 1990's, all this changed. I left to begin a full-time private practice. And because many of my patients had modest incomes and could not otherwise afford to come, I felt obliged to find ways to get my patients reimbursed.

In large part because of this, I enrolled in and graduated from Fordham. My MSW then entitled me to get what passed back then for a license. At that time, NYS social workers were not licensed to diagnose—let alone be reimbursed. Unless they acquired six years of post-graduate, supervised experience which added a letter "R" to your license number. This then entitled you to get these two things.

In effect, without this letter "R" tacked onto your license number, insurance companies in New York were not required to reimburse you or your patients for psychotherapy services. This was true even when a health insurance contract included reimbursement of qualified psychologists and psychiatrists. Knowing this, I chose to do the six years and acquired my "R" letter. Then eventually, those requirements were lowered to three years post-grad supervision. And in 2020, the need for this letter was dropped entirely.

Why all the personal history? I've included it to explain why I've always made diagnosis secondary to treatment. Critical in this is knowing that from my second week in the profession, I often did these therapies on my own. How could I possibly have done things like multifamily psychodramas—after only watching my supervisor a single time? To this day, I have no way to explain this—other than to say what I remember thinking back then. I recall thinking, this job felt like I was wearing my first pair of correctly fitting shoes.

My point?

I spent most of my first two years in the profession not only doing therapy. I also learned how to gather proper evidence. In part, this came from having to do charts for some seven hundred teens and several thousand family members. Not one hour a week, mind you, or even in single eight-hour days. Rather, I saw them in multifamily groups, eleven to fifteen whole days. And yes, my supervisor, Nancy, sat in with me in quite a few of those groups. Just as often though, I ran them alone.

Please take a few minutes to picture what this must have been like—and why it's affected my confidence. When I diagnose, most of what I draw on is experience no normal therapist is ever lucky enough to have. Indeed, I can't think of another therapist who has done so many multifamily groups—let alone multifamily psychodramas. At the same time, part of me is cringing even as I write this. I, in no way, wish to sound self-congratulatory or boastful. I include it only to explain my confidence when I diagnose. Every diagnosis is derived only after constellating an overwhelming amount of evidence.

So How Do I Diagnose?

To be honest, until this morning, I'd never considered this as being formative. As I look back though, I can see, I've never made diagnosis my main focus. From day one in the profession, I begin every session gathering evidence about the patient. Beginning where the patient is at always comes first. Diagnosis? Always second.

I'm also just realizing how different this is from other mental health professionals. Most mental health professionals begin cases—and sessions, by looking for, and deciding on, a patient's diagnosis. This diagnosis then determines the style of treatment they'll use, the goals they'll set, and how they'll monitor the patient's progress. And they do all this, all without the benefit of a real diagnostic manual.

The fact that they do this with no book to guide them seems downright crazy. Can you think of any other profession where a dictionary guides people's every move? How about writers? They rely on dictionaries for a bunch of stuff. Do dictionaries tell them how to write? Obviously, not. A dictionary can't tell you how to write any more than the diagnostic manual can tell you how to diagnose.

Questions are filling my mind. Is this why so many therapists tell me they feel unsure in sessions? It's not that they don't know how to do therapy? It's because they don't feel confident about what to treat the person for? Imagine how this would change if we had a proper diagnostic manual. My sense is that it would single-handedly improve and upgrade all mental health professions.

Then there's the thing about feeling like a fraud when I diagnose. I'm referring to having to give people diagnoses I know aren't real. If you're any kind of a practicing psychotherapist, I'm sure, you know what I mean. How then have I been deciding which diagnosis to use, given I so know the diagnostic manual is largely a sham?

Addressing this question will be a big part of what I discuss in this book.

So how do you decide on which diagnosis to give your patients? Does what you decide on then determine what you address in therapy? I openly admit that to know what to address, in theory, we should at least decide on a provisional diagnosis. But shouldn't this diagnosis be based on a science that you understand and trust?

Imagine if it was. A people-first, how-to guide? Wow.

At this point, you may be wondering if I will be offering you a completely revised manual. My answer? I will not be. As I write this, I'm 76 years old. I'm also just a very human, very busy person. Re-imagining what a better manual *would look like* will be enough of a goal, in and of itself.

The thing is, fortunately, even the existing manual can have great worth—given you learn to use **Visual First | Conceptual Second** methods whenever you consult it. This is how I'm able to use the existing diagnostic manual when I diagnose. I use what's in the drawing on the next page to guide the process. Doing this helps. A lot.

Please know, teaching you how to use this drawing will be my primary goal in this book's final chapter. For now, just try to picture what you see as an actual physical funnel. Want to be sure you are actually picturing a funnel? Ask yourself this. "What color funnel am I seeing?" No color? Then you're not picturing.

A First Look At The Diagnostician's Funnel

Now try it. Use the **Visual First | Conceptual Second** style of learning to explore this drawing. How? By focusing on the funnel drawing *without reading any of the words*. Know that learning to do this—to overlook words, can be quite disorienting.

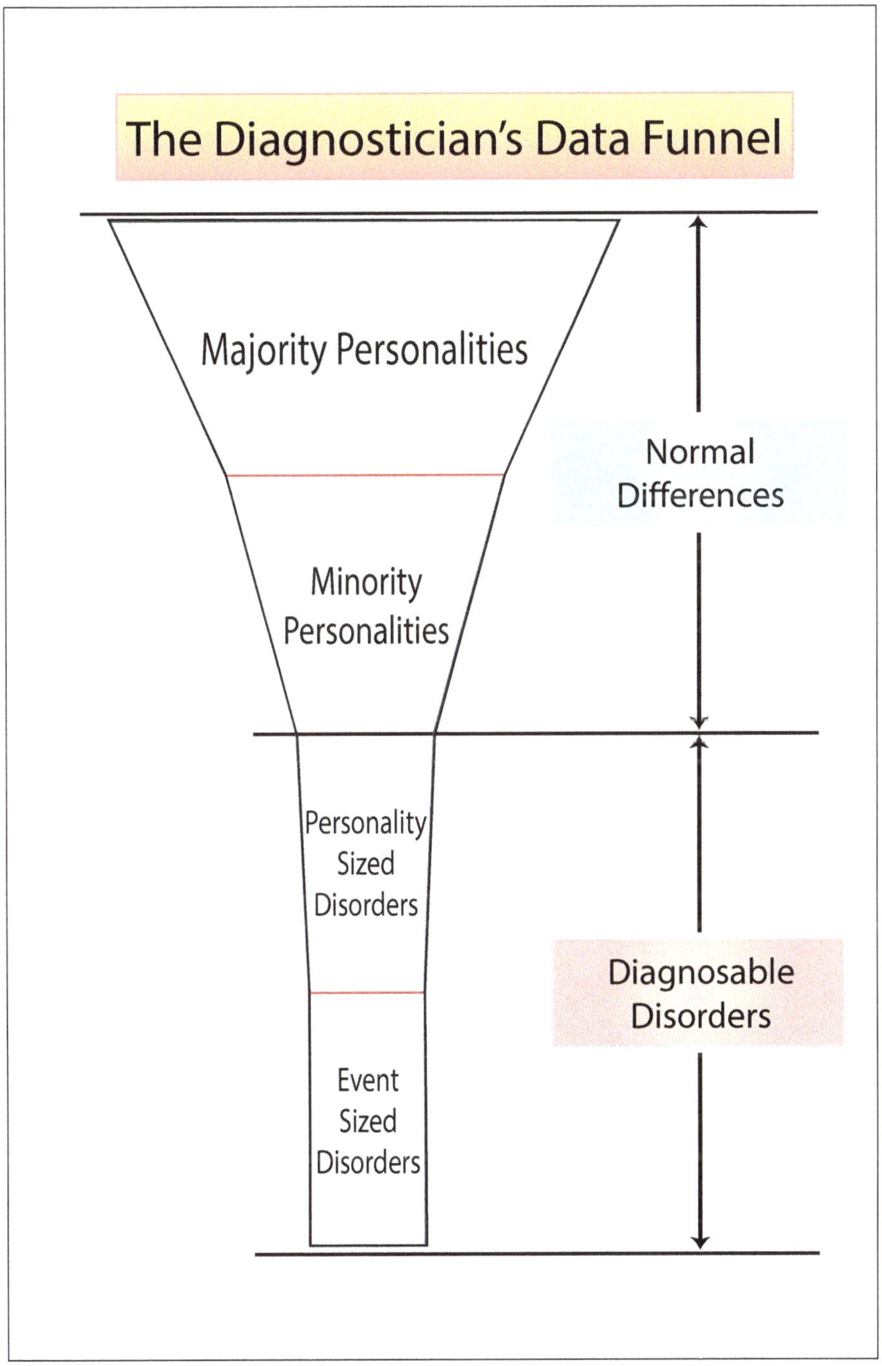

Most people barely see the shapes and focus only on understanding the words.

Unfortunately, if you do this, you'll learn very little—and retain even less. Why is doing this so hard? Because schools don't test people on drawings—they test people on words. This said, if you find this hard to do, please try again and take your time. And do your best to take in the shapes, without looking at the words.

Still finding this hard to do? Then know this. If all you've realized is how hard this is, then pat yourself on the back. Realizing this means you've taken your first steps towards becoming a master diagnostician. And if you were one, what would this look like? You'd be able to draw the entire funnel, in detail, from memory—all without recalling, let alone writing, a single word.

You'd also be able to treat what you'd drawn as if it functioned like a real evidence funnel. Not a cut-in-half drawing of a funnel, mind you. An actual, physical funnel. What would this be like? Like putting things into a real funnel. Master diagnosticians don't worry about what their evidence means. They just keep collecting evidence until the funnel makes it emerge.

Why draw a funnel cut in half then? Wouldn't what you put into it spill out? For now, just let this go. We'll have a lot to say about this later. What about the words in the drawing? Don't they matter too? They do. But if you focus on understanding words, you'll fall into what I call, "the Infinite-Meanings Trap." Meaning what?

To see, picture being in a first session with a new client. Do your best to make this scene come alive in your mind. Remember, to make things come alive in your mind, everything you picture needs to have a color. The chairs. The floor. The door and walls, and the windows, and even your new patient's face.

Now imagine you ask your patient the classic question—"What brings you in today?" I, myself, never ask this question. New patients already feel too much pressure. I also find I learn more by sitting quietly and letting the patient begin. Whatever they tell me, or do, then goes directly into a mental funnel.

It's twenty minutes in and you've just learned the problem involves someone she loves. Imagine you ask her what the word "love" means to her. Imagine too that you try to guess what she is about to say before she answers. Do this now. Try to guess what she might say. Make a note of this, then imagine you hear her answer.

Now comes the point of it all.

How many ways could your patient have responded?

What I mean is, how many meanings does the word "love" actually have? According to my god-awfully expensive, 23 volume, OED dictionary—the word "love" has, if I counted correctly, sixty-seven broad categories of meanings.

Did what she said at all match what you expected her to say? Probably not.

Now think about it. What are the odds you'd say the same things as your client? Know I've done this with clients many times. Even on my best day, I can't come close. Unless, of course, what's said is so vague, it's like newspaper astrology all over again. You know—that statistical stuff diagnostic manuals base their claims on—that worthless stuff.

Now try the thought experiment again, only this time ask your patient this. Ask her to ***picture*** the first scene that comes to mind when she thinks of the word, "love." Then do this same thing yourself. Try to see what you first picture when you think of the word "love." Then try to guess how close your two pictures will be.

Now ask her to describe what she pictured and compare it to what you imagined. Now ask yourself, how much more did this tell you compared to when your patient only used words. This is the essence of a real diagnostic process. Diagnosis IS "the art of becoming able to picture the patient's life." No picture. No diagnosis. Certainly not one rooted in the patient's actual, personal reality.

Asking patients to express their reality mainly in words guarantees that what you learn will be vague. And while most psychotherapy is done this way, doing this when you're diagnosing handicaps the process. For example, consider another case. This time, a new patient tells you she feels depressed. What exactly is she referring to? Sadness? Emptiness? A sense of loss?

Of course, in all likelihood, you'd then ask follow-up questions. But with every question, the vagueness would likely only get worse. In the end, all you'd have is a caricature of what she's going through. This is why—to properly diagnose—you must picture the client's suffering. The patient's picture is worth many thousands of words.

Does this sound like total bullshit? Then consider this. Would you want to be driving, blindfolded, to some place you've never been to before? Say your GPS was really articulate. Would those words be enough to make you feel safe? Each time you attempt to diagnose without seeing through a patient's eyes, you're driving blindfolded to a new place.

Your patients deserve the best, don't they? After all, each one is suffering in some way. Pigeonholing suffering patients into similar categories is yet another diagnostic manual atrocity. My guess though is—if you're reading this book, then you have a good heart. And all I'm saying is, pictures speak louder, and clearer, than words when you're diagnosing.

Could You Visually Teach Bipolar Mania to a Patient?

Before giving you a hopefully brief list of what's to come in the rest of the book, I want to first offer an example of the kind of drawing I find useful when teaching patients their diagnosis. In this example, you'll see visual representations of two similar, yet seemingly unrelated, experiences.

In one, you'll see an experience line which represents a bipolar episode.

In the other, you'll see an experience line which represents using crack cocaine.

Here again, to access this usefulness, you'll need to use the **Visual First | Conceptual Second** style of learning. This said, at this point, please don't try to understand everything in this drawing. Know we'll spend an entire chapter learning to recognize the kinds of patterns which are in these drawings. For now, just try to focus on the similarities in—and the differences between—the shapes of the two lines. At the same time, do your best to not try to understand the words.

Keep in mind, each of these two occurs over a different period of time. Obviously crack-based mania occurs more quickly than a manic episode. This said, would the ***shapes*** of these two lines change if we changed the overall time? Do you know? That's the beauty of these drawings—these shapes are fractal. So regardless of how long an event takes to complete, the shapes don't change.

More important still is how this drawing correctly identifies differences in the natures of these two conditions. Why? Because I've seen symptoms of these two conditions be diagnostically mistaken for one another. Considering you'll likely never personally experience either of these states of mind, this drawing can be incredibly useful—especially if you use these two lines to create visual experiences representative of these two events in your mind. How? By imagining you have to walk, crawl or climb on ground that's shaped like these lines. Picturing yourself doing this can give you a good idea of what it's like to experience these two things.

What Will We Address In This Book?

Finally let's briefly look at what we'll address in the rest of this book. Keep in mind, everything we look at will focus on how we might create a **Visual First | Conceptual Second** diagnostic manual. We'll begin with a chapter on **"The 4 States of Mind"**—the four basic fractal patterns of mental change. We'll then briefly look at the four algebraic formulas I've used to determine the shapes of these lines.

Next we'll look at why you must picture these shapes in a mental, three-dimensional space. Why? Because all life experiences emerge from some combination of these four patterns. Moreover, all three-dimensional mental spaces are governed by the same laws of physics as real-world, physical spaces. This means we can use the laws of physics to create mental pictures for any and all mental health diagnoses, giving us the ability to picture the workings of a patient's inner life.

Does this make sense? Instead of basing diagnostic evaluations on unscientifically vague word definitions, we get precise, accurate, visual definitions for all mental states. We then get to use these visual definitions to contrast, compare, diagnose, then explain things to our patients. For example, have you ever tried to explain the difference between mood swings caused by serious mental disorders and those caused by substance use disorders? It's hard. Having these shapes makes it easy.

In the next chapter, we'll expand on this as we visually define **"The Nature of Wounds."** Are symptoms really the best way to diagnose and if not, is there a better way? Is it even possible to know, with certainty, where and when an asymptomatic patient is reliving a trauma? Yes to all of this. All you'll need to learn is to watch for two simple, observable tells. No surprise, this involves watching your patient's face for some previously ignored, but important, movements.

Bipolar | Manic Episode

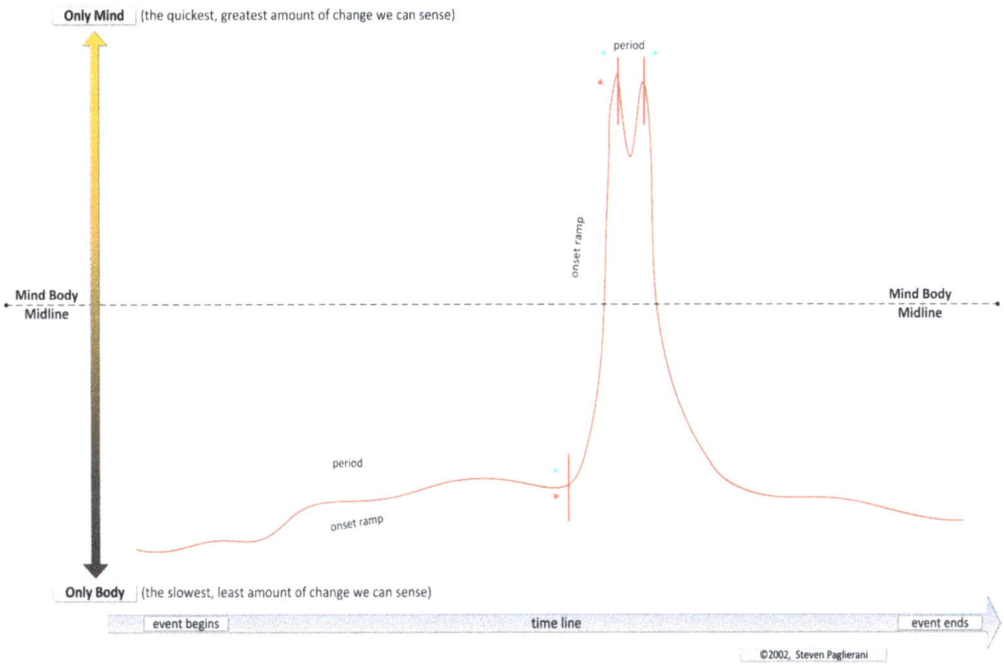

Crack Cocaine | Manic Episodes

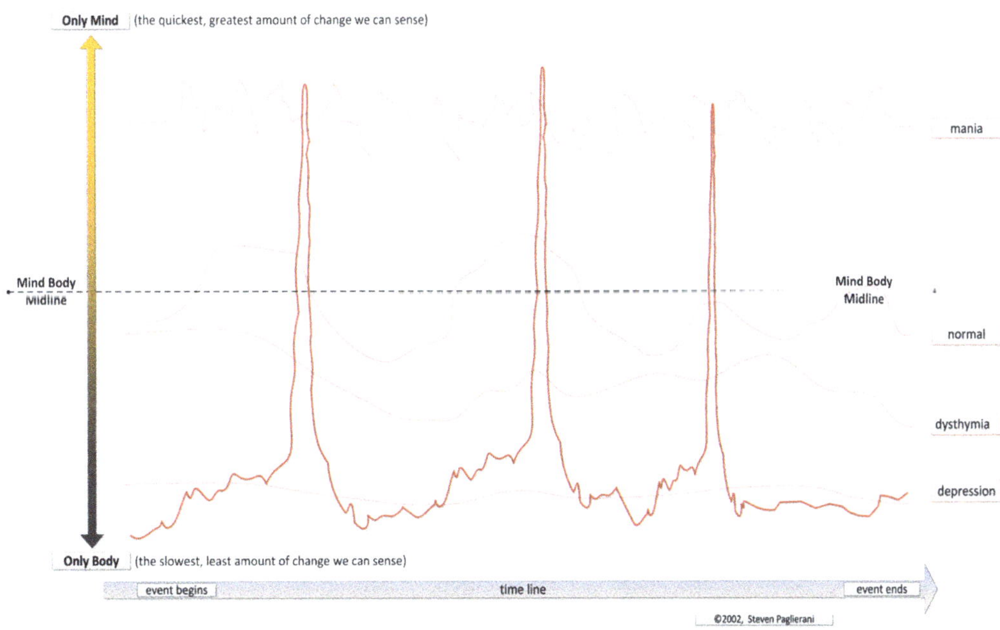

Then, in "**Evidence Gathering (a guide)**," we'll explore the heart and soul of diagnosis—**Funnel-Based Evidence Gathering**. Many current mental health service providers claim their diagnoses are evidence-based. But are they really? To begin with, have you ever seen a therapist scientifically explain what they mean by evidence—what qualifies something as evidence and what does not? Again, many readers may feel doing this is unnecessary—that these meanings are already self-evident. In this chapter though, you'll learn that much of what's been considered evidence is actually vague, meaningless, and useless. So what qualifies something as valid diagnostic evidence? Again, it's the funnel that determines this.

Next we'll spend a chapter exploring personality itself, as we ask, "**Can Science Measure People?**" Here I'll introduce you to Emergence Personality Theory's five fractal, real-world measures. These measures are what allow us to define baselines for "clinical insignificance." They also reveal the two kinds of normal personalities humans can have—"**Majority Personalities**" (where all five measures are present in smoothly varying distributions)—and "**The 4 Minority Personalities**" (where the distributions of two of these measures present as the kind of oddness people with OCD and Autism exhibit.) You'll learn these people aren't broken, despite what the diagnostic manual says. Why not? This is but one of the things we'll look at.

Having defined a proper baseline for clinical insignificance, we can now turn to what makes something abnormal. Diagnosticians commonly call this a "disorder." In this chapter, "**Classifying Disorders**," we'll explore the two kinds of disorders: "Personality-Sized" and "Event-Sized." What makes bipolar depressions different from clinical depressions? What makes schizophrenias different from PTSD flashbacks and hallucinogenic substance use disorders.

These conditions are all currently considered serious "disorders." But why? And what makes something a "disorder?" You'll learn that only by visually defining the word "disorder," can we design a proper diagnostic system. To do this though, we'll first need to question all those vague words we use, then replace them where we can.

Finally, I'll put it all together in a chapter titled "**The Diagnostician's Funnel | A How-To Guide**." Here I hope to arrive at something which can serve as a template for a workable how-to manual. What I will not do is polish the turds (the diagnoses) which together make up present diagnostic manuals. This said, since these manuals are likely not going away any time soon, I'll show you how you could use what's in this book to significantly improve your ability to use those manuals—so much so that your confidence should increase at least tenfold.

Is this a tall order? Does a bear do his stuff in the woods? Indeed, even reading this short list feels overwhelming to me. So can I accomplish all this? I am going to do my best to try. And if the realizations I've already had are any indicator, I expect writing this book will change my life in the process as well.

I hope reading this book will change your life tool. More important, I hope this book will make the world a better place for all of us, diagnosable or not.

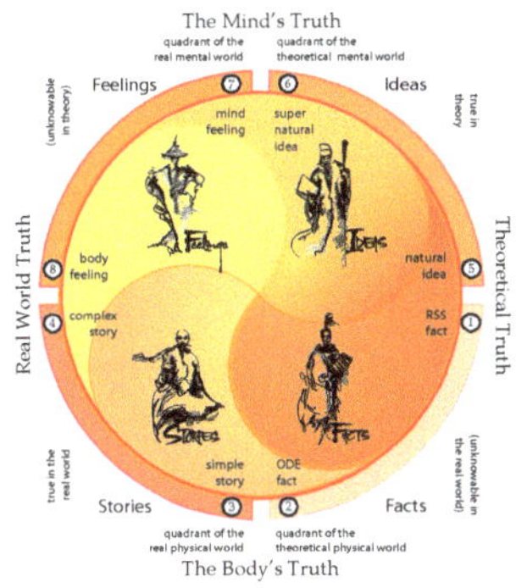

Chapter 1

The Invisible Mind
(what can we learn about . . . ?)

Can We Make What's In The Mind Visible?

As I've told you, this book will focus on how we might create a **Visual First | Conceptual Second** diagnostic manual. In this chapter, we will address what is arguably the most difficult problem we will face. Human beings cannot "see" thoughts and feelings—everything in the human mind is invisible. How then can we expect to properly diagnose the state of a human mind?

This is not to say our patients cannot mentally "picture" things—obviously, they can. Rather, because these mental pictures are not actual physical objects, they cannot be seen by anyone else. Nor will our patients ever have clear and precise ways to translate the inner workings of their minds into words. Do you doubt this? Then think back to a time when a patient told you she was depressed.

What did she tell you? Write down what you remember. Now pick another depressed patient and do this with her. Did the two women tell you the same things—did they use the same words? Did these words refer to the same exact life events? Probably not. So what does this word actually mean? What would you say?

Not coincidentally, diagnostic manuals treat the word "depression" as if it always means the same thing. If true, wouldn't both women have referred to the same inner experiences, using the same words? Not with a newspaper astrology level of vague descriptions, the kind which pervade the pages of all existing diagnostic manuals. Rather, with the same exact, scientifically measurable references to being depressed?

Science tells us that in the Real World, nothing natural ever repeats the same way twice. This not only includes snowflakes and rain drops. It also includes any two patients who both report feeling depressed. More important, were we to allow this was possible (even though it is not), a problem would still remain.

How could we accurately measure what is in these patients' minds?

What method could we use?

Some might now name one of the commonly used depression scales, for instance, the fabulously vague Beck Depression Inventory (BDI). This so-called "assessment tool" consists of 21 self-report multiple choice questions, takes about 10 minutes to complete, and claims to be valid and reliable across populations worldwide. But is it? Consider one of the questions it asks. I've placed it below.

0 I do not feel sad.
1 I feel sad.
2 I am sad all the time and I can't snap out of it.
3 I am so sad and unhappy that I can't stand it.

Seems like a simple question, doesn't it? Obviously, it is. But can this simple question ever result in what passes for a scientific outcome? Where's the definition of "sad?" Are we to assume the word "sad" means the same thing to all human beings? Perhaps you think these differences do not matter? If so, then picture this.

Imagine you've been tasked with creating a scientific definition for "sad." You decide to ask 100 people to ***picture*** the last time they felt sad. Already, you've done better than Mr. Beck—you're at least asking for pictures. This said, would any of these people report they had pictured the same exact thing? Probably not.

Then again perhaps you are thinking this question is good enough—or at least better than nothing? Would you want to bet your license on that it is? How about betting your patient's well-being? Setting aside this lack of a clear definition, a problem still exists. Mr. Beck claims this is a freaking depression scale. But if it was, wouldn't the word "sad" actually correlate well to "diagnosable depression?"

What do you think? Does it? If so, how well?

In truth, most sadness does not correlate well to depression. Sadness refers to an ***emotion***. Depression is not an emotion—depression is a ***state of mind.*** Also, sadness is ***a kind of change you feel***, whereas depression is ***an inability to feel change***. And sadness generally passes quickly and is more a momentary check-in. Whereas depression usually lasts far longer, even in cases where it's not diagnosable.

What if I now change the word "sad" to the phrase "feeling blue?" Imagine you now ask those 100 people to picture the last time they felt this way. How much better would this phrase correlate to being depressed than to the word "sad?" What do you think? I am betting a notable improvement would occur.

Why claim this? Because as I said, the sine qua non of depression is experiencing "the lack of change." When people picture themselves "feeling blue," this lack of change is the main thing they feel—that the emptiness will never end.

Would you see an improvement? What do you think? I can't imagine you would not. A phrase used in so many songs, books, and movies would surely help.

If you did see an improvement, how well do you think it would correlate to having added a commonly used, ***visual*** reference to your question? Similarly, what if you asked those 100 patients to picture the last time they "saw red." Would this simple reference to color correlate well to anger? And if you did see improvements, would they be enough? I, for one, think we can still do better. For instance, what if you unpacked the word "depression," similar to how I did with the word "diagnosis?"

Know I often do this with patients who feel depressed. I tell them the word "depression" means "*your feelings are being pressed into a small space.*" This helps me to determine if this depression is diagnosable or not—and improves their reporting. I then add, "You can know this is happening when you feel like nothing's changing—when life has no color—and when your sense of emotion feels small."

Can you see how these visual references to physical space could help patients to self-evaluate? *"Are your feelings being pressed into a small space? Do you feel like nothing is changing?"* And when diagnosing, can you see why a "space" would be better than a "color?" Also, did you notice my questions begin with a picture and only then, add words? And no, I'm not claiming these words are sufficient for a proper diagnostic manual—they're not. This said, they are a lot better than asking, "Do you feel sad?"—or worse, the dreaded, "How did that make you feel?"

What would be good enough? Consider the drawing you see below.

"Space" refers to a physical thing. Can you see how the depression line resembles something being "pressed into a small space?" Look at how much more space the normal line takes up as compared to the depression line. Can you see it? Are you beginning to realize we can make the invisible mind visible?

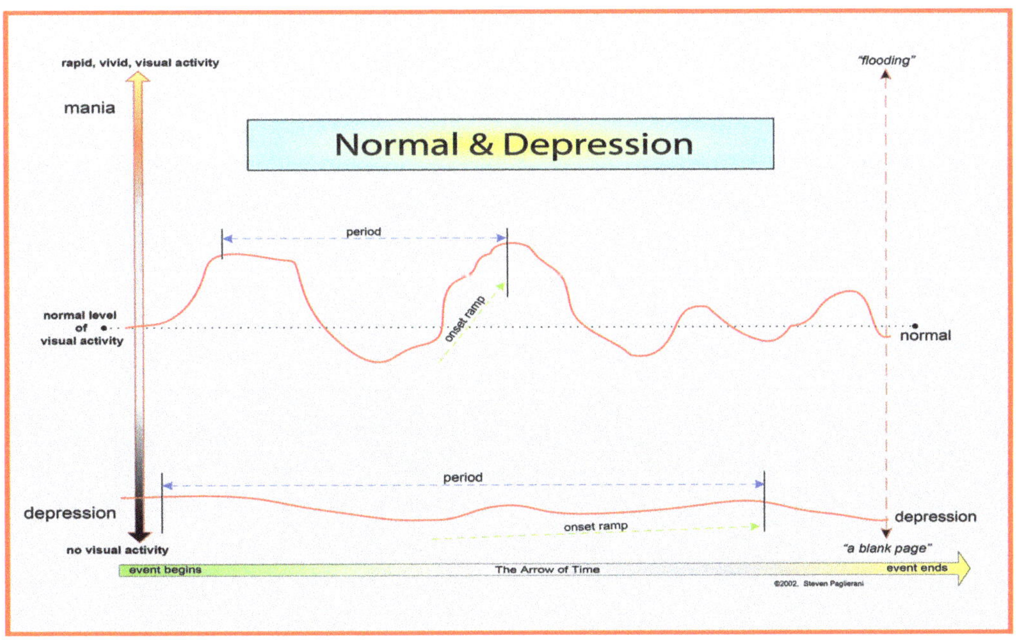

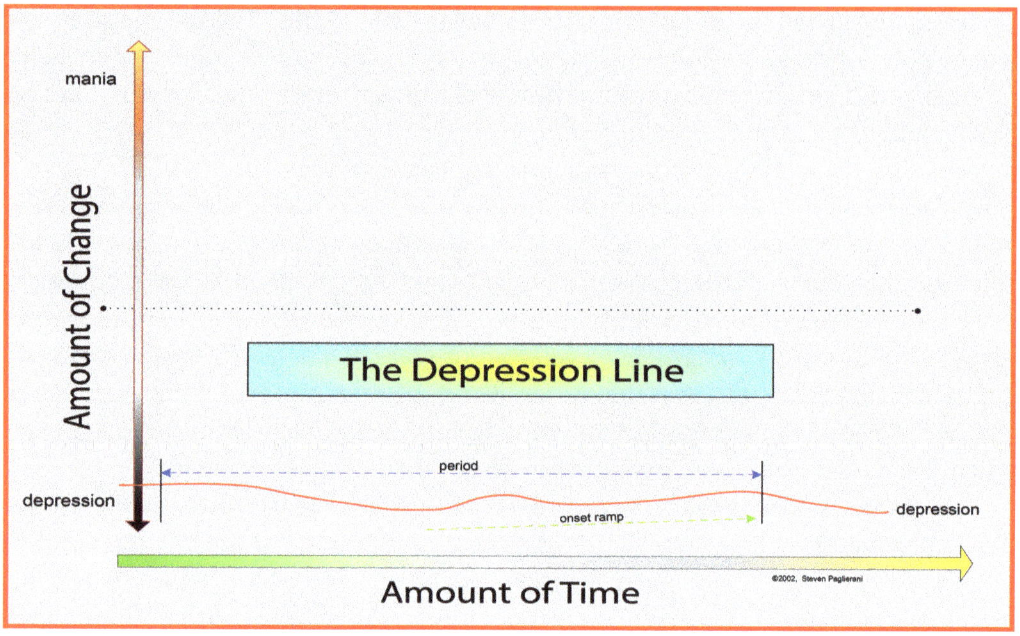

How Many Variables Do You See In This Drawing?

Now let's take a closer look at a similar drawing. Again, ignore the words and focus entirely on the shape of the line. Now ask yourself this. How can a simple line drawing do so much better than any amount of words? This power comes from one thing—do you know what it is? It comes from what this line creates—***a visual, physical representation of an invisible, mental experience.***

This sentence holds the entire key to creating a real diagnostic manual. Why? ***Because you cannot diagnose what you cannot see.*** This line makes an invisible thing—depression—visible. This visibility then makes the patient's depression diagnosable.

Now comes the critical question—can we create lines for everything in a mind? In this book, we'll do our best to start this process. Know you'll first need to learn to see this drawing's two measurement lines. Here the vertical axis represents the "amount of ***change***" the person experiences, and the horizontal axis represents the "amount of ***time***" in the measured event. And everything in this drawing derives from these two variables. Just these two.

Now try to picture these two axis lines as the two dimensions of a flat, physical space. This will give you a good idea of what the Depression Line represents. The Depression line is a picture of "how much change a depressed person perceives over time." Thus, *depression* is simply "the experience of very little change over time."

Now notice how much vertical space the overall drawing contains—versus how much vertical space the depression line takes up. Most of the "Y" axis space (the Amount of Change line) in this drawing is unoccupied. Empty. Does mental emptiness correlate well to what depression is and is not? It sure does. Are you beginning to see the diagnostic possibilities of these simple line drawings?

How Many Variables Will You Need To Learn?

At the risk of provoking any readers claiming to be "math phobic," I now need to introduce you to the four variables behind all my drawings. Please do not try to understand any of this yet. You will not need to learn algebra. You need only learn to picture the four symbols in this drawing. **M, I, T,** and **C.** That's it.

The Consciousness Formulas

M = Meaning	$M = I(T)$	Meaning = Information (Time)
I = Information	$I = \frac{M}{T}$	Information = $\frac{\text{Meaning}}{\text{Time}}$
T = Time	$T = \frac{M}{I}$	Time = $\frac{\text{Meaning}}{\text{Information}}$
C = Consciousness	$C = \frac{I(T)}{M}$	Consciousness = $\frac{\text{Information (Time)}}{\text{Meaning}}$

M I T C

Additionally, know we'll not concern ourselves with the **C variable** this book. You can look at it if you want to—but please don't linger. We'll only be using the first three variables— **M, I,** and **T.** These first three variables are all we'll need to create a science-based diagnostic manual.

What do these three variables represent?

- **M** represents **Meaning**—*how much* of it we have perceived. The first formula tells us, the mind perceives two kinds of Meaning. Can you guess what they are? If not, don't fret. This will soon become obvious to you.
- **I** represents **Information**—*what kind* we've perceived. The second formula tells us the mind perceives two kinds of Information as well. Can you guess what they are? If not, know this will soon become obvious to you as well.
- **T**, the third variable, represents **Time**—which is to say, *how long* we've been perceiving things in this event. Again, there are two kinds of Time. But here, I predict these two "times" will be impossible for you to guess. No worries, though. In a moment, I'll tell you about these two things too.

- Finally, for the terminally curious, we have the **C** variable. As I've said, we won't be looking at this variable in this book. **C** represents **Consciousness**, the thing which emerges in our minds—whenever we perceive the other three variables all at once. Does this tell you anything about Consciousness? It should. It tells us that Consciousness is neither a physical nor a mental "thing." Rather, Consciousness is an ***emergent*** property.
- What does this mean? It means that like rainbows, Consciousness is not a ***measurable*** property. Why? Because neither rainbows nor Consciousness exist in the usual measurable way. Similar to symptoms then, rainbows and consciousness become knowable only when certain conditions are met. And with Consciousness, the certain conditions are those I previously mentioned—the times we perceive a synthesis of the other three variables. When they merge and cease to be separate, then consciousness emerges.

What Does Any of This Have To Do With The Depression Line?

What do these variables have to do with what we see in the Depression Line drawing? Obviously, in this drawing, we see only two of the four variables. One is easily guessed. The Time line refers to the Time variable. And the other variable—the Amount of Change line? Which variable does this line refer to?

The Amount of Change line equates to the Meaning variable.

Know in this book, the Meaning variable will go by many names. Here the key to understanding why these names change lies in the phrase, "equates to." After all, this form of math—algebra—calls these kinds of formulas, "equations." Hence the equals sign does not mean "identical." It means "equivalent."

Now consider what is arguably the most famous equation of all time; $\mathbf{E = MC^2}$. Like all equations—algebraic or not, this one contains an equals sign. What does this equals sign tell us? As I said, that what's on one side of it is equivalent to what's on the other. In this case, Einstein is telling us that (in a vacuum) ***Energy*** "equates to" ***Mass moving at the Speed of Light squared.***

Said more simply, Einstein's telling us that ***Energy*** (patterns of matter moving) equates to "stuff moving very quickly." He's also saying that ***Matter*** (horse race, finish-line snapshots of these patterns) equates to "energy standing still."

Are you surprised? Did you think you could never understand this equation? Well, you can. Just as you can understand diagnosis, given someone makes it visual and clear. Nor are we diagnosing the entire Universe here. We're just diagnosing people. Either way though, the point is, that symbol in the middle—the equals sign—holds the key. In algebraic equations, the equals sign tells us that the things on both sides are functional equivalents. That despite having outward differences, beneath it all, these two sides are merely two versions (two forms of, two faces of, two names for) of the exact same *pattern*. In this way, the equals sign is the essence of the math we call, "algebra." What does it do? It allows us to make discoveries by contrasting and comparing two different forms of the same natural pattern.

In this book, all definitions will be based on these kinds of equivalent relationships. This is why we'll call them, "relative definitions."

What the heck is a "relative definition?" To begin with, let's look at "*what it is not.*" It's not a dictionary-style definition—a list of poorly defined, vaguely related single points. Rather, it's a succinct statement which describes the underlying natural patterns which make a thing this thing—where the word "succinct" means, this definition tells us both *what a thing is* and *what it is not* (its sine qua non).

My point? It turns out, we can know the nature of things (including the mind) only when we can see their relationships to other, equivalent things (such as the body). And when it comes to diagnosis, it's the Algebra of Consciousness which reveals the equivalencies in the human mind. With regard to Einstein's formula, he has given us a way to scientifically contrast and compare two equivalent physical world things: energy and matter. And this equation has led to all manner of discoveries about two of the most complex terms in all of physics.

Similarly, the four formulas which make up the Algebra of Consciousness give us the ability to explore and discover many things about the mind. These things will be the focus of this book. For example, take the Depression Line drawing. As you've noticed, the vertical axis is labeled the "Amount of Change" line. I've also told you this line equates to the Meaning variable. And since renaming this variable does not change any of the relationships—all the variables still apply, and all the equivalencies are still equivalent.

Why rename this variable then?

Because doing this opens up whole worlds of possible discoveries.

For example, in this book, you can assume that all vertical axes will be functionally equivalent to the Meaning variable, as in **M = IT**.

Meaning equals Information multiplied by Time.

By extension then, the Amount of Change in a given event must also equate to the product of how much *the Information changes* multiplied by how much *Time passes*. And yes, these relationships can seem complex and hard to remember at first. Then again, aren't all important things complex? Know it's this complexity that predicts how many discoveries we can make. Humans determine how much ***Meaning*** a thing has based entirely on how much ***change*** we experience—and complexity correlates to how things change.

For example, consider how much change you experience when you feel depressed? Literally, almost none. No coincidence, when you're depressed, life feels like it has little to no meaning. If we now juxtapose depression to its complementary opposite mental state—mania—we learn even more. When you're manic—such as when you've just fallen in love—you feel a whole lot of change.

This explains why manic experiences feel like they have so much meaning. We're experiencing major changes. And the Amount of Change is what gives us our sense of meaning. And there's more.

From this we can also discover where meaning does *not* come from.

If the mind assigns meaning only when we experience change over time, then things in the mind do not have inherent meanings. Why? Because Meaning is something which emerges in us only when we ***observe*** change. So, no observations. No Meaning. It's as simple as that.

Finally, do keep in mind, everything in my drawings is based on a mental to physical equivalence. For instance, in the Depression Line drawing, Time exists on the "X" axis and Change on the "Y" axis. As I've said, X times Y on any of my drawings is the mental equivalent of a physical space. So while this space is confined to the space in our minds, both spaces are governed by the exact same laws.

This tells us something else about depression. Based on the "Y" value of the Depression line, when we're depressed, our thoughts and feelings take up little to no mental space. And since all patterns in the laws which govern the physical world (physics) have mental equivalents in the laws which govern the mind, in the Depression Line drawing, most of the space in our minds is empty.

Are you beginning to see the importance of this equivalency thing?

What Part Does The Information Variable Play In All This?

Now comes the hard part. Are you thinking, WTF? That last stuff wasn't hard enough? The thing is, if you push through to the end of this chapter, you'll never have to feel the same anxiety about diagnosing ever again. Where do we start?

Start with this.

Imagine you have been tasked with creating a set of visual drawings. This set of drawings has to accomplish what no words have ever done before.

For one thing, you need to visually explain the differences between being Bipolar and being Schizophrenic. A lot, to be sure. But you're not done.

You also have to explain how the experience of having an epiphany—does and does not—resemble those two experiences. And you're still not done.

You also need to accomplish all these things in just one drawing of a single square frame. What does this square represent? In this book, all squares represent *a single moment of time* in the mind.

What must you put inside of this square? Three, and only three, vertical pairs of single points. No lines. No colors. No words. Only three vertical pairs of dots. Here each dot must represent *a single moment of experience* in this person's mind. So collectively, these six dots will represent six experiences. Two dots for Bipolar. Two for Schizophrenia. And two dots for an epiphany.

Now actually try to do this. Try to create your own drawing. I'm going to place mine on the following page. Before you look at my drawing though, do try to make your own. Know I'm claiming this is possible—and that once you know how to do this, that you'll be able to create physical representations of everything in the human mind. Can you imagine how this would change your ability to diagnose—and how you doing this could change the lives of every patient you ever see?

If you're still unsure, just simply allow for the possibility.

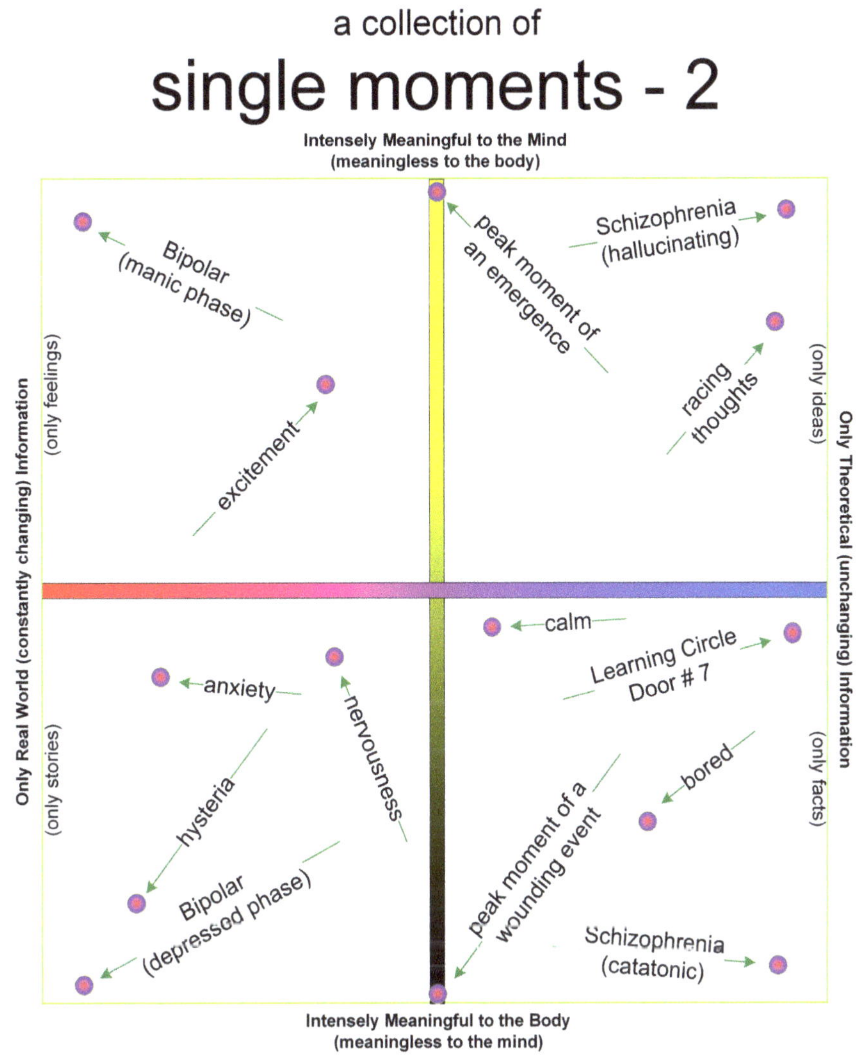

A Single Moment Square with Multiple Dots

Ok. I'm sorry. I seem to have lost my mind. Obviously, I've added in a few extra dots—well actually, quite a few. Then again, I did only use six dots to do what I asked you to do. Why the extra dots then? Because I love knowing that a single dot can explain so much. And yes, those extra dots can't possibly have much meaning yet. But as I've told you, they each represent single moments of life experience.

Now use your imagination. Can you see the hand of Descartes here? Cartesian Coordinates—two crossed axes dividing a square into four quadrants? Almost—but not quite. There are no scales. Do you realize what the vertical axis represents? You should by now. As always, it equates to—and this time is named—the Meaning variable.

What you should not know this time though is what the horizontal axis represents. This drawing is not a rectangular shape. So it can't represent Time.

What does the horizontal axis represent then? Information. Here, each dot is an "Information" dot—a relative measurement which tells us what kind of Information is in the person's mind in this moment. Know this applies to all square-shaped drawings. The horizontal axis in squares always represents the Information variable.

Now, if you look closely, you may be able to discover a few more things about the mind. For one thing, the four dots which define Bipolar and Schizophrenia function like the four corners of a table puzzle. Inside of these four dots lie all possible experiences in the mind. And separately, each condition occupies exactly one vertical half of the square—either the left side or the right.

Finally, if you pay attention to what is and is not on each side, you may learn a lot about what these two conditions do and do not affect. More on this to come.

Contrasting and Comparing The Rectangle and The Square

Now let's see if this visual "contrast and compare" stuff has been getting in. So far I've mentioned two "boundary shapes"; the *Rectangle* and the *Square*. Did you notice how each of these shapes represents a different mental state (one moment, or one event)? Also how the differences between these two shapes are based entirely in what's on the horizontal axis (Information, or Time)?

Let me say this again. For these two shapes, the vertical (Y) axis will always refer to the Meaning variable. But what's on the horizontal (X) axis will differ for Squares vs Rectangles. Squares represent one moment in time—so no Time variable is needed. Whereas Rectangles represent whole events—so time changes throughout the event. Thus the horizontal (X) axis has to tell us about this Time.

Said in still other words, the square represents a container for all possible things in a mind—in any given moment. Thus squares must have at least one dot in them. This dot is similar to what you discover when you ask a patient what they're experiencing in this or that moment. And since M=IT, if the Information changes, then the Meaning of this moment changes as well.

Rectangles, OTOH, represent whole events. And since M=IT here as well, any changes in the Time variable change the Meaning of each moment during this event. What about when Squares have more than one dot? Obviously any one person can have only one experience at a time. So multiple dots in a Square represent multiple people's experiences. And the same thing applies to seeing multiple lines in a Rectangle. Each line represents a different person's experience of this event.

Why use multiple dots or multiple lines? Because this enables us to contrast and compare different people's experiences. For instance, in the Square drawing on the previous page, the Bipolar side (the left side) has a set of top and bottom, single moments. These two moments show the two diagnostically necessary extremes (the manic phase and the depressed phase) of this diagnosis. Both must have been present at some time.

What about the dots in between these two points? These dots show that a person with Bipolar Disorder doesn't just go from the top to bottom or vice versa.

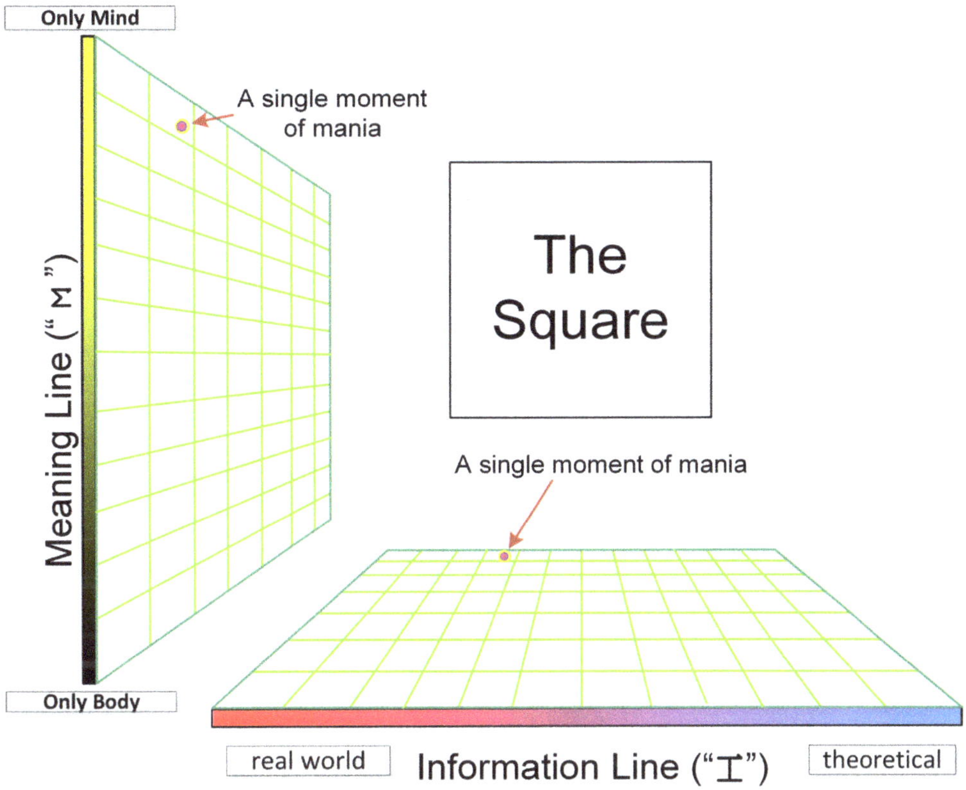
Only Mind
A single moment of mania
The Square
Meaning Line ("M")
A single moment of mania
Only Body
real world
Information Line ("I")
theoretical

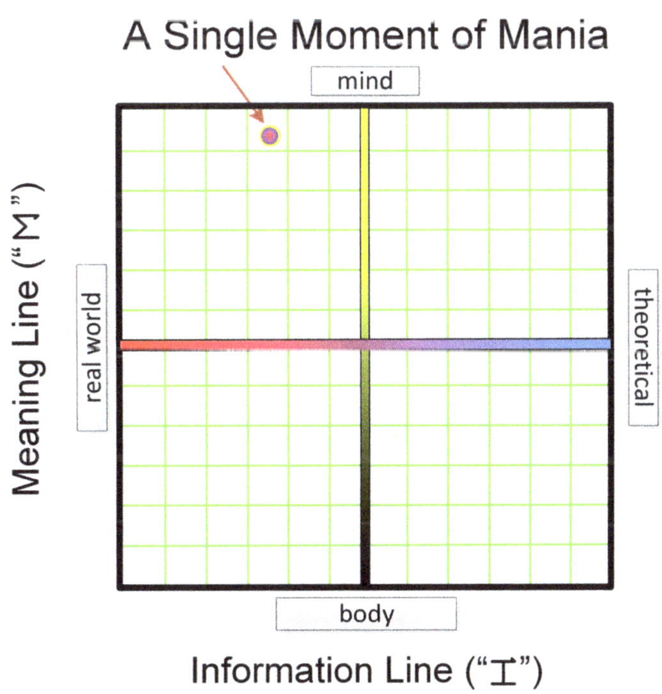
A Single Moment of Mania
mind
Meaning Line ("M")
real world
theoretical
body
Information Line ("I")

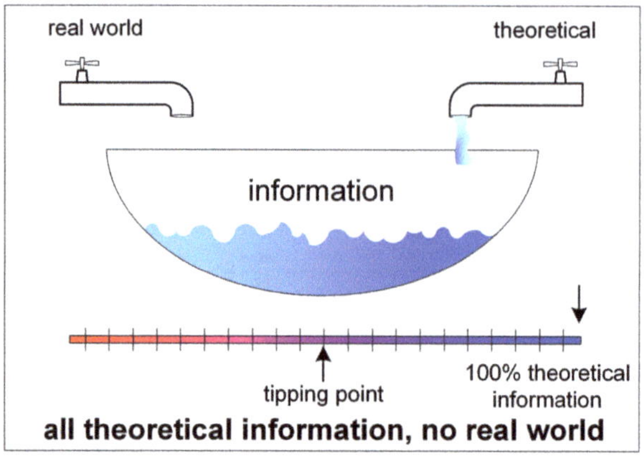
real world
theoretical
information
100% theoretical information
tipping point
all theoretical information, no real world

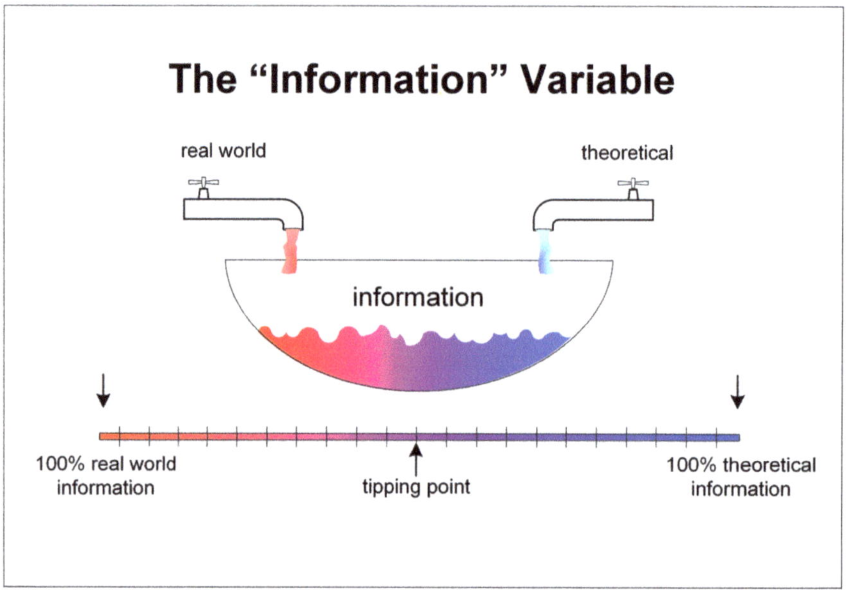
The "Information" Variable
real world
theoretical
information
100% real world information
tipping point
100% theoretical information

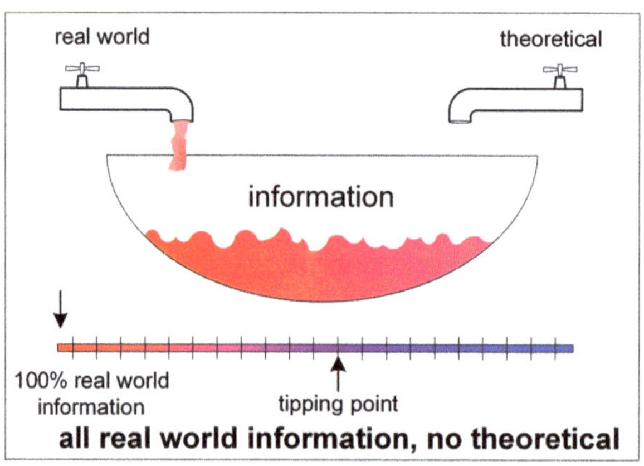
real world
theoretical
information
100% real world information
tipping point
all real world information, no theoretical

Here, on their way up and down, these folks can experience widely varying mood swings. These moods can include any of the possible states in between those two dots. Similarly, on the far-right side, we find the diagnostically necessary extremes for Schizophrenia (hallucinating and catatonic). However, in this case, rather than mood swings, the in between dots represent all the possible "thought" swings.

What's the Big Deal About the Space in Between Corner Dots?

Early in my career, I saw two women, both of whom had been diagnosed with Bipolar Disorder. Both had been hospitalized multiple times. Both were on strong medications and had been stable for years. This said, there were differences—one saw me for only a few months; the other, for seven years. The one who came only for a few months slowly went from being clinically depressed to having a manic episode. But the one who came for seven years, at age 70, became so normal that for that final year, I saw no hint of what was coming.

In the first case, I could see what was coming. That woman's moods incrementally went from clinically depressed to manically happy. But the second woman relapsed so badly in a single day that she then spent a whole year in a hospital and when she got out, she remembered nothing.

We'll look at both cases in depth in a later chapter—I mention them now for only one reason. Had I known about these drawings—and had I been charting their in between changes, I'd have done a much better job with them both.

Introducing the "Three Information Sinks"

If you now look over at the previous page, you'll find my favorite way of teaching people what the Information variable represents. In this drawing, Information is represented by water filling a sink. Like many old-fashioned sinks, this sink has two faucets—one hot and one cold.

Each of these faucets represents one of the two kinds of Information.

In the top sink—and in the middle sink, on the right side—you'll find ***Theoretical Information***. And in the bottom sink—and in the middle sink, on the left side—you'll find ***Real World Information***.

Theoretical Information is "cold" information and consists of some mix of the two kinds of cold information—***facts*** and/or ***ideas*** (logic and reasons).

Real World Information is "warm" information and consists of some mix of the two kinds of warm information—***stories*** (experiments) and/or ***feelings*** (intuitions).

Already, this is a lot to take in. So it's best if you focus only on the pictures. This is why I've taken the time to print this book in color. Now notice each kind of Information is a different color. Here, Theoretical Information is bluish in color—and Real World Information is a reddish color. Theoretical (bluish) Information represents information that is cool to icy cold. Whereas Real World (reddish) Information represents information that is warm to hot.

Why mention the water being different colors and temperatures?

How a Series of Single Moments Become an Event

(1) A Single Moment (one dot)

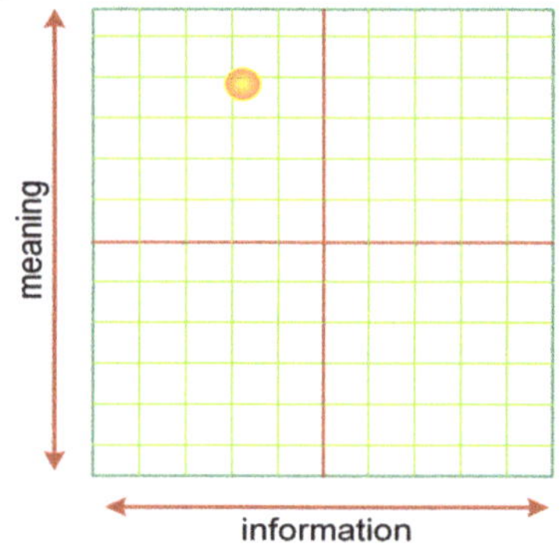

(2) A Single Event (Meaning times Time)

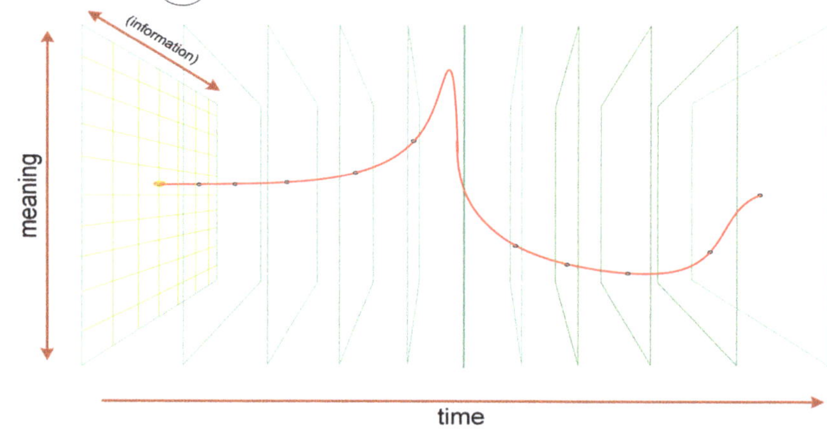

(3) A Single Event in 3 Dimensions

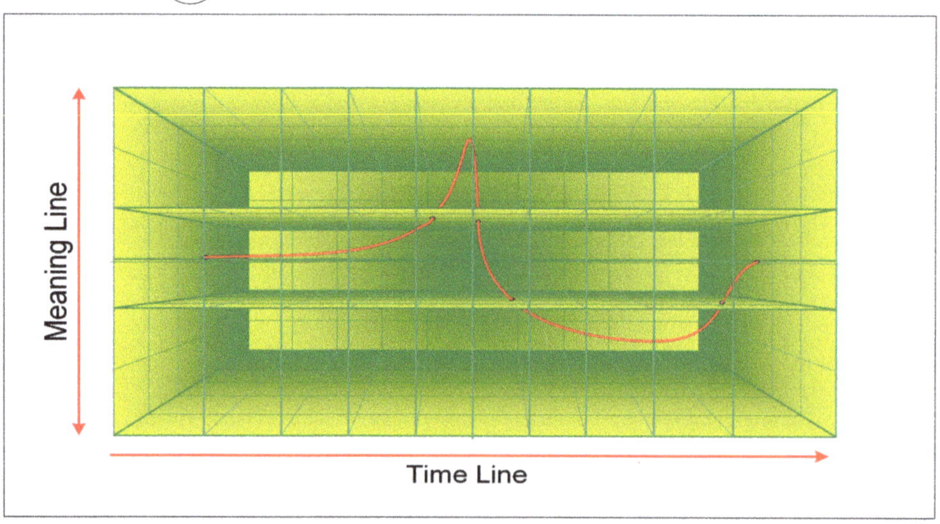

Because picturing real water flowing into a real sink can go a long way towards helping you to make sense of all this. In essence, there are only two broad categories of Information—theoretical (cold) and real world (warm). And below each sink, there's a tipping-point line which shows the current temperature in our mind—the changes in our perceptions, either from cold to warm, or from warm to cold.

Now take a moment to consider how these physical descriptions could help patients to describe all manner of mental changes in themselves or in others.

"My father was a hot-tempered man."

"My husband is never cold."

"My daughter is warm, even when someone hurts her."

"When I think of that, I feel hot under the collar."

What color is the Information in your mind right now? Perhaps you can try to picture what this would look like in color? Know the more you become able to do this, the more you'll retain these ideas, and the better you'll become at diagnosis.

Know we'll look at all this in more detail as we progress through the coming chapters. For now, I need to address something far more important.

How Does A Series of Single Moments Become An Event?

Please look over at the drawing on the previous page—the one titled, "How a Series of Single Points Become an Event." Remind yourself to avoid looking at the words. Just try to locate the three figure numbers—1, 2, and 3. In **figure 1**, you'll find a familiar shape, a single-moment ***square*** which contains a single dot.

Then, in **figure 2**, you'll see I've placed a sequence of eleven, single-moment ***squares***. Each square contains a single dot—a momentary check-in. I've then drawn a line which connects all of these eleven dots. Know ***this is how event lines get drawn.*** And it's these lines that then result in the easily learned, recognizable shapes.

Finally, in **figure 3**, you'll find a three-dimensional version of **figure 2**'s *event line* drawing. As with **figure 2**, **figure 3** is a front-facing, ***rectangular*** view. Here, the "Y" (vertical) axis variable is Meaning—and the "X" (horizontal) axis variable is Time. Then the "Z" axis (front to back) variable adds in Information, changing this rectangle into a rectangular cuboid.

In this way, together, the first three variables (M, I, and T) create a three-dimensional, physical representation of the space in the mind. All single moment dots and event lines exist within this mental three-dimensional space. They also all have recognizable shapes—and recognizable placements within this space. And together, these shapes and placements reveal the true nature of the mind.

Now, and for the rest of this chapter, we'll explore four of these recognizably shaped lines. The Four States of Mind—mania, normal, dysthymia, and depression. The skill of diagnosis becomes permanent and clear only when you learn to effortlessly recognize these four line-shapes. And yes, I know, this is a heck of a lot to take in. But please, do try to be patient. The reward is coming soon.

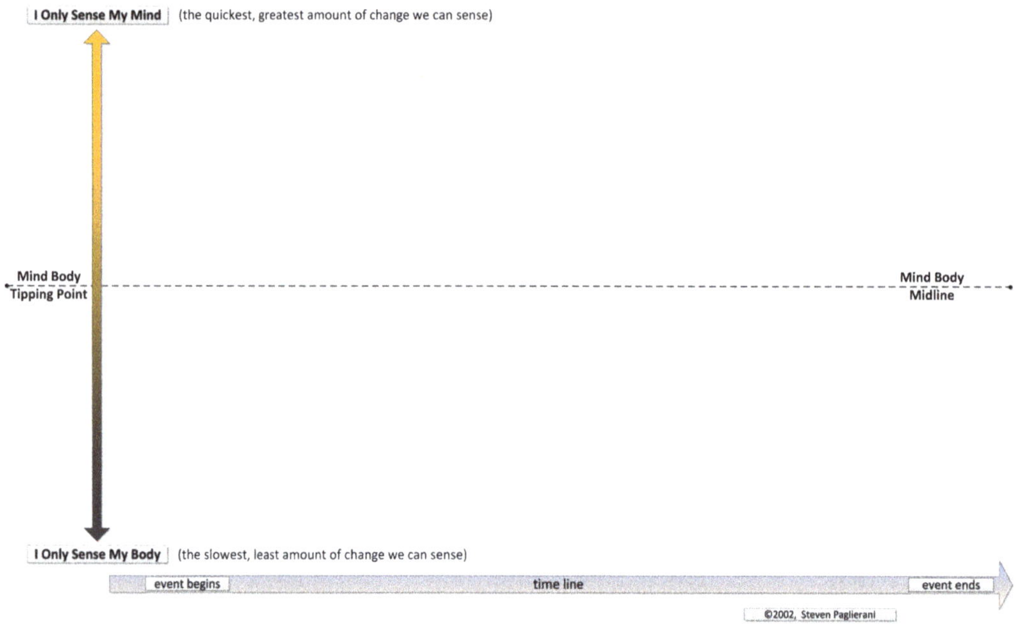

A Blank Event-Line Rectangle

From the shape of this drawing, you know it represents some kind of an event. But without a line being drawn in it, we have no idea what it was. I'm beginning here—with this empty drawing, because I want to familiarize you with the measures which define this space. As with all my rectangular drawings, a vertical two-headed arrow shows how the Meaning of this event varies up and down. And a horizontal, one-headed arrow tells us where in Time these up and down changes occur.

Please pay attention to the number of arrowheads on these two lines. All Time lines have one arrowhead, because this value varies only in one direction. Whereas all Meaning lines have two, as this value varies up and down as you move forward in time. This points to an important difference between the diagnostic process and doing psychotherapy.

Psychotherapists often revisit past events with patients, as historical knowledge is often buried in patients' minds. Diagnosticians don't do this kind of digging. Diagnosis focuses on how the patient is in the present moment. Thus psychotherapy is more backward looking, while diagnosis mainly looks forward. Why? Because looking too far back can alter the Meaning of the moment we are diagnosing.

Some may now ask—if this drawing represents a mental three-dimensional space, then where is the "Z" axis? Know it exists, just not in this drawing. This is similar to how an architect draws a front-facing view of a building in an architectural drawing. Only we do this in our event drawings so we can contrast and compare our recognizable lines to what patients are reporting.

This said, we'll now look at a dozen or so drawings of these shapes. All diagnoses begin with knowing the shapes of these 4 States of Mind lines. So go slowly and take your time. And remember, focus on line shapes, not words.

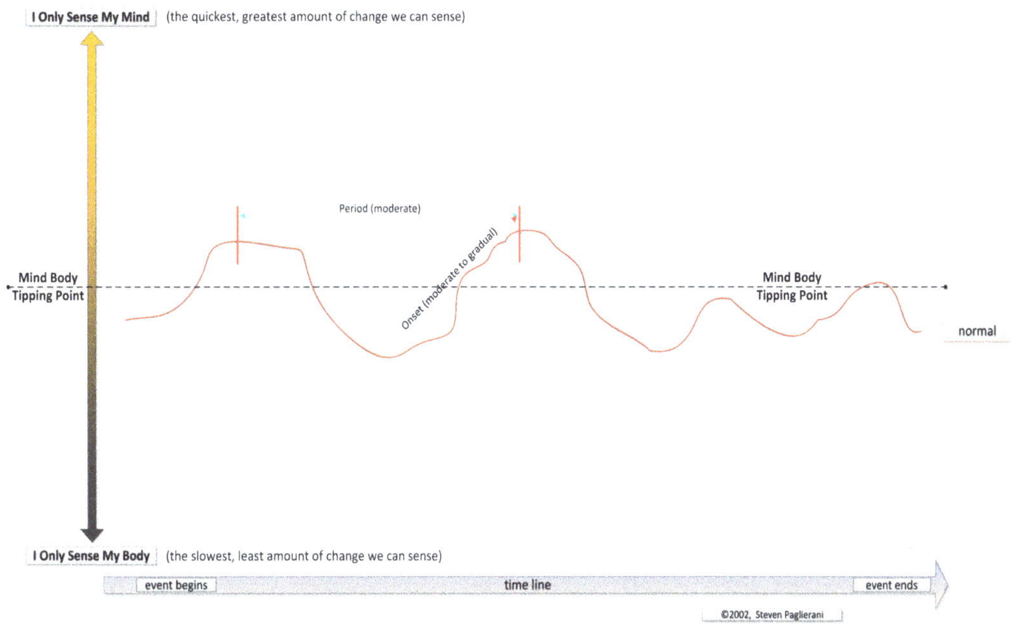

The "Normal State of Mind" Event Line

We'll begin our look at these lines with what I call the "Normal line." Admittedly, I wish I had another name for this line—I've already told you how I feel about equating the word "normal" to health. The thing is, this book is intended to be a bridge between what already exists and what a diagnostic manual could be. So I'll need to use some of the words diagnosticians already know and use.

At the same time, many of these words will need to be more accurately defined. This is the purpose of these lines. For example, when I use the word "normal," it doesn't refer to health per se. Rather, it refers to the placement and shape of this line.

Why doesn't the "normal line" refer to health? Because these four lines refer to States of Mind—not to diagnoses. Healthy people feel all four States of Mind. They feel depressed. They feel mania. And they feel dysthymic. So I'm only using the word "normal" to refer to the most-commonly experienced, ordinary state of mind.

Now let's explore the shape of the Normal line. Like all event lines, the Normal line has several observable measures. The first measure is called the "***period.***" It's the space between the two short vertical bars on this line. This space refers to the average amount of time it takes for this line to go from one peak to the next—in other words, the time it takes to go from peak-to-peak, or from upmost point-to-upmost point.

Know that the periods of all four State of Mind lines are recognizably different. So learning to recognize these differences is one way to identify each line.

And the second measure? This one is called the "***onset ramp.***" Think of this as the measure of how abruptly or gradually these lines rise upward. Know this measure will be of great interest to us in a later chapter, when we discuss differences in the risks for various addictions. Here, the steeper the onset ramp, the greater the risk.

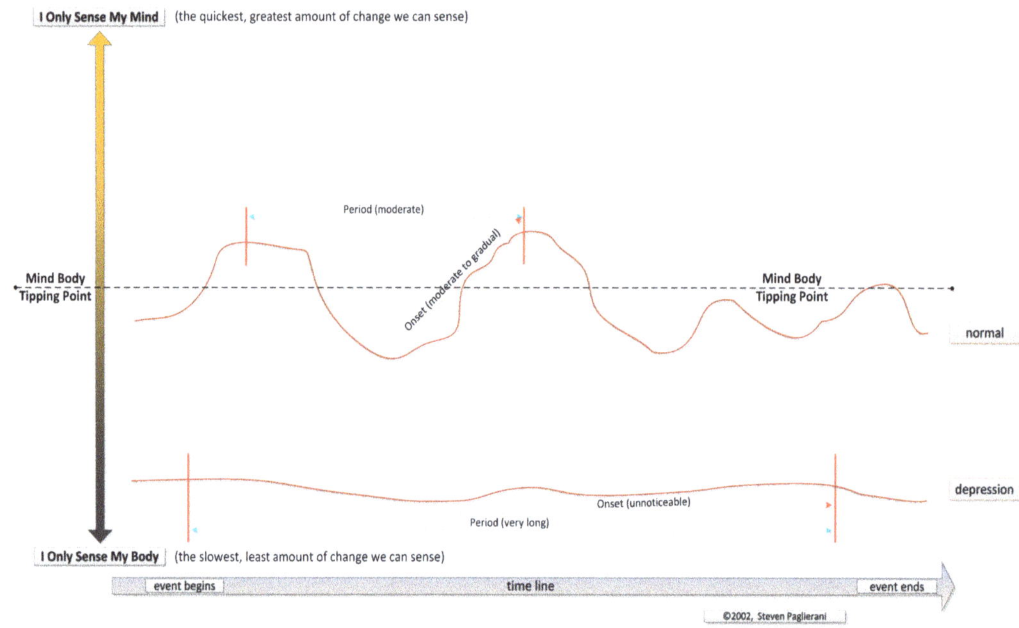

How Does Depression Differ From a Normal State of Mind?

Hopefully, you're beginning to see how this contrast and compare thing works. Please apply what you've learned so far to this drawing—by contrasting and comparing these two lines. Keep in mind, all State of Mind line-drawings occur in the same amount of time. So the only changes you need to focus on here are those which occur as you move forward in time.

Recall, these ups and downs refer to momentary changes in the amount of Meaning an event has—where *up* equals more meaning and *down* equals less. Can you see how the Normal line has quite a few ups and downs? Compare this to the Depression line, which has almost no perceptible ups or downs.

Diagnostically, we'd say the periods of Normal lines are a medium length—whereas the periods on the Depression line are extremely long. And the onset ramps of these two lines? How rapidly do these ups and downs occur?

Diagnostically, we'd say, the ups and downs on the Normal line are easily perceived. Whereas the ups and downs on the Depression line are almost imperceptible.

This means, on the Depression line, it feels like nothing ever changes. Whereas on the Normal line, it feels like nothing out of the ordinary occurs. Want to get a sense of what it feels like to be in these two States of Mind? Picture yourself hiking on ground shaped like these lines. Now imagine walking for long periods of time on ground that never changes. This is what depression feels like.

Contrast this to what hiking on ground shaped like the Normal line would be like. This hike would, at times, feel challenging, but doable, and interesting. This is the power of using shaped event lines to diagnostically evaluate what's in people's minds. Imagine how easily your patients could respond to how-are-you questions.

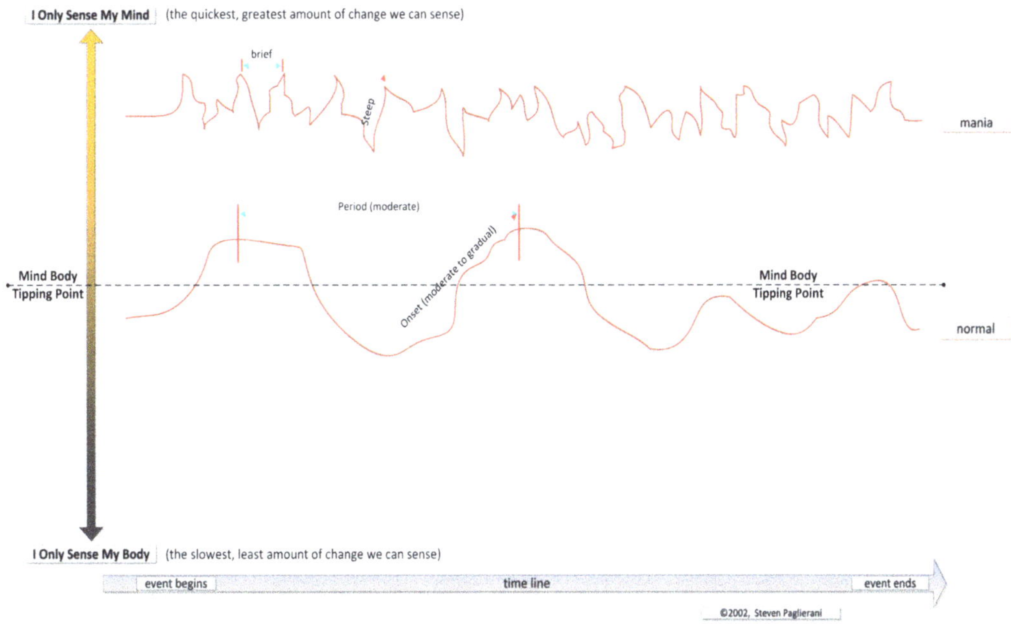

How Does Mania Differ From the Normal State of Mind?

Compared to what life feels like on the Depression line, life on the Mania line looks like it must feel crazy. And it does. For one thing, even compared to the Normal line, the Mania line has far more ups and downs. Also, these ups and downs occur unpredictably, and begin and end much more abruptly. They also change direction so quickly that it's hard to know what's coming next.

Diagnostically, compared to the periods on the Normal line, the periods in mania are much shorter. Of the four States of Mind, mania has the shortest periods. Also, in mania, the onset ramps are incredibly steep. Indeed, of the four States of Mind, these onset ramps are by far the steepest.

Taken together, these two measures (the period and onset ramp) make experientially recognizing changes on the Mania line harder to see than those which occur on the Normal line. To some people, this may sound counter-intuitive. Most people would think that mania would be easy to see. In part, this arises out of a mistaken belief that equates experiencing mania to feeling happy.

The Four States of Mind do not, as I've defined them, include references to emotions—or to the lack thereof. People who are experiencing mania can feel extremely happy, extremely angry, or extremely sad. Please keep this in mind then when diagnosing, as many diagnosticians make this mistake. A state of mind is not an emotion, nor is an emotion a state of mind.

Finally, I want to mention a third diagnostic measurement we need to make on these lines. This one is called, the ***Dynamic Range*** of the line. This term refers to the distance between the highest up and lowest low. I'll be telling you what this is and why it's important before the chapter ends.

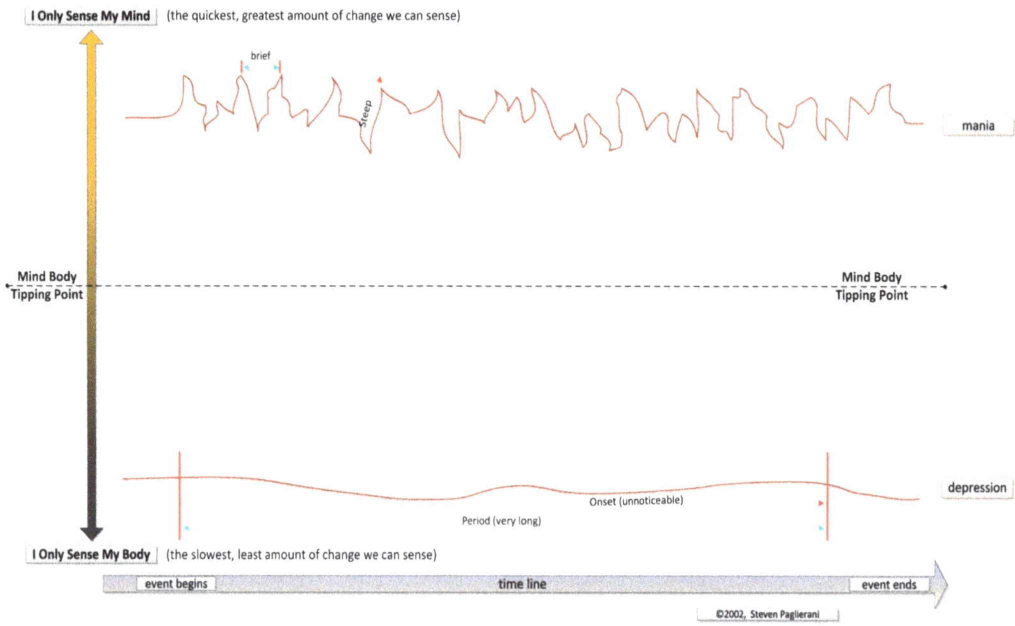

How Does Mania Differ From Depression?

Before reading any of this, please write down your existing impressions of how mania and depression differ. Literally, please do this. Not your impressions based on seeing these lines. Rather, your impressions before reading this book.

When you've done this, then spend a few minutes contrasting and comparing this drawing's two lines. Then—without thinking about what you thought mania and depression were, write down your impressions of these two lines. Only the lines.

Now let's talk about—and apply—the various measures I've previously mentioned to these two lines. Compare the ***periods*** in both lines. Compare the two kinds of ***onset ramps***. Compare the ***placements*** in this mental space, top to bottom. Finally compare the ***dynamic ranges*** of these two lines.

Periods? Mania has extremely short periods. The periods in depression are extremely long.

Onset ramps? Mania? Extremely sharp ups and downs. Depression? Close to imperceptible.

Placements? Mania is all the way up at the top of the mind's mental space. Depression? All the way at the bottom.

Dynamic Range? Mania has the second to the smallest of the four states of mind. Depression? The smallest.

Diagnostically, what does any of this mean? More than you could ever imagine. These four measures hold the keys to understanding the mechanisms of wounding and healing. They also reveal the mechanisms behind memory problems—including why people can't remember what they did during clinical depressions or diagnosably manic episodes. All this from just four easily remembered, simple line drawings.

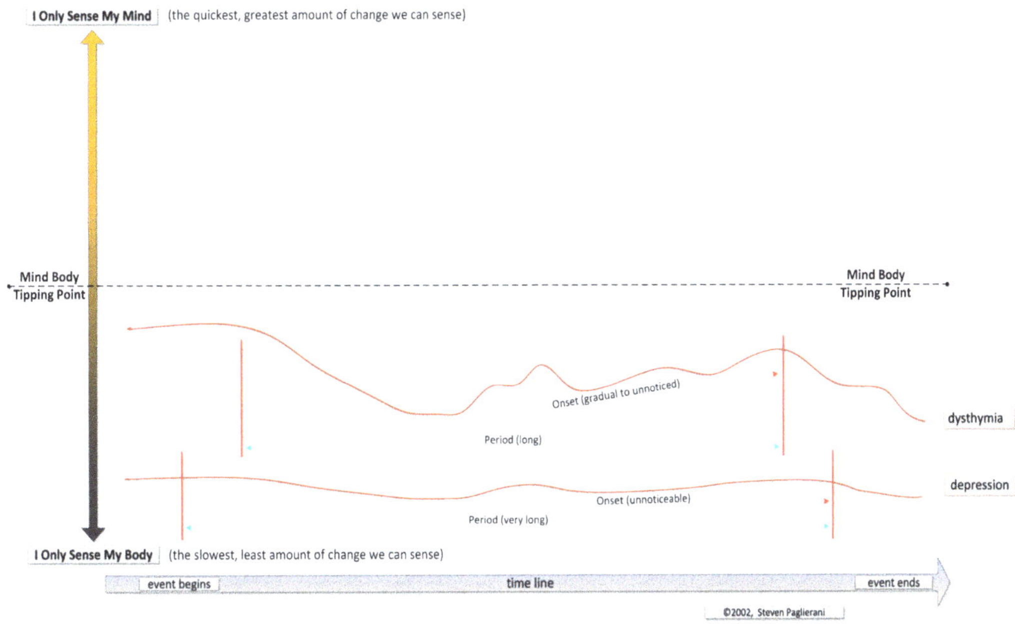

How Does Dysthymia Differ From Depression?

Every time I look at this pair of lines, I recall not understanding the word "dysthymia" back in college. I remember being told it was *sort of* like a low grade depression and feeling confused as to why I was paying to learn unscientific nonsense like this. Is dysthymia a low grade depression? No. Dysthymia is a distinctly different state of mind from depression. Likewise, a diagnosis of dysthymia is even more distinctly different from the diagnosis we refer to as clinical depression.

Now imagine you are back in college, taking a test. On it, you're asked to describe these differences. What a crock of BS that would be, now wouldn't it? How many words would you need to scientifically do this? Compare doing that to drawing these two lines, in their proper places, in this rectangular-shaped mental space.

Which would be more doable for you?

Do you have to think about this?

Probably not. Hopefully, this difference is beginning to sink in.

Ok. Now do a diagnostic assessment of these two lines. Contrast and compare the periods of these two lines, the two onset ramps, the two spacial placements, and the two dynamic ranges.

A simple response might go something like this.

The State of Mind I'm calling "dysthymia—"as compared to the state of mind I'm calling "depression"—has somewhat shorter periods (changes come more often), has somewhat steeper onset ramps (these changes are somewhat more noticeable), is placed notably higher up with regard to the Meaning line (it has more meaning), and it has quite a bit more dynamic range (these changes feel stronger).

Now consider how what I've just written compares to what you'd have written back in college. Any different? Any clearer? Any easier to access?

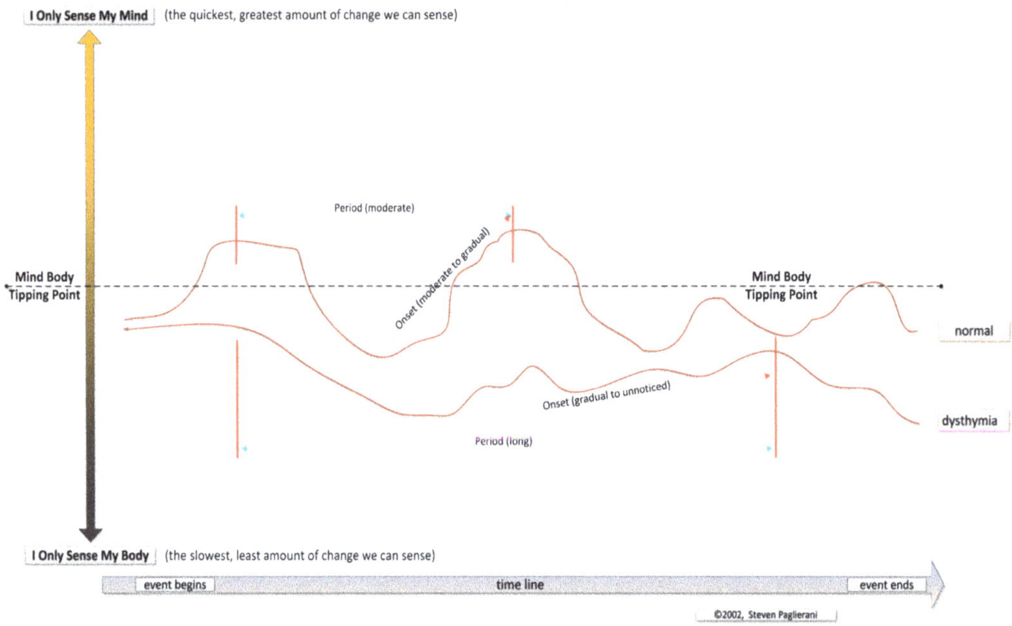

How Does Dysthymia Differ From the Normal State of Mind?

To most people, the State of Mind I'm calling "dysthymia" is the least familiar of the four. Keep in mind, I am not referring to the diagnosis by the same name. This drawing refers only to the fractal pattern of this line. Also, the diagnosis requires a much longer Time line. Short periods of dysthymia are not diagnosable.

This said, it's not surprising that people who *should* get diagnosed with dysthymia often do not. Why?

Because even well-educated people can diagnostically mistake dysthymia for "low normal."

Then again, I've also often heard therapists call dysthymia, "functional depression." Word-wise, either of these descriptions could fit—and at times, be useful. However, compared to what we gain by seeing how the Dysthymia State of Mind line compares to the other three lines, these vague descriptions fail miserably.

Which is it?

Functional depression?

Low normal?

Something else?

Is this any way to ground diagnosis in science?

Obviously, not.

The thing to pay close attention to here is where dysthymia lies meaning-wise. Specifically, it rarely rises above the midline, and this can be diagnostically helpful. Clearly, people feel changes when they are experiencing this state of mind. However, while these folks do accomplish tasks in life, they rarely if ever enjoy having done them. These accomplishments are more just things they've checked off a list.

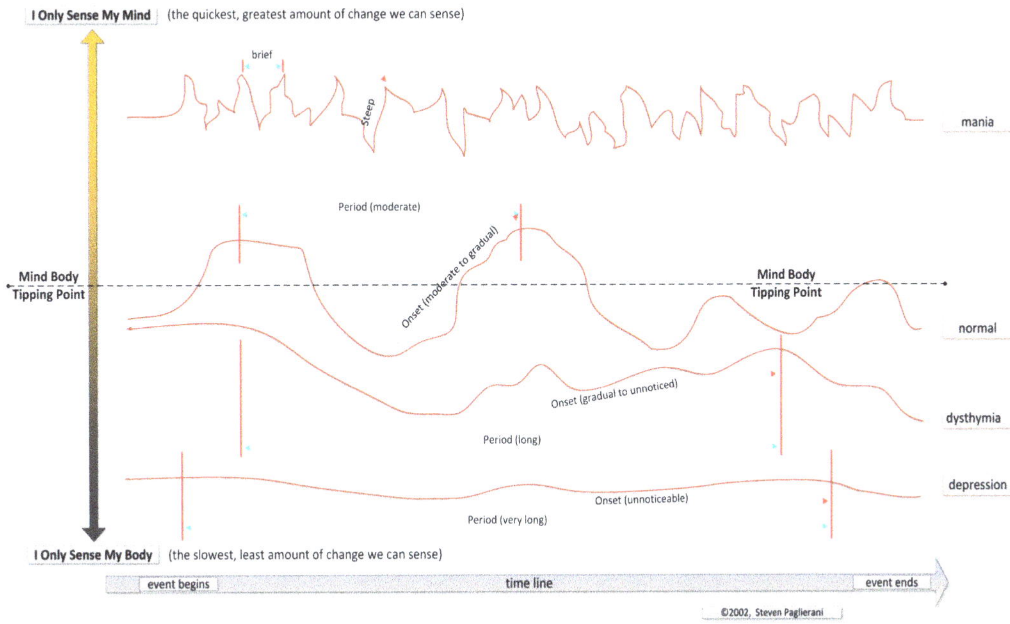

Can You Possibly Have Trouble Telling These Four Lines Apart?

Ok. Take a few minutes to contrast and compare the diagnostic points on these lines. Look closely at the length of the periods of each line—could you possibly not see these differences? How about where these lines have been vertically placed in this mental space? Could you possibly miss how many peaks each line has?

How about the four onset ramps of these four states of mind? Could they be any clearer? Is it now beginning to make sense to you how these simple lines could communicate proper diagnostic data? Imagine drawing a line in a patient's chart as opposed to writing all that pathetic, unscientific, technically accepted psychobabble? How about how you might gather better diagnostic data from your patients were you to teach them to recognize these lines? More important, could you possibly mistake any one of these four States of Mind for any of the others?

Is the candle lit?

Is the client depressed?

Is this way of diagnosing easier?

Duh!

What do you think?

Should You Believe This Stuff Without It Being Peer Reviewed?

In the Introduction, I commented on how everything in diagnostic manuals is based on assumptions about personality. Despite this, no references to these assumptions are ever made. More specifically, no actual personality theory is ever mentioned. Why? Because diagnostic manuals are created by committees.

According to the APA—the latest diagnostic manual was created by over 160 Work Group members and over 300 outside advisors.

Obviously, getting this many people to reach a consensus is a monumental task.

Getting them to agree on aspects of personality theory is even harder.

To solve this, the authors agreed to leave out all possible mentions of personality.

As my Jewish friends might say, this was truly a "shanda"; a scandalously shameful act. This means the included diagnoses have no actual baselines. The thing is, while this, in and of itself, is an egregious problem, there is another problem which is far worse. Know this worse problem becomes visible only when we dissect the word, "consensus."

Here, the "con" part means "with," and the "sensus" part—well, I'm guessing you can see it.

The point is, all existing diagnostic manuals were created by taking a census. Not coincidentally, most of those polled in this census were untrained in personality and psychotherapy. Some might say, since neither personality nor psychotherapy are ever mentioned in these books, this doesn't matter. But even if we were to correct this by polling only those well-educated in personality and psychotherapy, we'd still be left with a glaring problem.

Can you guess what it is?

Based on what I just said, clearly, it's not education.

The problem I'm referring to can be found even in the most educated people. I, myself, came to learn about this problem only later in life. I learned about it from one of those tiny-sized books often found in people's bathrooms. You know, those books which offer simple explanations for everything on a particular topic?

The topic and title of the book I read?

"The Forty False Arguments."

Truly, this book opened my eyes to much of what couples say to each other in their worst fights.

More important, it helped me to understand how so many otherwise smart scientists can make false claims which to many people do sound possible.

How?

Because they arrange their words to fit certain patterns.

These patterns were the actual focus of this little book, the title of which should have been, "The Forty Patterns Smart People Use When They Want To Bullshit Themselves and Others."

The false argument that applies here?

That "popularity equates to truth."

That voting on an idea or belief can prove an idea is sound.

This brings us back to that word again—consensus. So what is a *consensus* really?

It's simple. A *consensus* is a "statistical popularity contest."

The false argument I'm referring to here?

"Argumentum ad populum."

This argument claims that if most people believe something, that this proves this something is true.

The world once believed the Earth was flat. Did this mean this claim was true? Obviously not. Yet everything in existing diagnostic manuals has been created similarly—by consensus.

Guess what this means about these sacred texts?

Is this why "statistics" is mentioned in all of the titles?

Clearly, this is not something I'd risk mentioning if I'd been asked to choose the title. In truth, it's one of the best ways to prove a book about diagnosing *individuals* is based on bad science. Statistics does not apply to individuals.

Then too, there's the fact that arguing to popularity isn't the only problem. The opposite false belief is also seen as true.

The belief?

That if less than a consensus (and especially, if just a single person) believes something is true, then this something must be false.

This is the oft-used argument which supposedly proves Freudian therapies are scientifically false.

Know I'm not claiming they are true. I'm only claiming this way of proving them false is nonsense. Smarter people might add, this claim only means we cannot know if something is true. And when it comes to words, this is often the case. But when it comes to pictures of fractal things—such as candle flames and cumulus clouds, this is not true.

With these kinds of things, a single visual experience—made by a single person, can be known, with certainty, to be true.

For example, can you ever not know if a candle is lit or not? Or if the sky has clouds? Or if a tide is coming in or out?

Based on a single experience, a five-year-old could be certain of these kinds of things.

All this is to say, in this chapter, I have offered you a shitload of single, visual fractal experiences.

Everything in this book will be based on similar single, visual fractal experiences. This means, nothing in this book will be claimed to be true because people voted on it and these ideas won.

Peer-reviewed?

Agreed on by consensus?

10,000 psychiatrists say it's true?

All these things are complete and utter bullshit when it comes to proper science. And lest you disagree, I suggest you consult Dr. Google on this phrase.

"Argumentum ad populum."

What Will We Look At Next?

In this chapter, we asked, **Can We Make the Invisible Mind Visible?** In the next chapter, we'll expand on this with a first look at what should be the main focus of all diagnostic manuals—**The Nature of Wounds**. Like all things in the mind, wounds are also invisible. Ironically, no existing diagnostic manual has ever directly referred to—let alone, defined wounds. All they've done is vaguely define categories of similar symptoms. And this really runs off the rails when several diagnoses all refer to the same symptoms.

Which is the right one? All of them? This can't be right.

So how will our diagnostic manual be different?

To begin with, we'll explore the previously unknown nature of getting wounded. All existing diagnostic manuals address "mental" wounds. Yet none of these books explain or describe what actually occurs in the mind—what a wound actually is. What happens to us when we get wounded? Is there an underlying fractal pattern?

You're about to learn that there is such a pattern, and that it's easily recognized. This is one of the things we'll visually explore in the next chapter.

We'll also discuss something no mental health professional ever speaks about—let alone, gets right—the idea that the size of the symptoms you can see and observe *never* matches the size of people's wounds.

How do these sizes of wounds and symptoms differ?

The symptoms of any and all wounds are actually exponentially greater than those present in the original event.

Why?

Because each time you relive a wound, regression and transference form a feedback loop. And like all feedback loops, this one amplifies the symptoms similarly to how auditory feedback occurs in an auditorium.

Symptoms are like auditory squealing? Who knew?

Then there's the idea that all medical professions conflate the wounds themselves with the observable symptoms and painful events. Here, by "conflate," I mean they speak about these two things (wounds and symptoms) as if they are interchangeable. This means ***any attempts to address these wounds will be based on erroneous assumptions***, the main one being that the size of the symptoms indicates the size of the wounding event—another being that if you eliminate the symptoms, then the wound is healed.

Neither of these things are ever true. Not even once.

Finally, we'll look at how you can use event lines to diagnose specific "disorders." Do know that like many other medical words, we'll be redefining this word as well. So what is a "dis-order?" We'll have a lot to discuss. Just know, like the things we've previously looked at—where what I show you makes things clear—redefining the word *disorder* will likely change your entire practice.

Curious?

I certainly hope so.

See you in the next chapter.

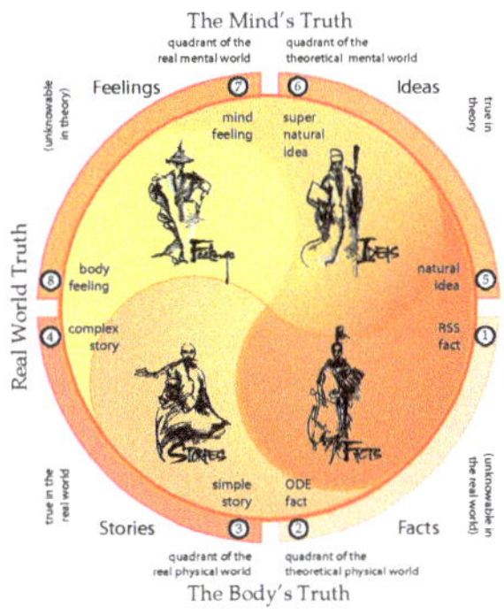

Chapter 2

Wounds or Symptoms?
(what can we learn about . . . ?)

What Should Diagnosticians Be Looking For?

As I begin this chapter, I'm smiling at what just went through my head. I just thought, "I'm going to define *wounds*. I wonder what you, the reader, would write if I asked you to define this word." Know I'm not smiling because I think you'd do badly. I'm smiling because of how short I'm guessing your definition would be. A few sentences? A few paragraphs? A page or two? More?

Please realize, in my thought experiment, I haven't asked you "how you find" wounds. Nor have I asked you how you assign a diagnosis to what you find. All I've asked for is a quick and dirty blurb which, to other professionals, would scientifically describe what wounds ***are*** and ***are not***. Oh. You didn't realize I was asking for a scientific definition of the constellated variety? If so, please don't feel bad.

It can take some time to get used to this more rigorous type of science.

How about this. How about if you write a brief description of what it is you look for when you diagnose. Add to this how you know these particular things refer to a wound. Your proof. When you're done, please set what you wrote aside. We'll return to it later. Now let me ask. Are you at all curious as to how long my definition of *wounds* will be? A hint. I am going to claim I can scientifically define the word *wounds* without using a single word. Further, I am going to claim that it will not be possible for you to forget this definition—after seeing it even once.

Are you curious now? I'm excited. Scientific diagnosis, here we come.

What Will We Talk About In This Chapter?

Before we begin, I want to ask that you do an exercise as you read through this section. I'm going to ask you to stop reading at several points. Each time you stop, I'd like you to do two things—in this order. One. Try to literally picture an example of what I've just said. Literal pictures have colors. Two, ***if you can't***, then ask yourself this. How many times did you feel overwhelmed by the things I'd just said?

Please know, you'll still gain from what you read here, even if you do not do this exercise. But not doing it may prevent you from acquiring the personal experience necessary to retain what you read. For this reason, please, do your best to self-examine as you read through this section. And remember, when diagnosing, you shouldn't ask patients to look at, or try, things you yourself won't explore.

∞

Ok. I'm sure you see it. It's on the next page. An event line drawing of the shape of all wounding events—complete with that nasty looking, spiky black ball. Of course, to know what this line means, you'll first need to correlate it to a sufficient number of real world, professional experiences. And to do that, you'll need to know what this simple line represents.

This said, having read Chapter 1, you should recognize a few things in that drawing. The Meaning and Time lines should be easy to spot. The series of connected single-moment plots which create that line too. Even the shape of this line should tell you something about what is going on. The places it moves through inside the rectangular space. Its onset ramp. The number of periods. Its dynamic range.

I'm curious though. The words? Did you have trouble not looking at them? Did you even remember to try not to do this? If so, don't be hard on yourself. Learning to focus on event line shapes—and not on words—can take a bit of time as well. This said, clearly we have much to discuss before we explore this line.

I first need to ground this chapter in something you hopefully already know.

To start with, I'd like to know what you look for as you begin with a new patient. What do you usually focus on? The person's face? Appearance? Their mannerisms? Something else? Whatever you just answered, let me ask you this. Did any of what you thought of involve some variation of "I look for *symptoms* and *signs*?" If it did, do you think you could scientifically define the difference between these two words?

What the heck is a sign anyway? I recall back in school being told, a *sign* is something only those trained in diagnosis could know to look for and recognize. As opposed to *symptoms*, which even laypersons can supposedly identify.

I now need to tell you something. Please read this sentence slowly.

To gather scientifically sound data from your patients, you'll need *to teach them to see both of these things*.

How? And doesn't doing this violate that secretly implied mandate you were given back in school—you know, the one that says you should assume patients are "fragile morons" who need to be protected from needing to know such things?

Obviously it does violate that mandate. Then again, your patients aren't morons.

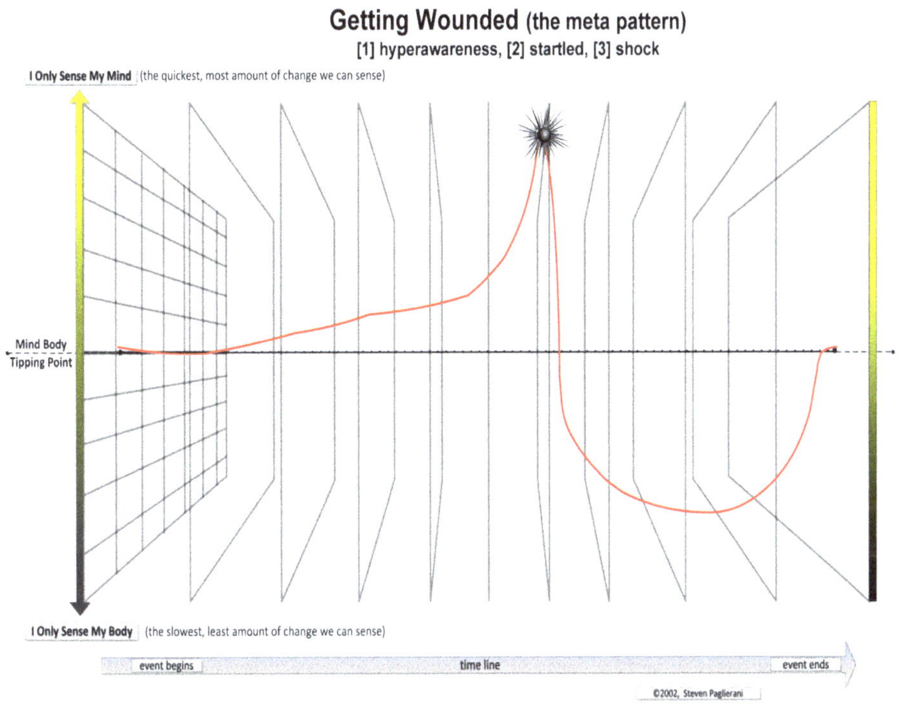

They're human beings who deserve respect, regardless of their diagnosis.

Also, patients can—and should—be taught to partner with you in the diagnostic process. To be blunt, being treated as an equal human being by a therapist can be a life-changing experience for them. And shouldn't they always be treated like this anyway? I, for one, think so. How will this affect the diagnostic process though? Are there any downsides? This is a great question.

For one thing, many patients—when asked how they are—feel afraid to express the wrong words. After all, you may laugh at them for doing this badly. You may see them as dumb. And patients frequently feel inhibited and embarrassed by things. So they voice the symptoms of these things in guarded ways.

They also don't want to feel stupid or small because they don't know as much as you. And in some cases, they feel afraid you'll say they need serious medications or worse, that they need to be sent to a rehab or hospitalized because they're crazy.

What about you? Have you ever gone to a therapist? If so, did you feel any of these things? If you did, how did those feelings affect your work in therapy?

In my lifetime, I've been to many therapists. Some were kind. Some were cold. One was even as mean as a junk yard dog. Regardless, when it came to being diagnosed, I never completely opened up. No surprise. None of them got me to feel like an equal—and this affected my openness in sessions.

One—the junk yard dog woman—in the final minutes of my last session with her, screamed at me and said, "I feel sorry for your patients if you stop seeing me." Talk about a bad therapist. The "C" word comes to mind.

Then again, I did gain from that suffering. To this day, I consider my patients in ways only that experience could teach.

Mainly, I never ever want them to feel like they are less than me.

[STOP, get up from your seat, and do a standing self check-in]

So what will we talk about in this chapter? A whole lot of things. I'll first introduce you to another set of four event lines—*the Four Kinds of Mental Changes*. This set of 4 lines describes and defines the ways changes happen in the mind. Here, two of these kinds of changes are temporary—and two are permanent.

Can you guess what the two kinds of permanent changes are?

A hint. One involves symptoms, but only after the fact.

Another hint. Both involve being suddenly surprised.

A third hint. One of these kinds of changes is the shape of all experiences which teach you to love.

A final hint. Used together, these kinds of two permanent changes form the scientific basis for all diagnostic inquiries. One rules things in. One rules things out. And together, nothing gets omitted or overlooked.

Am I driving you crazy? If so, know I am doing this on purpose. Learning does not occur until what you already know gets challenged in deeply troubling ways. No surprise, one of the times people get deeply challenged is when they get a diagnosis.

Does this explain how even just diagnosing patients can change their lives?

[Please STOP and do a still-seated self check-in]

The second thing we'll look at? Something I'm sure you've known about for years. *The nature of Regression and Transference*. Why look at this? Because you cannot diagnose properly without knowing how to determine the true size of your patient's wounds. Know I'll claim in this chapter that "the present-day sizes of your patient's symptoms" are *never* the same as "that which existed in the wounding events." In other words, the suffering present during wounding events will always be magnitudes smaller than the size of the symptoms these wounds later cause.

Please realize, exploring this topic took four chapters in my previous book. Does that tell you how much more you might learn from what we'll be looking at here? Know that when I discovered how these two things interact, I felt blown away.

In truth, before that, my ability to diagnose depended a lot on intuition.

At the time, like most of you, I'd known those two words for my whole career. Somehow though, I'd never thought to ask if and how they might interact with each other. So do they? The surprising truth? They cannot exist separately. Not ever. And together, these two things distort your patient's symptoms almost to the point of being diagnostically useless. Every single time.

Because of this, your patients' symptoms cannot tell you the seriousness of their wounding events. Thus many of the things you've been using to arrive at a diagnosis have never, not once, scientifically correlated to any of your patient's wounds. Obviously, we have a lot to discuss here, and I'll have a lot to prove.

[Please STOP and do a self check-in. Are you overwhelmed?]

What else will we discuss? A simple, but really important topic. Something we'll explore in depth in a later chapter, and one of the main words you encounter each time you diagnose. The word? ***Disorder***. What makes this word so important? A belief that most diagnosticians have about it.

That the presence of any notable amount of disorder requires a diagnosis.

Sadly, assuming all disorder is diagnosable is an unscientific crock of shit. A "notable lack of order" can exist in both normal and abnormal life events. What makes ***disorder*** clinically significant then? This is what we will discuss.

Why does this matter? Again, we'll have a lot to talk about and more to prove.

Then there are those two words again—*signs* and *symptoms*. And yes, as I've just said, you likely already know a lot about these two words. Trust me though—not in the ways we are about to discuss here. For one thing, did you know there are only two *primary* kinds of symptoms—and that signs are the visible kind?

The first kind of symptoms? They're always physically visible, but only to diagnosticians who are trained to see them. The second kind? They're sometimes mentally visible, but only to patients and sometimes, even patients cannot see them.

Know the first kind of symptoms are better called "signs," as they involve easily read, visible evidence which occurs only in the patient's body. Unfortunately, few diagnosticians ever get taught to look for, let alone read, these signs. And no, they don't involve "body language." In fact, learning to read these signs more resembles learning to see a magician's sleight of hand trick. This said, personally, I know of no better way to scientifically identify wounds. Period.

The second kind of symptoms? They derive entirely from patient reporting. But to make this reporting diagnostically relevant, you'll need to teach your patients a new skill. This skill involves asking them to divide what's in their minds into two piles. "Can you picture yourself doing such and such? Yes (pile 1)? Or No (pile 2)?

If the patient answers—"Yes, I can picture this thing"—then it's clinically *insignificant* and you've just ruled it out. If the patient says—"No, I can't picture this thing"—then it's clinically *significant* and you've just ruled it in. Know at times, you'll need to advise patients to just try to imagine this thing. No need to recall an actual example. And if they can't even then? Then you can rule this thing *in*.

Obviously, you've never been trained in either of these skills. Indeed, I'd bet you've never thought to divide diagnostic assessments into what's *visible only to you* versus what's *visible only to the client*. Did you notice, both things involve the ability to picture things? This makes picturing things an important diagnostic tool.

The last thing I'll mention here is how these two skills can form a baseline for determining clinical significance. Used correctly, they let you scientifically test for whether or not wounds exist. Know these tests will work regardless of whether symptoms exist or not. And yes, by themselves, these two skills are not enough to arrive at a diagnosis—you'll also need to learn a lot about *measuring* personality. But learning to do that will come much later in this book.

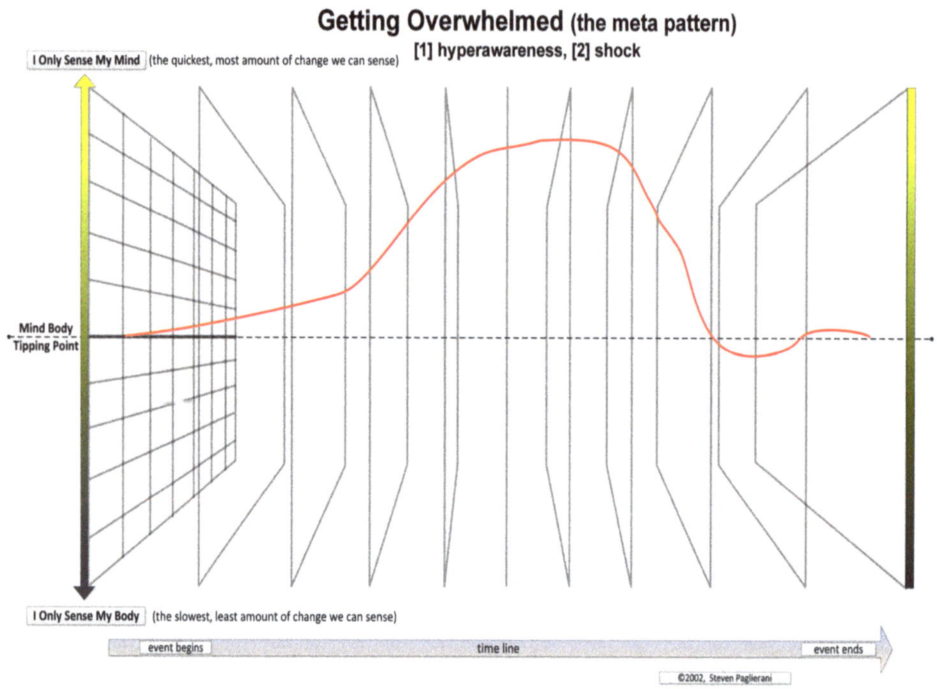

Change Type One: Getting Overwhelmed

Imagine hiking on ground shaped like this line. Can you see that much of this experience would be hard? No coincidence, experiences like this one can occur when you exert yourself physically—especially when you don't realize you're overdoing it. More often though, they occur when you try to take in too much information—like in the previous section.

There, I listed a bunch of new ideas, but with no explanations.

Know I deliberately did this as I wanted you to have recently felt this feeling. This is why I asked you repeatedly to pause and check in with yourself. And if you didn't feel overwhelmed? Then in all likelihood, you skimmed rather than pictured my words. People who skim words tend to think they already know what's there, especially when reading a relatively unknown author.

Know some of this also correlates to folks who have above average IQ's. They hurry through words, looking to get to the salient part. Others rush though, thinking there's nothing important to be had—that whatever's there is just rehashed old news. Still others simply wish to bypass the hard part, thinking they're not going to get it anyway. So why bother. And others realize there is a lot there. So they put it on their to do list for later, knowing all too well, that is not likely to happen.

What does any of this have to do with diagnosis?

Whatever you felt as you read that previous section, realize, new patients often arrive feeling these same things. This is why, when I sit with new clients for the first time, I begin by assessing them for how and why they're overwhelmed.

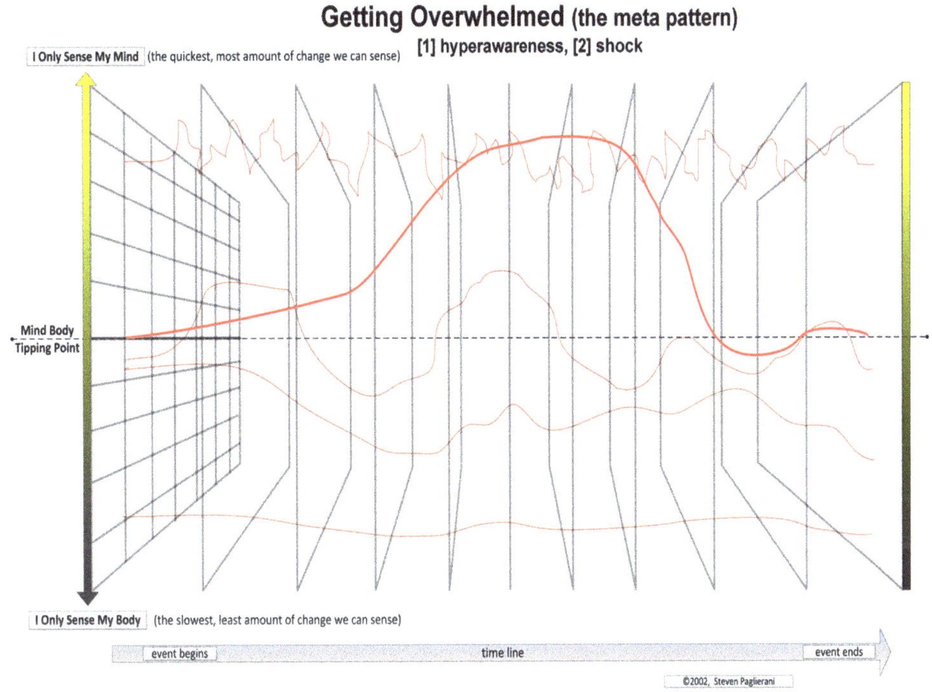

No one enters therapy because they're feeling fine. So new patients often present as having more wrong with them than is actually wrong. They also often arrive feeling they've had too much on their plates—but no one to listen to them. This means you get tacitly nominated to hear weeks, months, or years of their backlog. The upside? You get a lot of data without having to work too hard for it. The downside? It can feel like trying to keep your hair neat in a windstorm.

Picturing the Getting Overwhelmed event line—when you start with a new patient—can help, especially if you pay attention to how this line intersects with parts of the four States of Mind lines. These intersections correlate well to moods, and this can tell you a lot about your new patient's mental state. Then again, to do this, you'll first need to learn what each of these intersections mean.

We'll be looking at this throughout the chapter.

Now focus on the two axes which together define the rectangular space in this drawing. Here I'm referring to the Change line (the vertical axis) and the Time line (the horizontal axis). Recall, I've previously told you that the Time variable in all of the **Four States of Mind** represents the same amount of time. Know this is also true for the Time variable in all of the **Four Kinds of Mental Changes** as well.

This said, obviously, there must be differences between these two classes of event line drawings. Can you see any of these differences yet? One difference is the number of periods. All of the Four States of Mind lines have a different number of periods (mania/manic depression/one). Whereas all Four Kinds of Mental Change lines, including the Overwhelmed line, have the same number of periods—one.

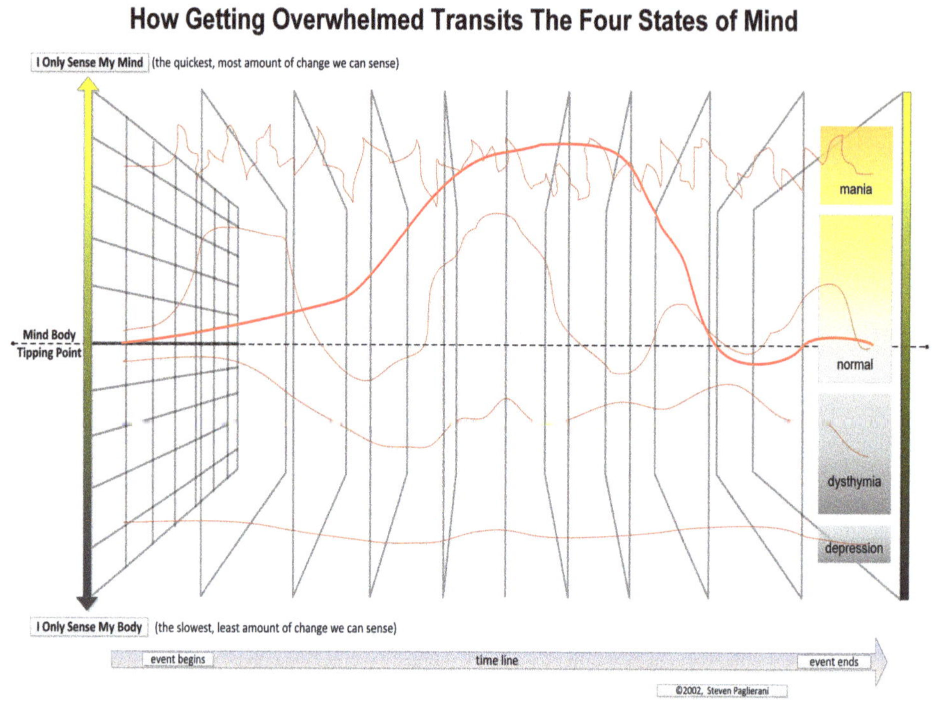

Why point this out? Because if the Time variable doesn't change—and if **Meaning = Information times Time**, then any differences between the Four Kinds of Change lines must derive from the Information changing. This leaves us with two factors we could chart here—the ***kind*** of Information (warm or cold), and the ***amount*** of Information (less or more). Event line drawings do not specify the kind of Information present. So we're left with one possibility. Any differences between the Four Kinds of Change lines must derive from changes in the ***amount*** of Information.

[Please STOP and go take a break. This stuff is extremely dense.]

The last thing I need to point out is how each of the Four States of Mind exist in a mildly overlapping, but different, "zone." Here, by *zone*, I mean a different stripe of horizontal space—*low* (depression), ***low-mid*** (dysthymia), ***high-mid*** (normal), and ***high*** (mania). This is similar to how ocean fish live in different zones. Some live closer to the surface. Some live in deeper water. And when it comes to the Four States of Mind lines, each line lives in a different zone as well.

All this is to say, all four of the Kinds of Change lines transit differently through these zones. For instance, notice how the Overwhelmed line passes through only two of these four zones. At times, it passes through the high-mid (Normal) zone—at others, the high (Mania) zone. Know it rarely exists in the low-mid (Dysthymia) zone and never in the low (Depression) zone. We'll have more to say about this line as we proceed. But it's the next line that holds the key to this entire book.

Getting Wounded (the meta pattern)
[1] hyperawareness, [2] startled, [3] shock

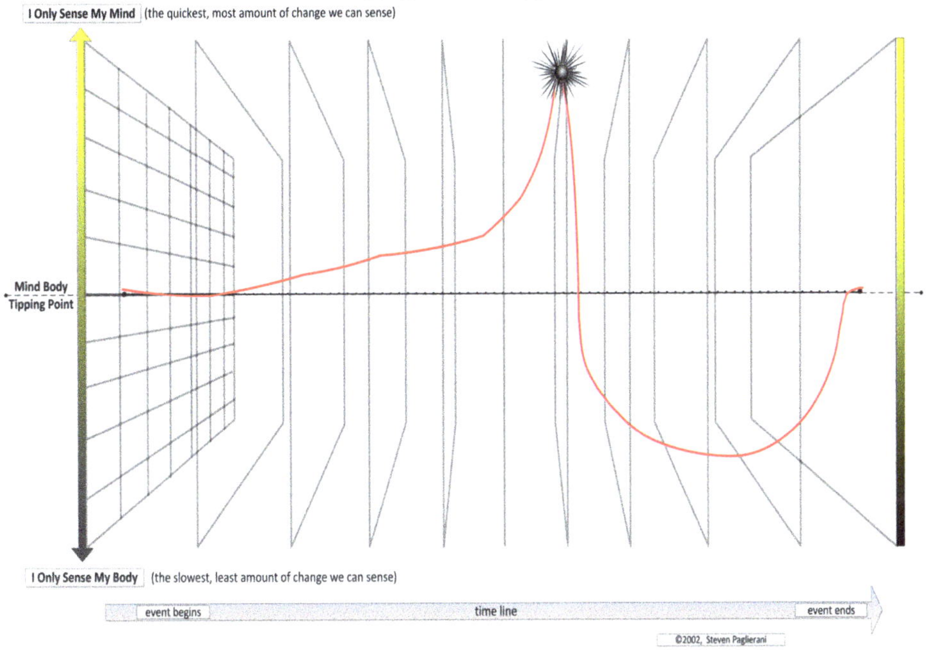

Change Type Two: Getting Wounded

Of all the things I present in this book, the Getting Wounded line is by far the most important. Every discovery I've made since 1996 has emerged from understanding this line. In particular, that spiky, black orb. Can you guess what it represents? From the zones this line passes through, you might guess, this experience involves getting overwhelmed. And it does. But the position of that spiky black orb tells us, the overwhelming part of this experience must happen suddenly, abruptly, and then quickly end.

What exactly is that spiky black orb? A sudden instant in which taking in too much information causes us to blow a mental fuse. In everyday language, we call this experience, a ***startle***. As usual, I'll need to redefine this word. In this book, a "startle" is "a three to five second pattern where taking in too much information leads to a period of sudden-onset, mental blankness." Know this blankness can last for minutes or days, or even dominate a person's mind, ***in these situations***, for years.

Regardless of the duration though, from then on, any similar life experience will permanently and involuntarily cause the person's mind to suddenly go blank. What triggers this reliving? That three to five second pattern. Moreover, any time the person relives this pattern, they will relive the startle. No exceptions.

Worse yet, because this trigger is pattern based, the situation need not look anything like what occurred in the original event. This idea—***that people relive patterns, not events—is the most important thing to know about all event lines.***

How Getting Wounded Transits The Four States of Mind

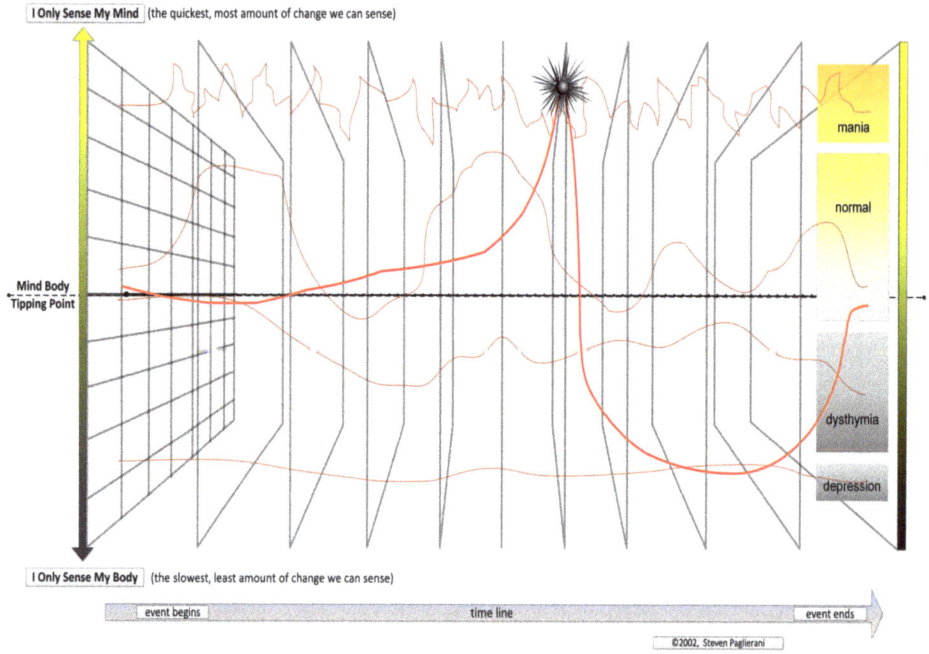

Do you want to diagnose properly? Then you must understand this idea. People get wounded because they experience a sudden jolt of too much information. That's it. It's this jolt which programs the three-to-five second pattern into the person's mind. From then on, this pattern functions like a mental cookie-cutter mold. Any life experience which can fit into this mold triggers the reliving.

Can you now see why using symptoms alone to diagnose can never result in good science? The wound itself never literally correlates to the symptoms. The wound is a pattern into which present day life events do or do not fit. These present day life events may be similar to, or completely different from, those in the original event. But if they fit the pattern, they will trigger this wound. And since the present day details will always be different from the original event, the symptoms will change.

Keep in mind, the event line in this drawing only represents the event in which this pattern got programmed into the person's mind—and not a reliving. Also recall, both the Getting Overwhelmed lines and the Getting Wounded lines represent the same amount of time, and the same number of periods—one. The key to seeing how these two lines differ then lies in noticing which zones these lines travel through. Most times, the Getting Wounded line travels through parts of all four zones—whereas the Getting Overwhelmed line travels through only two.

This means the dynamic range of Getting Wounded is roughly double that of Getting Overwhelmed. And since wide dynamic range is what causes memories to record permanently in the mind, this accounts for why Getting Overwhelmed is a temporary state. It only goes through two zones. So we forget it and move on.

	Getting Overwhelmed	Getting Wounded
# of periods	One	One
onset-ramp	Gradual	Extremely Steep
placement	Between Mania & Normal	Between Mania & Depression
dynamic range	2 Zones - 3 Mood Changes	4 Zones - 7 Mood Changes

Getting Wounded is a four zone line though. So this pattern is permanent. Like scars, it exists in us even after we heal the wound. Another part of this permanence involves the differences between the two onset ramps. The Getting Overwhelmed line onset ramp is gradual—the Getting Wounded line onset ramp is very steep.

This explains why people can see themselves getting overwhelmed, whereas no one can know they're about to get wounded. This also explains why *most wounds occur in otherwise ordinary events*—and not during what diagnosticians would call "traumatic events." Another outrageous claim? WTF. Admittedly, most diagnosticians will find this hard to believe. Isn't trauma the source of all wounds?

Actually, no, it's not. Any time a person gets startled, they will get wounded.

My proof for this? The diagnostician's two main signs—wincing and flinching. Oddly, despite years of searching, I've not found a single mention of how these two things indicate that people are reliving wounds. Mentions of the idea that regression and transference can't exist separately are similarly missing. As are mentions of the idea that without transference, a therapist cannot have empathy. So much for that shit about boundaries. Making people cold doesn't make them safe.

Yet another difference between these lines is where they exist in the drawing's space. This placement points to the kind of moods people will feel during these events. The Getting Overwhelmed line exists almost entirely above the mid-line. It usually begins in the Normal zone, then gradually ascends into the Mania zone. Whereas the Getting Wounded line also begins in the Normal zone. But then it suddenly and unpredictably ascends into the Mania zone.

It then precipitously falls into the Dysthymia zone and at times, falls into the Depression zone before gradually ascending back to the Normal zone. **[Note: Aren't you glad you have a drawing?]** More important, the Getting Overwhelmed line does not have a startle, and the Getting Wounded line does. In a way then, while both lines begin in a Normal State of Mind, then rise to somewhere in a Mania State of Mind—when you get overwhelmed, this happens *gradually* and you can see it coming. Whereas when you get wounded, while you also get overwhelmed, this happens *suddenly and painfully* and you can never see this coming.

Realize, the word "overwhelmed" is just a fancy way to say the person experiences "too much information." This happens on both event lines. But with wounds, this happens so abruptly that the person suddenly goes blank. This means what actually wounds the person is sudden onset TMI. Who knew it was this simple?

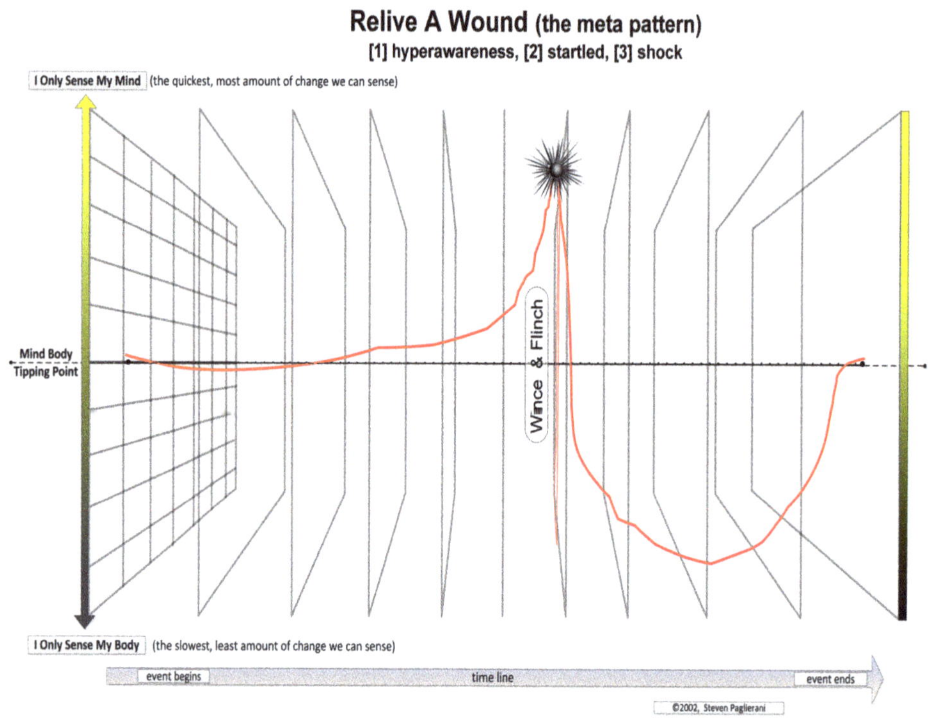

Change Type Three: Reliving a Wound

Before going into detail as to what this next line represents, please take a minute to contrast and compare it to the previous two lines. Here, focus your attention on the shapes of the onset ramps—and on the fact that there is now an additional, precipitous drop. Now let's look together.

The onset ramp of the Getting Overwhelmed line is gradual and fairly smooth.

The onset ramp of the Getting Wounded line is fairly steep and smooth.

The onset ramp of the Reliving a Wound line is steep and bumpy, and it now has a hard to see, very thin, almost imperceptible, sudden drop and rise from the peak.

Now notice the two words to the right of this new drawing's onset ramp drop. And yes, I'm pointing out words—something I rarely do. The two words? I mentioned them a moment ago—***Wince*** and ***Flinch***. Here, I'm sure you know the gist of what these words mean. However, as I'm sure you've noticed, I often tweak the meanings of already existing, but important, words.

Diagnostically, these two words: "wince" and "flinch," are beyond important. In fact, I call these two words, "the diagnostician's friends." Why? Because they offer a rarity in diagnosis—they offer a diagnostic certainty. Specifically, they are the only two *visible* ways to be diagnostically certain you've seen a patient relive a wound.

And the scientific definitions for these two words? First, I'll offer what they both have in common. Both of these things are, "An involuntary, sudden anticipatory response to the expectation of pain." How are they different then?

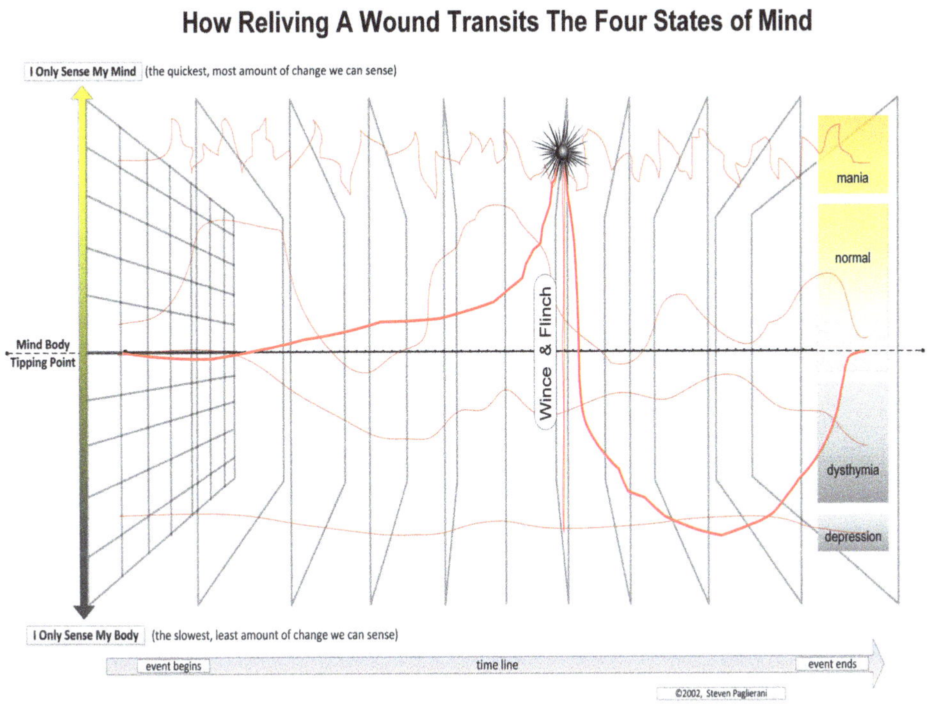

A wince is how the mind responds to the anticipation of pain.

A flinch is how the body responds to the anticipation of pain.

Winces cause the patient's *eyes* to tighten and stiffen.

Flinches cause the patient's *body* to tighten and stiffen.

Can both things happen to a person at the same time? Sometimes, yes, they can. Most times though, it's one or the other.

What determines which it is? Often this depends on the person's Mind Body Orientation. Here ***Mind First*** people mostly wince (their first reaction occurs in the mind), and ***Body First*** people most often flinch (their first reaction occurs in the body). Know we'll look at ***Mind First*** and ***Body First*** in depth in a later chapter. But diagnostically, when looking for wounds, this difference is of minor concern.

What is important to know is that, without exception, each time you see a patient winch or flinch, the person just relived a wound. Keep in mind that prior to being wounded, people often find it hard to believe they will suffer in a situation. Whereas once they've been wounded, they will find it hard to believe they will not suffer in this situation.

Clearly, we have a lot to discuss about this difference. For now, try to focus only on learning to see the shape of this new line. Here, pay special attention to that thin, hard to see, sudden dip and rise from the spiky ball. Imagine trying to hike on land shaped like that? I can. No way do I ever want to have to do that again.

So what does that dip in that line represent?

It represents what happens to you whenever you winch or flinch.

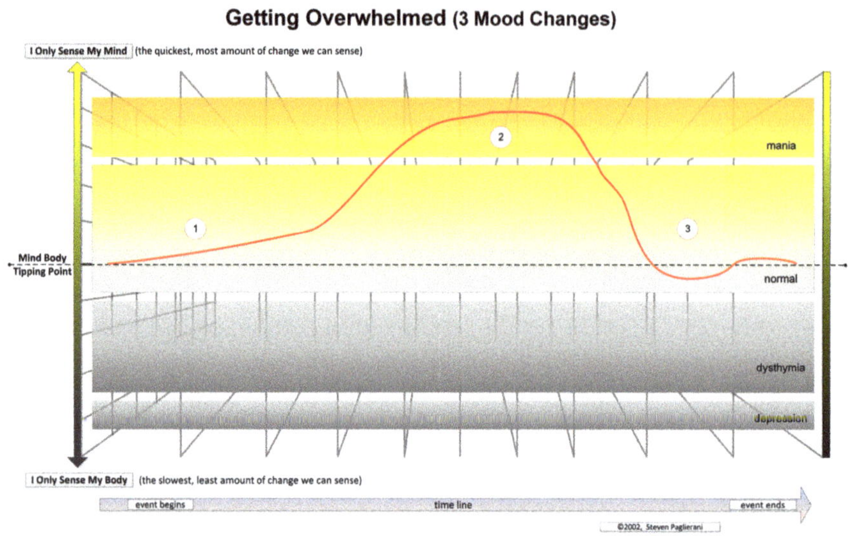

What's the Most Painful Change? A Hint. It's Not Getting Wounded

Now we come to a rather simple, but important, set of four drawings. In each of these drawings, you'll see a sequence of between three and thirteen numbers. Each of these numbers represents a mood change you go through when you experience these event lines. And the thing to pay attention to here is the total number of mood changes in each drawing.

What does this total tell us?

How complex each kind of change is.

For instance, look at the drawing I've placed at the top of this page. In it, you'll see the number of mood changes you go through when you get Overwhelmed.

This drawing tells us, you only go through three.

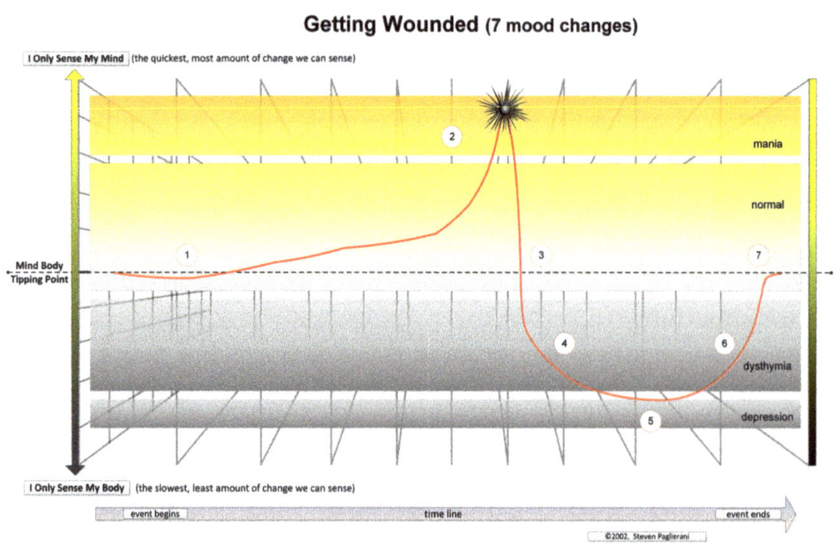

Relive A Wound (13 mood changes)

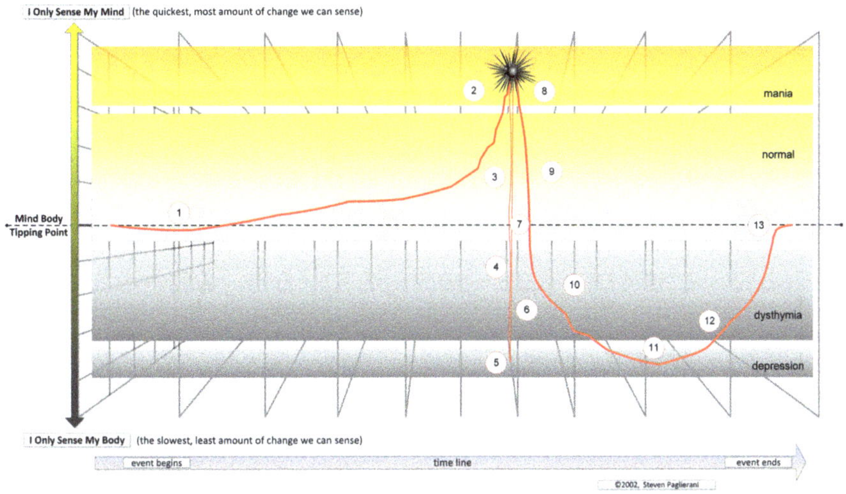

Contrast and compare this to the number of mood changes you go through when you **Get Wounded.** Here you go through *seven* mood changes. This number increases to *thirteen* when you **Relive a Wound**—telling us, this experience is far more complex. Take a moment to consider this last idea. Has this ever occurred to you before? That **Reliving a Wound** is far more complex than **Getting Wounded**?

According to the drawing, reliving involves almost twice the number of mood changes. And when you consider what this makes therapy like, this makes sense.

Finally, while we're at it—and despite my not having described the Healing line yet, we might as well include that drawing here as well. Here, when you **Heal a Wound,** you go through *nine* mood changes.

Who knew Healing a Wound was simpler than Reliving a Wound?

Healing (9 mood changes)

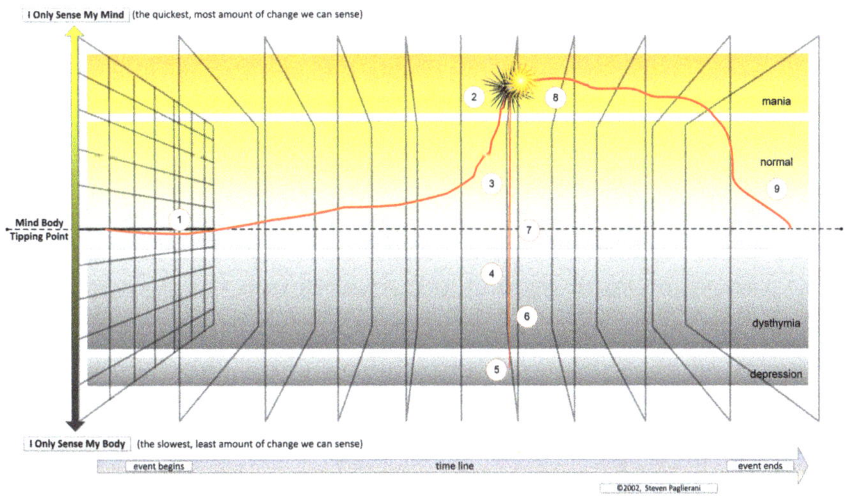

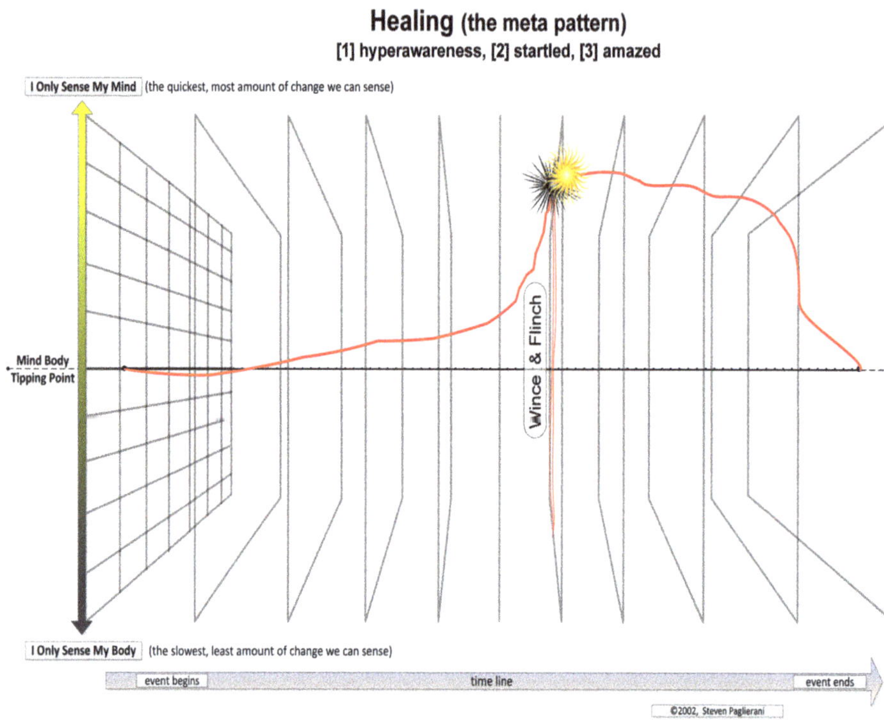

Change Type Four: Healing a Wound

Finally, we arrive at the fourth and final drawing in this set—the **Healing a Wound** event line. Not surprisingly, the latter parts of this line look a bit like an upside down version of the Relive a Wound line. Also, the front half of this line looks like it has things in common with all the other three lines. And if we ignore that dreadfully steep, down and up bit (the wince and flinch part), parts of this line look similar to the Getting Overwhelmed line as well.

The big deal here is that together, these four lines form a comprehensive foundation for diagnosis. And yes, it's taken us a lot of work to arrive here, beginning with having to learn the Four States of Mind lines. Hopefully, you can see why we had to do that first. The Four Kinds of Mental Changes describe the basics of all thought and mood changes human beings can have. So while there's a lot more to discuss, at this point, you have all the basics necessary to read these drawings.

Are you beginning to see how these drawings could teach you to diagnose in a scientific way? If not, don't worry. Along with an incredible amount of old stuff to let go of, I've given you an incredible amount of new things to take in.

What you can't deny though is how these four lines make it hard to mistake one life experience for another. Impossible, really. So what's next? A first look at how Regression and Transference form feedback loops.

Can you guess which lines these loops exist on and where they occur on those lines? A hint. Only two lines include feedback loops. This is what is coming next.

Getting Overwhelmed (the meta pattern)
[1] hyperawareness, [2] shock

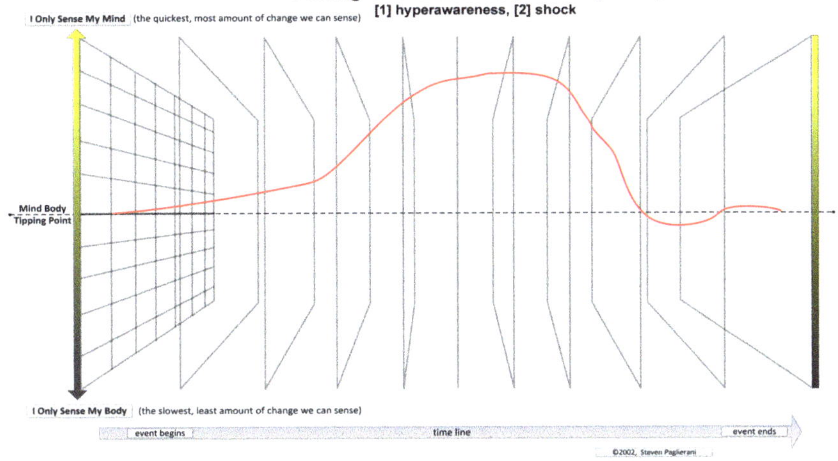

Getting Wounded (the meta pattern)
[1] hyperawareness, [2] startled, [3] shock

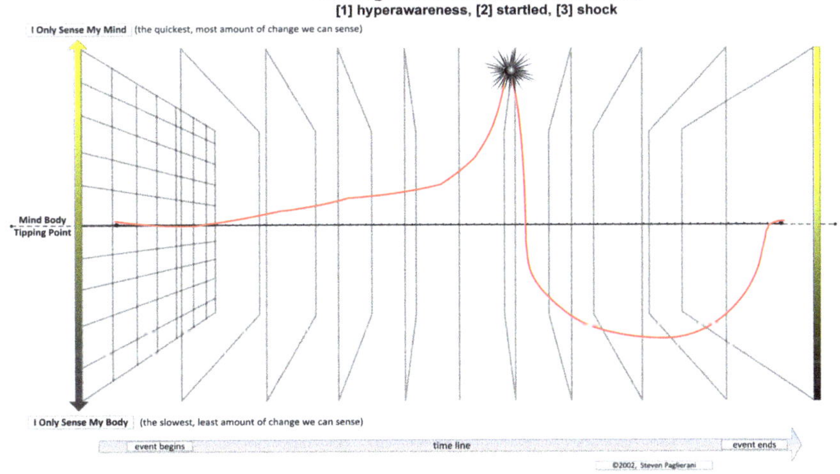

Relive A Wound (the meta pattern)
[1] hyperawareness, [2] startled, [3] shock

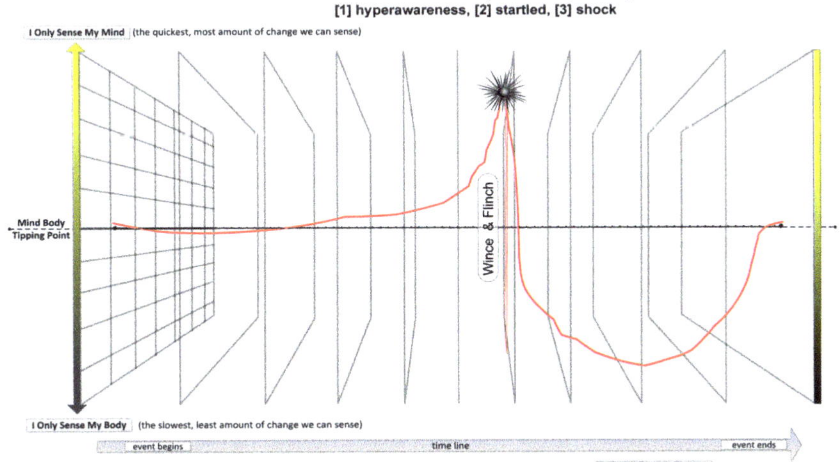

How Regression/Transference Feedback Loops Exacerbate Symptoms

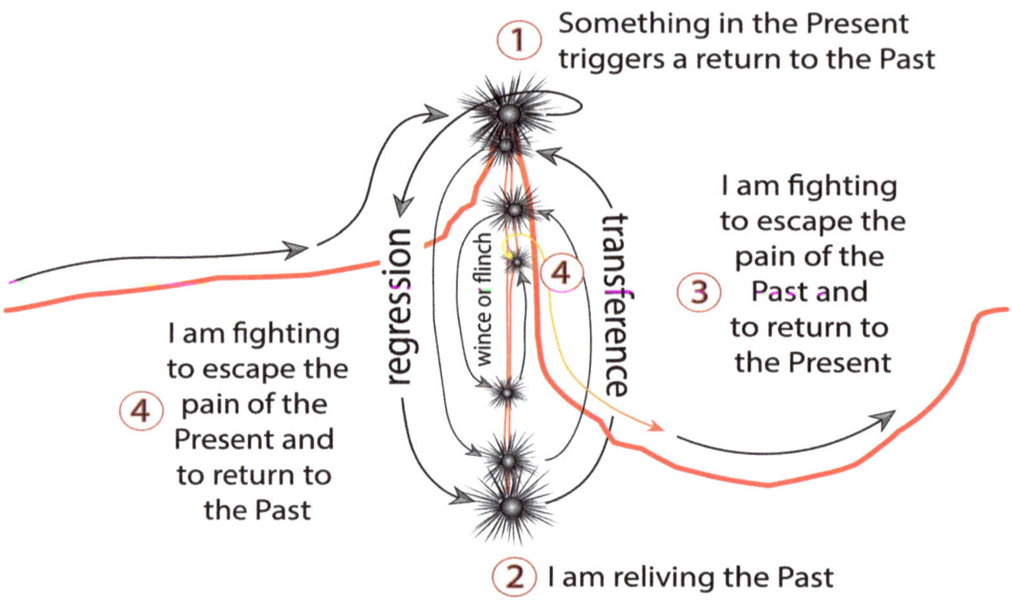

Regression and Transference: the Symptom Making Machine

In my previous book, explaining regression and transference took four entire chapters. Here, we only have time for a 5-cent tour. This said, the Regression Transference feedback loop drawing you see above may help. As compared to the drawing in that previous book, it's far more complex but vastly improved.

What's different and what does this drawing have to do with diagnosis? This is what we're about to explore. As usual, please try to only look at the drawing—not at the words. Admittedly, in this drawing, doing that can be especially hard. Try hard though. Everything we're about to do requires that you see how the ***Relive a Wound** event line* and the ***Regression Transference Feedback** loops* interact.

Ok. Now imagine someone is shooting an arrow at you. [Oh, boy. He's at it again.] Obviously, you'd try to avoid getting hit. So where would you focus? On the writing on the archer's hat—or on trying to predict where his arrow will go?

Me. I'd focus on the path of the arrow every time. Otherwise I'd likely get hit.

No coincidence, this is what we do each time we Relive a Wound.

We focus on the arrows, trying to predict where they will land.

The thing is, these arrows function a lot like the rings of arrow-headed Regression Transference loop lines. BTW, did you notice, those lines go counter-clockwise? Know this choice was deliberate. Unlike the Relive a Wound event line—which goes forward, we're talking about a process that causes us to go back in time. Ergo, the Regression and Transference feedback loops go counter-clockwise.

What about those spiky "startle" balls at the ends of those counter-clockwise lines? What are they? First, notice, they all begin at, and descend from, the highest point in the line. This spot tells us that this person has been triggered by the latest iteration of a wounding pattern. And the first ball on the Relive a Wound line represents a startle which has occurred in the present day.

Why say "iteration?" Because no wound exists in isolation. Each time we get a new wound, an earlier wound made us vulnerable to getting this wound. In other words, all wounds come from having pre-existing precedents. And the thing that makes us vulnerable to getting these new wounds?

Getting caught in one of these Regression Transference feedback loops.

This is why finding these loops is a large part of what good psychotherapies are all about. Emergence Psychotherapists call the act of retracing these "going-backwards" paths, "finding the wound chain." Admittedly, this topic is complex, and in this book we won't explore therapies. So for now, focus on learning to see how these feedback loops distort and exacerbate the symptoms of already existing wounds. And to do this, I need to ask you to do yet another thought experiment.

This time, imagine you're entering a beautiful park—onto an oval-shaped walking path. Now imagine, after walking ten feet or so down that path, a vicious dog leaps out of the bushes at you. No doubt, you'd rush past those bushes. Imagine you do and you get away. No doubt, you'd then breathe a sigh of relief.

Can you picture this happening to you? Please try. Now consider what you'd do next. Likely, you'd keep walking forward, wanting to get as far away from that dog as you could. But imagine, as you reach the far end of this oval-shaped path, a second dog lunges out from the bushes at you. How would you feel this second time? Even more flustered? Worse? Angry? WTF.

This sequence of two dogs jumping out at you is a lot like what it feels like to Relive a Wound. But you're not done yet. Now picture how you'd run past that second dog. Of course, this time, you'd run even faster. You'd also likely head towards the park's exit point. Now imagine that just as you're about to reach that exit, the first dog lunges out of the bushes at you again. What would you do then? Would you run past the exit, back into the park? What would you do then?

Perhaps you'd think, "If I can reach the far end of the park, maybe I can wait until those dogs are gone." At the same time, consider what your intuition might be telling you. I'm sure you'd by now be expecting more trouble. Sure enough, when you reach the far end of the path, that damn second dog is there, waiting for you at the far end of the path.

Imagine if it was to keep happening until at last, you feel totally exhausted?

Welling up, you sit down mid-path, not knowing what to do or where to go.

Now imagine, a man comes along who is not afraid of dogs, and he stops to ask you if you're alright. Almost magically, as soon as he does, you feel all grown up and back to being yourself. Now imagine you and he then walk back to the park's exit point. Now imagine you thank the man, then say goodbye and leave.

If you were actually able to do this thought experiment, try to recall all the things you just experienced. Your positive expectations at the start of your walk. Your relief when an adult showed up. If you were able to do it, then you know what it's like to relive a wound. These feelings include the idea that none of what happened felt like you were making choices. This is one of the worst parts.

And if this was hard to imagine?

Then it's likely you've never been wounded by a dog. Lucky you. If you had been, then you'd know all too well what a shitshow this walk would have been. The first time you escaped? The symptoms? Not so bad. The second time? A little worse. The third time? Hope's fading and your inner world has begun to collapse. And in the end, everything you thought you knew about life would have begun to disappear—leaving you with a desperate need to get away.

So Where Do Symptoms Come From?

Physicists call this kind of a loop—where things feed back on themselves—a "feedback loop." An example most people have experienced is when feedback occurs in an auditorium. Here, the specifics are different. But the pattern is the same.

- Someone speaks into a microphone *(you enter the park)*.
- This microphone sends the signal to an amplifier, making the volume of this sound louder *(the dog leaps out at you, and your awareness of life gets amplified)*.
- This amplified sound comes out of a speaker *(you shout as you run)*.
- The microphone then "hears" the sound coming from that speaker, and this sound gets sent to the amplifier a second time *(the second dog jumps out at you)*.
- This re-amplified sound comes out of the speaker a second time *(you shout even louder)*.
- This sound keeps passing through this loop. Each time, it gets louder. Until at last it's so loud that all that's left is an awful sounding squeal *(you sit down, exhausted, hoping it will all just go away)*.
- Finally, someone arrives and turns the amplifier off, at which point, the squealing thankfully stops *(the man arrives and walks with you out of the park)*.

This is where symptoms come from.

They come from feedback loops. These loops amplify the pain which existed in the original, wounding event. This means, no diagnostician ever gets to witness the original event. All they get to see are the amplified versions of the original suffering.

You burn your finger on a stove at age three. It hurts like hell. You move your finger close to a lit stove at twenty-three. You relive an amplified version of the original burn. Here, you do relive the original hurt—but only for the first few seconds. After that, you relive the relived hurt—over and over again. Until your mind finally blows a fuse and you mentally and physically shut down.

Can you see how, when you relive wounds, this feedback loop amplifies the original pain—telling you over and over what will happen if you touch the lit stove? Moreover, since thoughts move at close to the speed of light, these painful repetitions quickly merge into one big painful event. Diagnosticians then assume this amplified accumulation indicates the nature of the original event.

Obviously, you can *relive a wound* within minutes of getting wounded. But even these symptoms are larger than what you felt in the first painful moment. Not that the first moment didn't hurt. Of course, it did. But the mind creates an early warning system within seconds of the first pain. After that, even thinking about that first pain causes reliving loops to form. And within minutes, these loops distort and exacerbate the symptoms of the original event.

Where's My Proof That The Mind Does This?

When I was writing my previous book, I searched far and wide for any mentions of this idea. As far as I know, there are no other sources which mention feedback loops as the cause of symptoms. The implications? That most therapists, psychiatrists, and diagnosticians believe, symptoms match the sizes of the original events. Thus to most professionals, big symptoms mean the original wound was a big event—and no symptoms means there is and was no wound.

Can you see how the Relive a Wound drawing makes these assumptions fall apart? And yes, I know you'll need to see more proof. It's coming. Being this book isn't only for therapists though—and being as most normal people diagnose each other and themselves almost daily—I'll limit my evidence to one example.

If after this, you wish to see more evidence? Then I suggest you explore that series of four chapters on Regression and Transference in my previous book (*Therapy for Therapists - a guide to changing lives, 2020*). Now, my one example.

Imagine you're four years old and standing in a line with a bunch of your relatives. You're about to get your picture taken for an older cousin's wedding photo. Further, try to imagine that you've never done this before.

If you haven't, then this will work. If it has, then doing this will be hard.

Now imagine you hear the photographer tell everyone to say, "cheese." Please try to picture this, including hearing his voice. Now let me ask you. In this example, you've never done this before. So what will be different about you as opposed to everyone else? Everyone except you will wince. They'll all expect to be blinded by the flash. But not you. You won't wince. Why? Because at age four, you've yet to be wounded by a blinding wedding photo flash.

Fast forward thirty years. You're now thirty-four. Picture yourself in another wedding photo line. This time, when the photographer says, "say cheese," you wince right along with everyone else. How could you not? You're reliving an injury.

Now imagine, for some reason, this time, *the flash fails to go off.*

Now let me ask you this. Would you have winced anyway? Go slow. Would you have? Think about it.

Of course you would have. You couldn't have prevented it, if you tried.

Your anticipation would have triggered your mind's early warning system.

Realize, too, you'd still have felt as if you'd just been blinded. And this would have happened despite there not having been any flash. This is why I love this example—it's so easy for most people to test for. It also shows that once you've been wounded, these reactions never go away. Both the feedback loop—and the three-to-five second bit of programming which triggers the reliving—last forever.

At the same time, the exact nature of the reliving will be different every time this happens. Why? Because the details of the present day situation will always be different from the original events. And yes, some parts of what's being relived will be coming from the original event. But the small details from the present day situation will go into the mix as well.

This means, while the content of the feedback loop will in part be coming from what you expect to happen, since there will always be differences, the symptoms will never be exactly the same. To see why I'm saying this, consider that auditorium feedback situation again. How many people might speak into that mike? Will any of them say the same things—in the same way?

Admittedly, the details of a present day event must be similar enough to trigger the feedback loop. But no speakers or microphones or auditoriums or halls will ever be identical to the original event. So each time the squealing sound occurs, ***the parts which get fed into the feedback loop pattern will change***. And these changes will confound any and all diagnostic attempts to quantify the wound.

How Much of What Patients Remember is a Reconstruction?

This points to something every aspiring diagnostician must know—the idea that while the *patterns* underlying wounds never change, the *symptoms* of these wounds change every time. Here the only thing the patient's mind actually records is the three-to-five second triggering pattern just prior to the startle. This means ***the patient's mind does not record any of the literal details of this event.***

When you burn your finger on a stove at age four, what does your mind record?

Only *the pattern underlying the experience* in the three to five seconds just prior to the startle. Nothing else.

An example of what gets recorded might be "feeling excited about seeing a beautiful flame." Another might be the shapes, colors, and sizes of the pots on the stove. It could also be things like the feeling of standing next to your mother in a white apron. Or that it was morning. Or that it was Christmas. Or that she'd just asked you to pass her a spoon.

All these little patterns would then coalesce into the constellation diagnosticians call a "wound." And from then on, anytime you experienced this constellation of little patterns, this would trigger a winch or flinch.

What present day situations might this constellation of patterns then affect?

Standing to the left of tall women, if your mom was standing to your right.

Or to the right, if she was standing to your left.

And of course, seeing flames of any kind—campfires to birthday candles, especially if this involved cooking.

And certainly you'd come away with a fear of touching hot things.

Realize, this would happen to you even if these things only looked like they were hot. They might actually even be frozen. This is how we acquire associations between colors and temperatures—as well as how we come to believe brightly colored red things are likely hotter than lightly colored blue things.

Now add to this that the more these underlying patterns were present, the more intensely you'd relive the wound. And this difference would be a prime driver for how intensely or weakly your symptoms would become.

Are All Wounds, "Context Independent?"

Of all the crazy-sounding ideas in this book, the one in this subhead may be the hardest to accept.

The idea?

That the only thing the mind records is the tiny, underlying patterns—and never the literal details.

Is this true for all of life's situations?

This I can't say.

What I can say with certainty is, this idea universally applies to getting wounded.

Sounds crazy?

I know it does. But it's true nonetheless. How? Because the point I've been trying to make here is simply this.

All wounding patterns are *context independent.*

What do I mean by this? To see, ask yourself this.

What does it mean when someone says, "How are you?"

Most people would quickly say, "It's a greeting."

As you'll learn in the chapter on measuring personality, though, to a small but significant portion of human beings, "How are you?" is a question.

You might now add, "Yes, it can be," and of course it can. But how do you know which it is?

To most people, obviously, the answer depends on the situation—the context. For example, if your doctor is the one asking, then likely, he's asking a question.

Know this distinction is something people with **Majority Personalities** make automatically. Thus they never notice they do it. Then again, there is that small portion of humans—those with one of the four **Minority Personalities (Physical Autism, OCD, Mental Autism, ADD)**—who almost always hear "How are you" as a question. To people with **Majority Personalities** meeting a casual friend on the street is a different context than sitting in your doctor's office. But to some people, such as the folks I just mentioned—***and to all people reliving a wound***—the context rarely, if ever, matters.

What Does It Mean to Say Wounds Are "Context Independent?"

As I've just said, all wounds share the Minority Personality person's view of this idea. All wounds are entirely pattern-based. This means, they're sort of like constructing something shaped like a square—only the patterns wounds use are not geometric.

Would making a square object from different materials make it any less square? Wound patterns are the same. Reliving a wound is reliving a wound, regardless of how the details change. Unfortunately, most helping professionals treat wounds as if these details do matter, because the context is part of the wound.

This is why most diagnosticians, in their examinations, ask a lot of questions about the details present in the original event. This presumes those details are part of what injured the person. In truth, the patterns the mind records are never linear patterns. Thus they're never identical. Rather, these patterns are always "fractal patterns."

These kinds of patterns are what four-year-olds learn to recognize when they see flames. Or cumulous clouds. Or carrots. Or ocean waves. Once learned, these fractal patterns then generalize to all things which look the same. Moreover, they never need to be relearned.

Does it make a difference whether that first flame was on a birthday cake candle or on a kitchen stove? Obviously, not. Once the mind records that first example of a fractal pattern, you will effortlessly recognize it for the rest of your life.

This same idea applies to wounds. The mind records the first example, then generalizes this pattern to any and all similar things. Then, because wounds are patterns, not events, these constellations of little patterns function like cookie cutter molds. Any life experiences that can fit into that "mold" will trigger the person.

How Does Healing Alter Regression Transference Loops?

How does healing affect Regression Transference feedback loops? This is what we'll look at next. Please note, in the language of Emergence Psychotherapy, an event in which you heal a wound is called, "having an emergence." Most laypersons call this, having an "aha moment." Many therapists call these moments, "having a breakthrough."

Words aside, if you now look over at the next page, you'll see the line drawing which explains what happens during this kind of event. To begin with, contrast and compare the Relive a Wound drawing to the Healing a Wound drawing. Perhaps you can look back and forth a few times, then write down any noticeable similarities and differences.

Obviously the big difference is, the healing drawing uses the Heal a Wound event-line. Whereas the relive a wound drawing uses the Relive a Wound event-line. Now try to focus on the Regression Transference feedback loops. Can you see that on the Healing a Wound drawing, five sun-shaped balls have been added and placed on top of those spiky balls?

How Regression/Transference Feedback Loops Exacerbate Symptoms

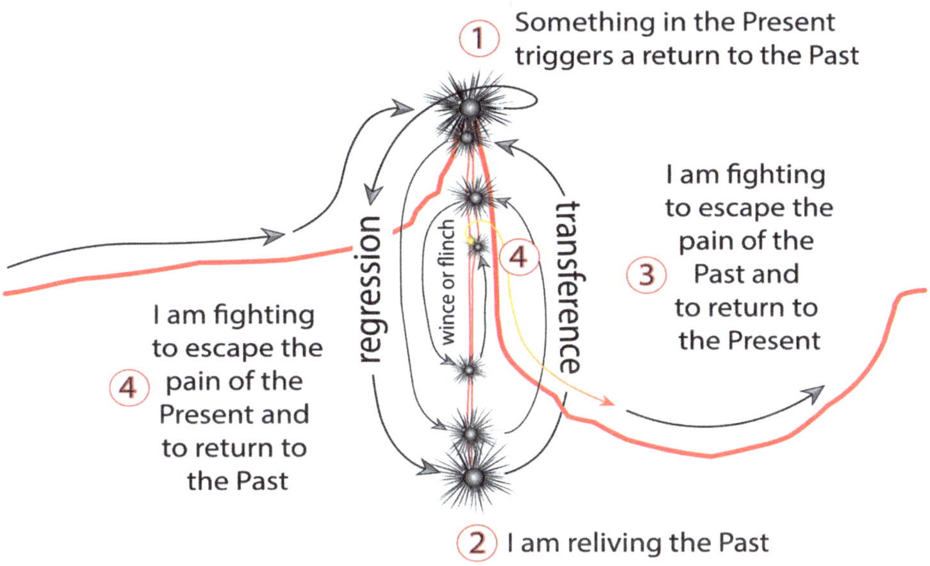

How An Emergence Alters the Loop (Healing)

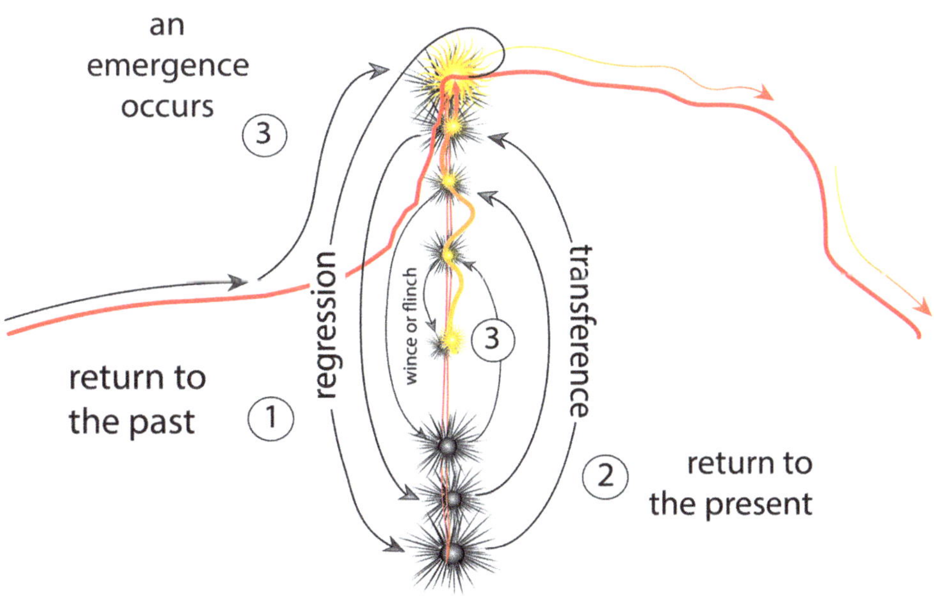

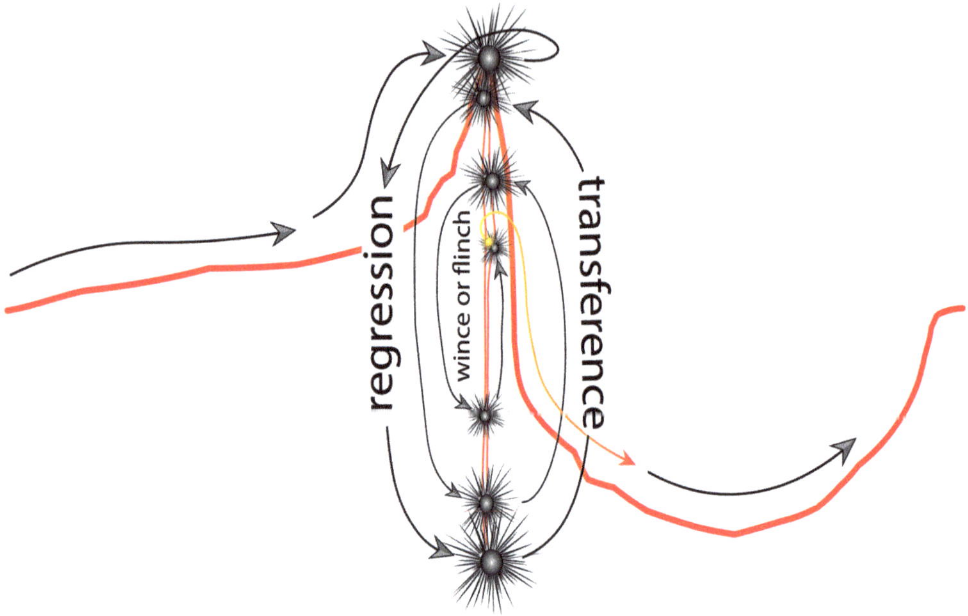

Know that if you are looking at the color versions of these drawings, you'll see that these sun-shaped balls are bright yellow and look like suns. No coincidence. When people experience an emergence, their dispositions suddenly and permanently become sunny in these situations. This doesn't mean they now want to get wounded again. No one is that dumb. Rather, once healing occurs, people become curious in these situations.

Contrast this to what people are like when they relive an unhealed wound. The last thing they feel is curious. All they want to do is look away. Finally, did you notice in the Healing a Wound event line drawing, there's a snake-shaped loop which climbs upwards towards the aha moment? Realize, even after healing, people still regress to the past, then transfer to the present.

But these regressions now include regressing to the healing moment as well.

This means now, whenever they relive that wound, they will momentarily relive a tiny bit of the original pain. However, they will also, almost instantly, then relive the joy of the emergence moment. From then on, they will feel excited about the possibility of learning more about these situations. No surprise, these kinds of experiences are what drive many, if not all, people to choose their careers.

This includes the folks who become therapists and diagnosticians.

To see this, consider how healing might affect the situation with you and the dogs in the park. Remember that man who stopped to check in on you, then walked you out of the park? Well after healing, you might feel curious to know what it would feel like if you saw him on another day, and perhaps this time, he would teach you more about dogs and how to not be afraid.

For instance, imagine that this man handed you a dog bone.

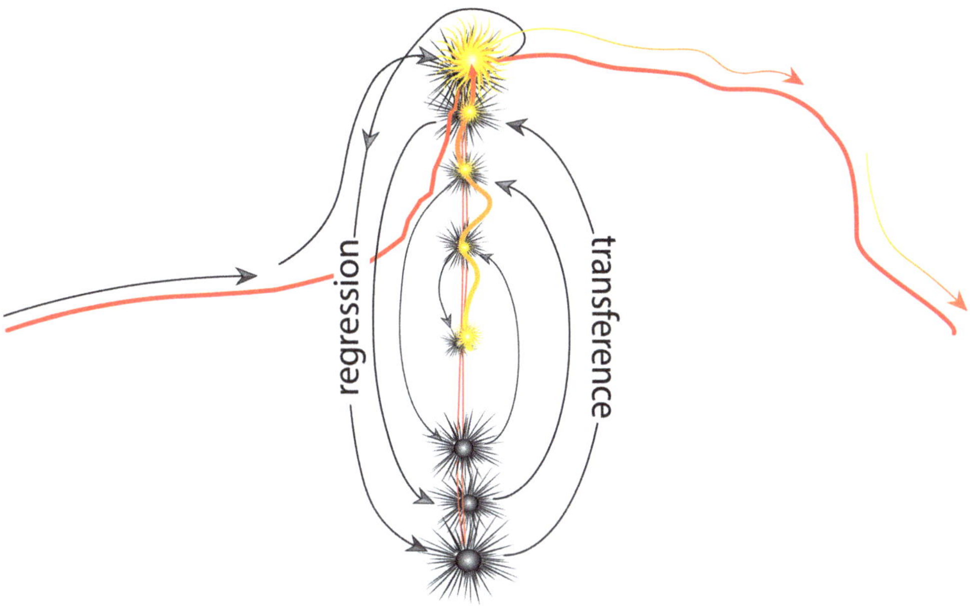

Then imagine he told you to call the dog to come out of the bushes. Can you picture that previously angry dog coming out, wagging his tail? Can you then imagine how this new experience might change your life? Certainly, from then on, each time you went to the park, this altered Regression Transference feedback loop would add positive versions of this event to the loop.

Now it would be the joy you felt in the healing moment which would get amplified, over and over again. Add to this how your curiosity and positive anticipation would change your out-in-the-world behaviors. You might try to always remember to bring dog bones with you, and you'd actually look forward to the dogs jumping out of the bushes at you. Imagine that? This is healing.

How Do You Diagnostically Discern Clinical Significance?

Now comes the useful part—being able to, with certainty, diagnostically differentiate between clinically insignificant and clinically significant symptoms.

Diagnosing the presence or absence of a wound will become easy.

Recognizing a wound that's already been healed will become easy too.

What will you need to look for? There are three things. I call them, "meta-symptoms." Meta-symptoms are symptoms which are universally true.

Here, the word "universal" refers to them being context independent. Like what it's like to have learned to recognize flames and cumulous clouds as a child, once you learn to see meta-symptoms, you know them for life. And this is true regardless of how your clients and their specific situations may change. Diagnostically, these three meta-symptoms will always scientifically indicate the presence, or absence, of a wound.

What are the three meta-symptoms?

- Wincing and flinching.
- Sudden-onset mental blankness.
- Being unable to picture things, even when asked to make them up.

We'll address each of these things—one at a time.

The First Kind of Meta-Symptoms: Wincing and Flinching

People often hear me say "the body never lies."

Much of my confidence in this statement comes from knowing the nature of wincing and flinching. The fact is, the only times you will ever see a patient wince or flinch is when they are *reliving* a startle. And the only time you'll ever see a person relive a startle is when they are reliving a wound.

This makes watching for these two things a seriously important diagnostic tool. This said, obviously, both are important. But how do they differ?

Wincing is the mind not wanting to look at or see something mentally painful.

Flinching is the body not wanting to relive physical pain.

Either way, if you monitor your patients for either of these things, you will know exactly what to focus on.

Either you will rule *out* what you see—as it is clinically insignificant. Or you will rule *in* what you see—as it in some way indicates a wound.

Clearly, flinching is the easier of the two to learn to recognize. We've all flinched at times—so we know what this is like. In truth, it's kind of hard to miss, especially when compared to recognizing wincing. Why? We'll look at this next.

Have You Ever Noticed A Client Wincing?

One way to describe what causes people to *flinch* is that they are "physically bracing for pain." But technically, when you *wince*, your eye muscles flinch as well. The thing is, wincing is far more complex than merely tensing eye muscles.

It also involves an unnatural act—the eyes cease to move.

How long are the eyes still for?

For anything from forty milliseconds up to several seconds.

Why is this stillness significant?

Before I answer, let me ask you this.

Have you ever noticed that all people's eyes, including yours, are in constant motion? Do you know why eyes do this?

Warning. Brain-breaker coming.

One—because **"sensation"** is **"the experience of change."** And two—because **"the mind very quickly goes blank anytime we do not see or sense change."**

This is a large part of why we feel uncomfortable whenever we see people stare. If you stare at something and that thing does not move, then either you must move your eyes to keep seeing it, or you will go blank and stop seeing it.

Don't believe me? Then try testing this idea for yourself. Try looking at yourself in a mirror without moving your eyes. Literally, try to not move your eyes for a minute or more. While doing this, try to keep seeing your eyes.

The truth is, I doubt you'll be able to last for an entire minute. In less time than that, you'll either move your eyes, or you'll find it hard to keep seeing them.

All winces cause the eyes to momentarily stand still. And this stillness causes the mind to suddenly go blank.

It also causes us to be unable to see out into the world. So for a moment, technically and literally, we are completely blind.

Confused? Think about it.

Even when you close your eyes, your mind doesn't necessarily go blank. But when you wince, it does. You see nothing.

In the case of reliving a wound, this is why you can't see what it is you are reliving. It's this blindness that makes healing so hard. If you can't see the problem, how do you know what to work on, let alone heal it?

This is where meta-symptoms come in. They always tell you when and where to focus on the small details. And once healing occurs, a small opening appears in this mental wall. Over time then, curiosity drives you to see what else you can discover. And the more you discover, the more curious you feel.

To Diagnose, You Must Learn to See Winces

Ok. So learning to see winces in patients is a critical part of being able to diagnose. And learning to see winces is harder than learning to see flinches. Is this why so few people ever learn to notice winces in themselves? I'm not sure. Just know, if you're patient and put your mind to it, you can learn to see them.

What should you be focusing on as you try to learn this?

For one thing, a sudden-onset stillness in the eyes—a sudden lack of movement.

Keep in mind, people wince to avoid seeing something in their minds—and the mind is much quicker than the body. So this stillness can come and go in an instant.

Indeed, some winces—the ones I call, "micro-winces"—come and go so quickly that they become almost impossible to see. With practice though, you can develop what I sometimes refer to as "physical intuition." Here, you learn to notice your own body reacting to things like the patient's breath pausing and momentary stillness in their eyes. So even if you miss seeing them, you can know when they happen.

Something else that can help is to treat this process like learning to see a magician's slight-of-hand trick. At first, it feels like you'll never get it. But keep at it and eventually, you'll get so good at it that like learning to recognize candle flames, when your patients wince, you'll be unable to miss this.

Yet one more thing which may help you here is to Google videos of people wincing and flinching. Like all visual material, these videos are far better than any words I can offer you. Watch. Rewind. Watch again. While doing this, look for as many details, in and around the eyes, as you can—especially stillness.

Each new detail you learn to see will then add to your diagnostic skill set. And of all the diagnostic tools you could learn, seeing winces is probably the best.

Ok. So to review. With wincing, look for stillness in the muscles around the eye and in the eye itself. With flinching, look for shoulders raising, head pulling back or away, hands or arms raising to shield the body or eyes, and so on. In either cases, when you see these things, you can know with certainty, your patient has just relived a wound.

Finally, one last thing.

I mentioned earlier, there are two kinds of symptoms—those only the diagnostician can see and those only the patient can report.

Wincing and flinching fall into the first category—only the diagnostician can see them. This said, patients can be taught to feel themselves wincing and flinching, in effect, to develop their own physical intuition. In truth, most people can already easily sense when they've flinched. Conversely though, most people do not realize when they wince. However, I've often taught patients, in a single session, to see themselves wincing. All you need to do is to persistently point it out to them each time it happens.

The Second Meta-Symptoms: Sudden-Onset Mental Blankness

The second class of meta-symptoms falls into the patient-only category—the stuff only patients can see. This is because it's invisible to diagnosticians, as it occurs entirely in the patient's mind. This means you'll need to ask patients to watch for this in themselves. And since no one is normally taught to pay attention to their mind going blank, some patients may struggle to comply.

On the other hand, no one winces or flinches without their mind also going blank. So you can gather indirect, but reliable, evidence using the first class of meta-symptoms. More important, you can use your own physical intuition to, with certainty, tell patients they just winced or flinched—even when you yourself didn't see them do it.

Also, like all proper diagnostic signs, there are two opposite kinds of mental blankness. Like what you've learned to see in the Getting Overwhelmed versus Getting Wounded event lines, one type comes on gradually, and the other, suddenly. Gradual onset blankness rules things out. It's just patients feeling overwhelmed. Whereas sudden onset blankness is always a clinically significant sign.

Realize, the best of all worlds occurs when you can combine what you, the diagnostician, see—along with what your patient reports. For example, if your patient reports suddenly going blank when you see this patient wince, then you've gathered evidence from both categories of symptoms.

The Third Kind of Meta-Symptoms: Being Unable to Picture Things

Obviously, the third kind of meta-symptoms also go into the patient-only category. And to be honest, this topic is yet another extremely complex one.

As such, exploring it here is far beyond the scope of this book. But if you are interested, you may want to read about it in my previous book. I've included a lot of information about it there.

Know that learning to help patients to see themselves going blank is the basis for one of the principal kinds of Emergence Psychotherapies—the one called—Visual Dialogue. This said, I'm going to offer you a simple way to begin learning to see this.

How simple?

Asking yourself one question.

The question?

Try to think of a food that you hate.

Eggs? Fish? Lima beans? It doesn't matter. Most people have some kind of food they hate.

And if you can't think of a food you hate?

Then try to think of something ordinary you hate to do or say. Having to ask people for help. Saying you're sorry for something you're not sorry for. And in case none of this rings any bells, I've excerpted the following descriptions from that earlier book.

> • In its simplest form, this block marker can consist of anything which causes you to become acutely aware of any of your five physical senses. For example, hating being touched, hating the taste of liver, hating the sight of blood, hating the sound of chalk on a blackboard, hating the smell of mold. It can also refer to having an acute dislike for certain feelings. For example, hating crying, hating when people are angry, hating when you're afraid. Here even simple responses can indicate scenes in which a wound exists. Thus if you hate feeling sad or excited, or being touched on the head, or smelling leaves in the fall, this hatred points to a wound.
>
> • Any negative prejudice towards large groups of people or towards non-violent beliefs or ideas. In truth, human beings can dislike many things. But when you hate things like religions or religious people, politics or politicians, certain countries, certain nationalities, all men or all women, all children, all people who are old or young, all teachers, all poor or rich people and so on, this hatred indicates a wound.
>
> • Hating compliments. Some people hate getting compliments. Two's are especially vulnerable to this kind of wound.
>
> • Hating certain subjects in school such as math or English. Babies love learning all things. Wounds kill much of this love of learning.
>
> • Hating the sound of a certain word.

Once you think of something, write this thing down. Then set this paper aside and sit quietly for a few minutes. Then, when you're ready, try to picture doing this thing. Eating eggs or fish. Saying you're sorry to an enemy. Getting a compliment. And so on.

Keep in mind, if you are picturing things, these things will have a color. Knowing that they exist as an idea is not the same as picturing them. This makes seeing color an easy test for picturing. Can you see this thing in color?

If you can't then you've just discovered a wound in yourself.

Lastly, a Brief Look At The Word "Disorder"

In coming chapters, we'll talk a lot about the word, "disorder." I know I've mentioned this word before. For now, all I want to do here is to add something to what we've discussed in this chapter.

Most diagnosticians assume that all clinically significant symptoms are caused by a wounding event. This is not true.

My point is, there is a second cause of clinically significant symptoms. Existing diagnostic manuals refer to these conditions as personality disorders. For now, all I'll say is that there are two classes of disorders, because disorders come in two sizes.

One is the small size. These disorders are caused by the wounding events we've spoken about in this chapter. I call these disorders—***event-sized disorders***. Here, the disorder these injuries cause is limited to specific situations which trigger regressions. The rest of the person's life is reasonably well ordered.

The second category of disorders is the large size category. These disorders come into being somewhere during the first year-of-life. I call this second category of clinically significant disorders—***personality-sized disorders***. Here the disorder affects most, if not all, of the person. Thus this disorder knows no limits. It is personality sized.

Know we'll explore this rather important distinction in depth in Chapter 5. The thing to keep in mind will be this. Personality-sized disorders are NOT caused by wounds. More important, all people with personality-sized disorders, like people who do not have them, also have numerous event-sized disorders.

Obviously, we'll have a lot to discuss here.

As for what's coming next, we're going to look at Evidence Gathering. Realize, this is coming on the heels of just having learned how and where to focus most of this work. This is, however, a visual process which can organize what you gather.

This is what we're about to explore.

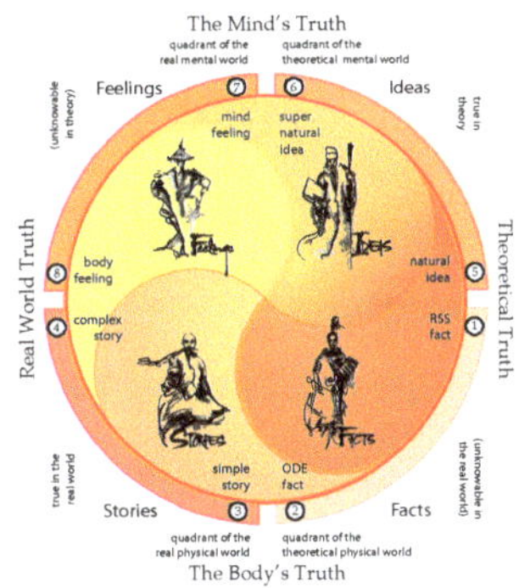

Chapter 3

Measuring Personality
(what can we learn about . . . ?)

How Many Drawings Should It Take To Define Personality?

As I begin this chapter, I have to admit, I feel overwhelmed. Can you picture the hill-shaped event line which describes my current state of mind? Hopefully so. Event lines aside, I am concerned this chapter may discourage many readers. It's quite complex. Know I honestly wish there was a simpler way to quantify human nature.

As of this morning, I know of none.

My point? To diagnose properly, we must begin from a measurable baseline. All scientific measurements require two things, in this order. One—a proper way to define the terms being measured (qualities). Two—a proper way to quantify the presence or absence of these qualities. In prior chapters, I've done my best to begin to address the first of these requirements. Clearly, using event line drawings—wherein the laws of physics visually describe and define the patterns present in the mind—addresses much of what's been missing in prior diagnostic manuals.

For example, consider yet again the shape of the depression event line.

If something is scientific, it must lead to new and better knowledge.

The proof for this line being scientific? It tells us things most people, including diagnosticians, haven't known.

For one thing, the idea that sadness ***is not present*** in depression.

For another, a scientific explanation for ***why*** sadness is not present in depression.

Something to also consider here however is ***how*** this line can accomplish all this. Taken by itself, it could not. Rather, this line's power comes from more than its own qualities. What gives this line its power? The presence of the three other lines. Together, these four lines describe what depression is and is not.

This then is one of the principles we must adhere to in the present chapter. We must describe and define personality similarly, making clear what it is and what it is not. This new form of science— known formally as "constellated science"—is what everything in this book is based on. It says that to scientifically know something—we must meet two requirements. One, tipping-point based inclusion. We must use pairs of logically perfect (complementary) opposites to define what a thing is *and* what it is not. Two, that together, each pair of opposites must address all possible cases of what this thing is—and is not—defining. All things must be considered.

Are you ready to throw this book at a wall yet? If so, know I understand. After all, it's taken me close to three decades to discover, and find the words to describe, what I've just written. I hardly expect you—and hope you won't try to—grasp the meaning of these opening words in a mere few minutes. But I also hope that by the end of this book, I will have permanently awakened your scientific curiosity.

How Many Qualities Will It Take To Define Personality?

As I've just said, Constellated Science uses two forms of scientific measurement—Visual Definitions (qualities) and Tipping-Point Based Measurements (amounts). Together, these two things describe and define the entirety of a new form of science. Of course, to see this claim as valid, I'll need to offer professionally useful examples of this science in action.

In this chapter, I hope to give you more than enough proof to support this claim.

Arguably, the subject I've chosen to focus on here is one of the more complex to define and measure. Based on how many books have tried and failed, clearly, personality is far beyond the grasp of mere words and numbers. Fortunately, we will not rely on words or numbers to do the main portion of our work. Rather, we'll build on an idea so simple that I still find it hard to believe no one's used it before.

Base all measurements on tipping-point based measures of perfectly defined pairs of opposite qualities.

An example?

Imagine a perfectly constructed and balanced schoolyard seesaw. On this seesaw sit two six-year-old girls, giggling and excited, and rocking back and forth.

Now imagine you've been asked to scientifically measure which girl is currently sitting higher up in the air. Could you possibly not determine this, with scientific certainty? Obviously, not.

Keep in mind, these two girls are in motion, rocking back and forth. In other words, during the measurement, these girls are moving. This movement is a critical thing to consider. Most scientific measurements assume something has to stand still in order to make an accurate measurement. Despite this movement, obviously, in this case, it would be impossible to not accurately measure this. Moreover, the results would be 100% accurate, every single time.

Another example?

Imagine you and a friend have decided to go out to see a movie. Imagine you each have a different movie in mind. Being you're close friends, you decide to toss a coin to choose which movie to go to. Imagine your friend pulls out a silver dollar, the one he always carries with him for good luck.

Now imagine you're both standing in your living room and he hands you the coin. Imagine tossing this coin into the air and seeing it land on the carpet.

Now comes the same sort of question.

Could either of you not know which movie you two were going to see?

Granted, it is possible for a coin to not fully land, given the carpet pile was thick and the coin landed on its edge. Know I know this from personal experience. I was once demonstrating tipping-point based measures to a group and the coin landed on edge and stuck upright in the carpet.

Like all failures, this one taught me something quite valuable.

Scientific measures which do not account for all possible outcomes cannot be called proper science.

Given the coin landed properly in this case, it could only result in being heads or tails. Why? Because these two possibilities comprise the only possible outcomes.

No other outcomes exist.

So how many tipping-point based qualities will we need to account for to comprehensively describe personality?

With confidence, I can say five.

How many pairs of opposites will these five qualities entail?

I'm going to skip this question for now.

What I will tell you at this point is the level of accuracy these five measures can attain. Given the tests are administered properly, they can tell you which group of roughly 200 people you are in. Out of how many people? Eight billion. The entire current population of the world. And that 200 people will share the exact same personality as you.

Realize, "wounds"—the quality you learned about in the previous chapter—is not one of these five measures. So even in that group of 200, you will be unique. This points to something important. Wounds are not part of personality. But personality effects how people respond to wounds.

This explains why diagnosticians must be trained in personality.

Equally important, no human being incurs the same wound pattern, even in the same event. A wound is a three-to-five second pattern of experience which imprints in the mind just prior to a startle. The odds that people will experience a startle at exactly the same moment is small. But the odds that people will be focusing on, and thinking of, the exact things just before a startle? Astronomically against.

This aside, does it seem unbelievable that five measures will do? How is any of this possible? This is what you're about to find out.

Can Human Beings Ever Become Fully Conscious?

Most readers will have heard some variation of this story. I tell it because it may help you to see how my claims of accuracy could be possible. How can five simple qualities create such a diverse, but accurate measure of something so complex? I'll begin by listing the sequence of five measurable qualities I'm claiming we can use to arrive at this astounding level of accuracy.

- The Person's Mind Body Orientation (2 root possibilities)
- The Person's Character Type (4 root possibilities)
- The Person's Social Priorities (24 root possibilities)
- The Person's Decision Tree (4 root possibilities)
- The Person's Gender Identity (65,536 root possibilities)

Setting aside the testing methods, we can now calculate the number of possible, scientifically-measurable personalities. Here we can arrive at this total simply by multiplying this sequence of five numbers, in this order. The total number of tipping-point based outcomes is equal to 2 x 4 x 24 x 4 x 65,536. Thus there are 50,331,648 possible outcomes.

How many people have the exact same personality as you? Divide the current world population—eight billion—by this number. This means there are currently about 160 people who have the same personality as you. Compare this to any other personality theory and you begin to see the value of this one. Add to this the idea that all of these measurements are tipping-point based measurements of living people.

What does this have to do with human consciousness? To see, look over at the drawing on the next page. In it, you'll see a large vertical rectangle which represents a single moment in a person's mind. Now notice the five progressively smaller rectangles inside of this big rectangle.

What do these rectangles represent? The five measures of personality. The largest is the first bulleted measure I've listed above—Mind Body Orientation. The smallest is the fifth measure—Gender Identity. If you now look closely, you'll notice there is also one dark colored space without a number. This dark area is part of a photo of something this person is currently looking at.

Clearly, from what you can see, you cannot tell what this is a photo of. This small area represents how much of this photo you would normally be conscious of. In the next few pages, I'm going to remove those five rectangles, one at a time. Each time I do, please try to guess what's in this photograph.

Keep in mind how each of these five measures of personality functions like a filter—each one blocking out parts of what's in that photo.

Can you guess what's in that photo yet? Try. Then turn the page.

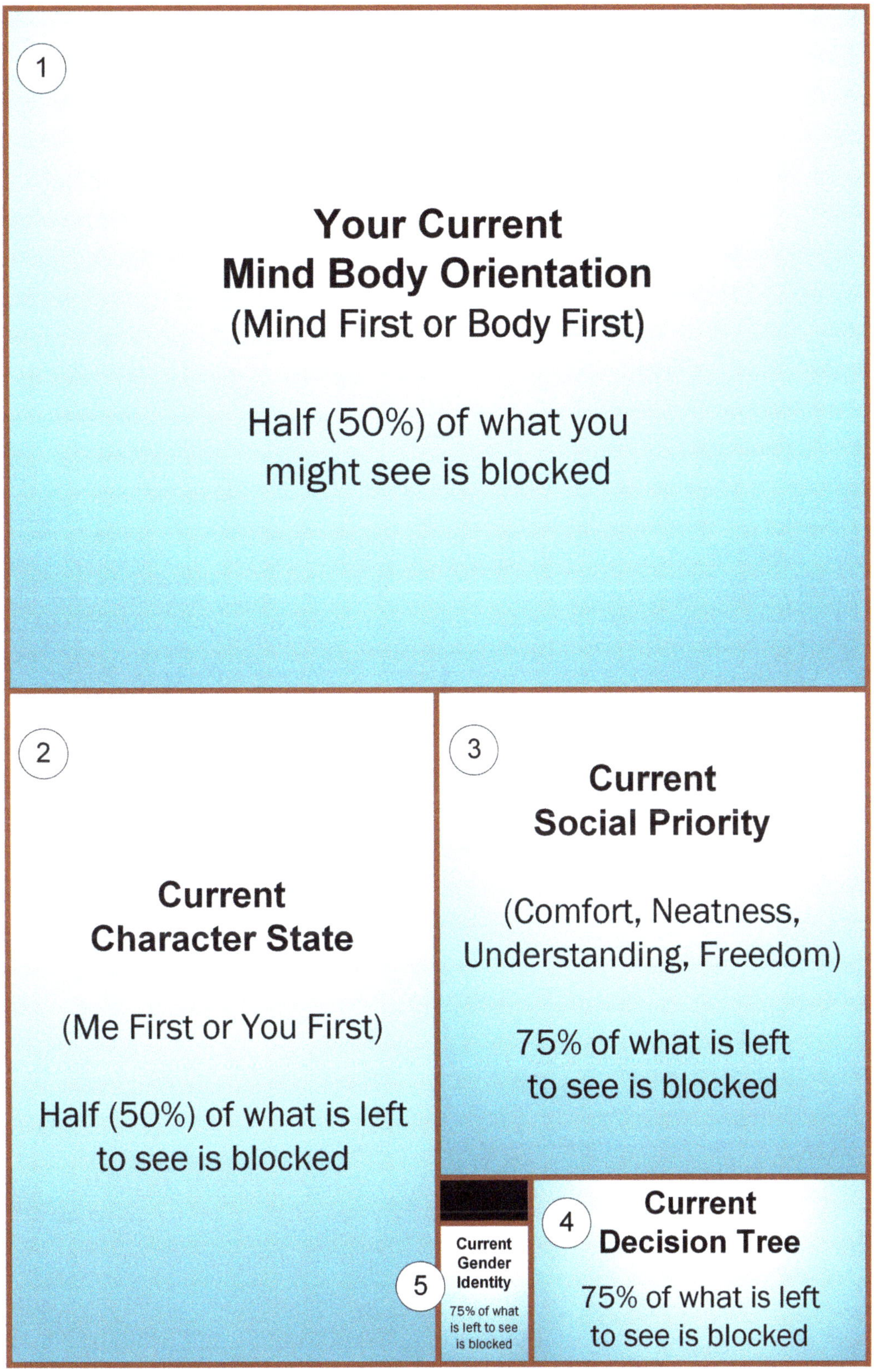
1
Your Current
Mind Body Orientation
(Mind First or Body First)
Half (50%) of what you
might see is blocked
2
Current
Character State
(Me First or You First)
Half (50%) of what is left
to see is blocked
3
Current
Social Priority
(Comfort, Neatness,
Understanding, Freedom)
75% of what is left
to see is blocked
4
Current
Decision Tree
75% of what is left
to see is blocked
5
Current
Gender
Identity
75% of what
is left to see
is blocked

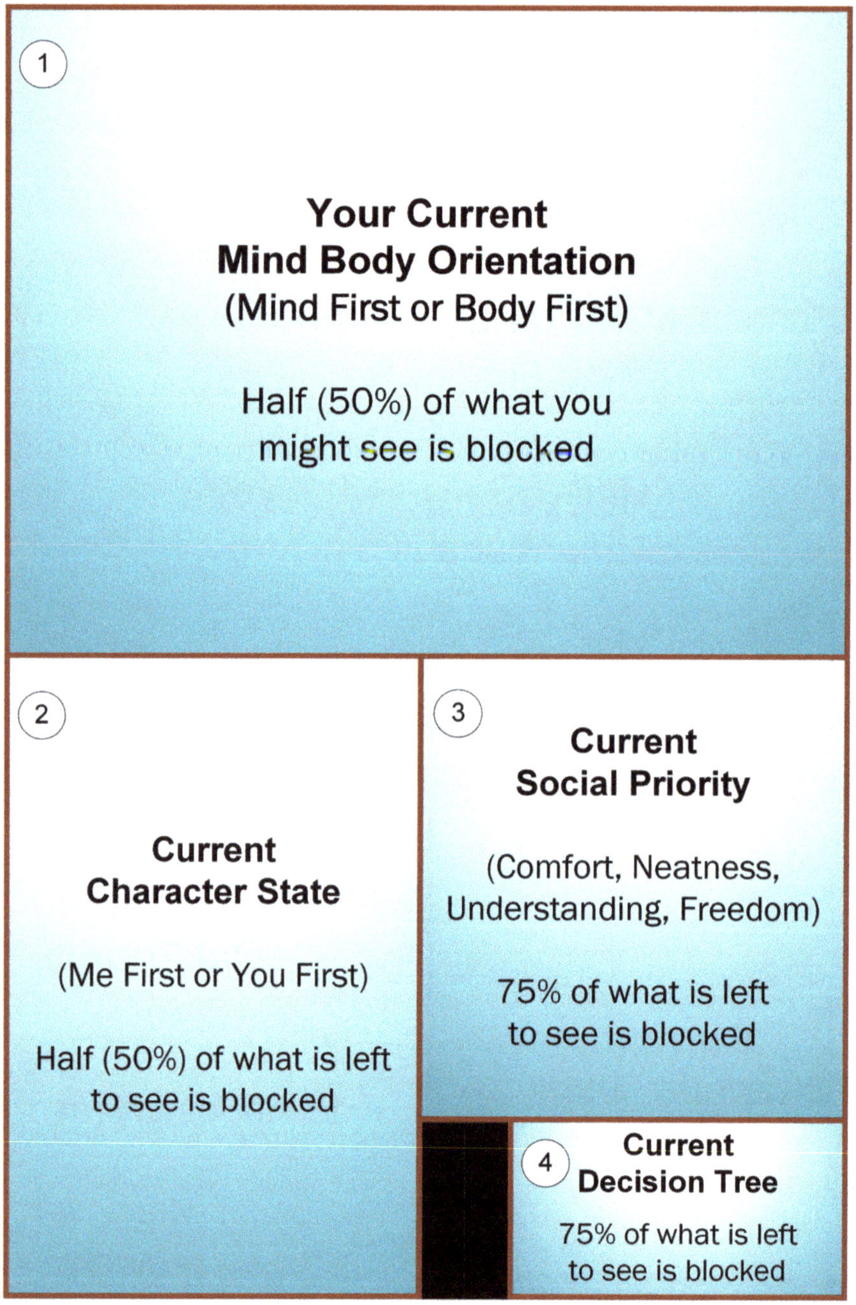

OK. One personality filter removed—this person's Gender Identity. Not much more to see yet, this despite the fact that we see gender as a big deal. And it is. But in the scheme of things, it's the smallest of the five filters. At the same time, it's also the most complex. There are 65,536 possibilities.

What does this filter represent? The *direction* (outward/assertive or inward/receptive)—and *degree of force* with which we execute the 4 kinds of decisions. Physical, sexual, psychological, and social decisions. More on this in a bit.

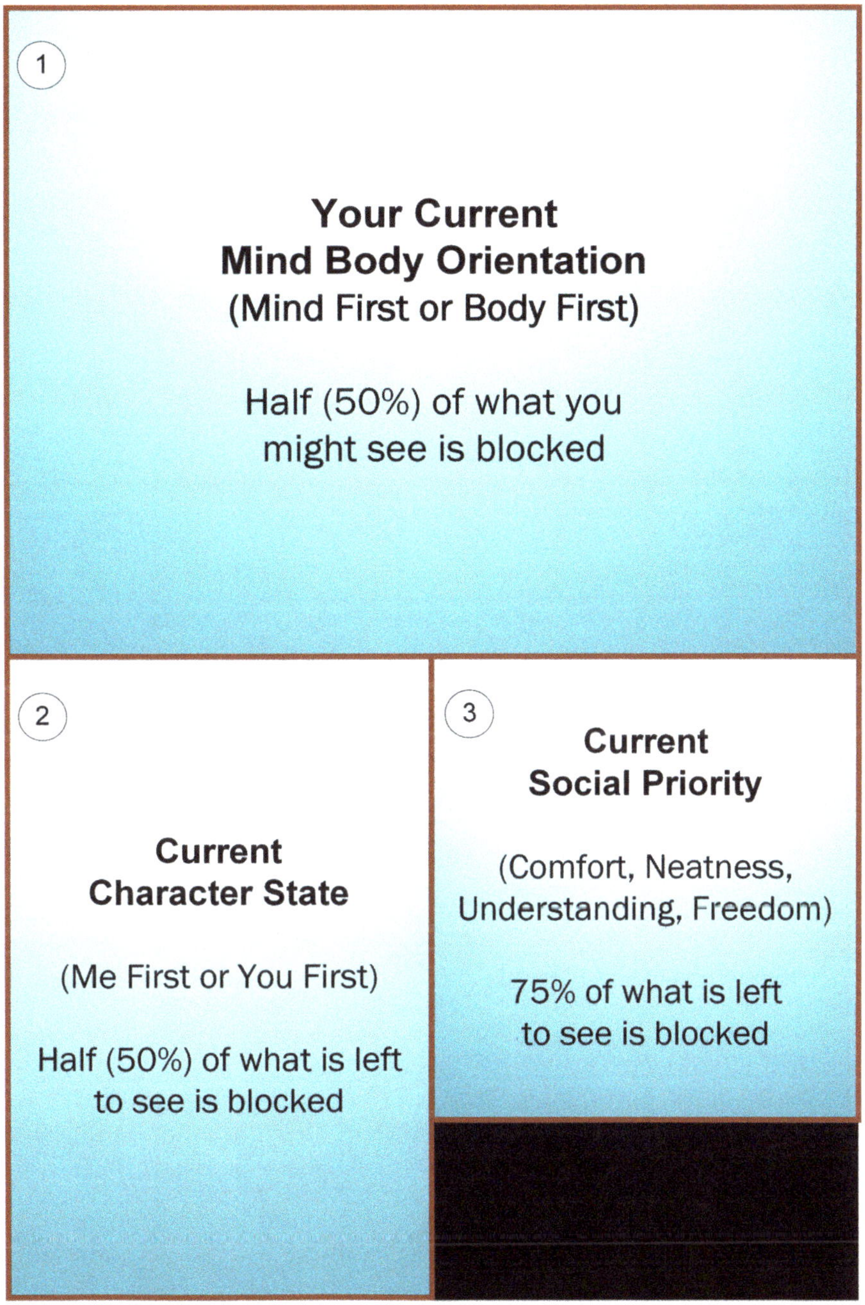

Now I've removed a second filter—this time, the person's Decision Tree. Seems like we should be able to begin to see something. But nothing so far.

What does this filter represent? One of four possible sequences of decision-making styles. My tree is Precision, Correction, Digression, and Bluntness.

All human beings employ *one* of these four Decision Trees. This leaves 75% of this filter in place. But even removing this entire filter doesn't reveal much. From the looks of the next one though, perhaps you'll be able to guess the photograph.

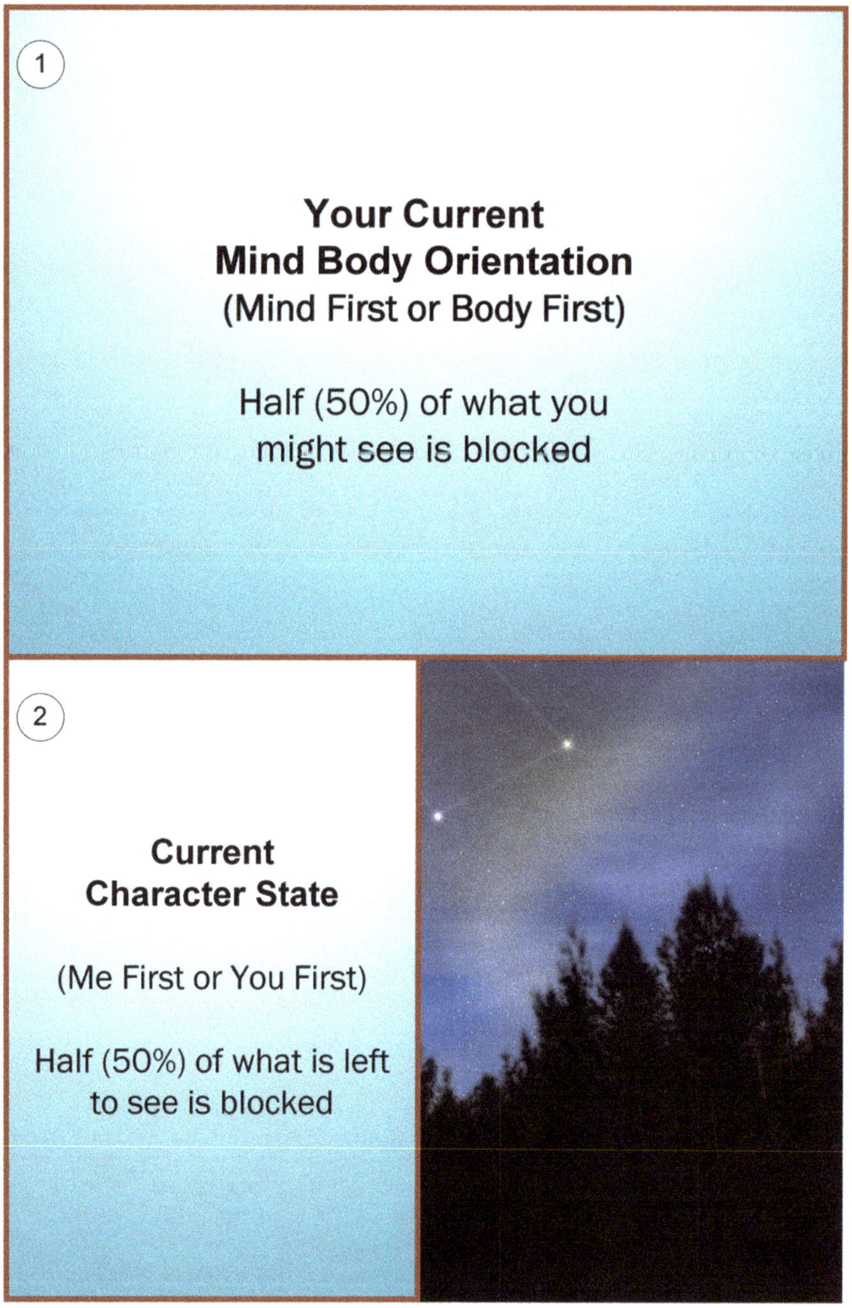

Ah. Finally. By removing a third filter, you can see trees, and sky, and a couple of stars. This filter—Social Priorities, determines the kind of urges you are currently sensing. Here, "urges" equates to unresolved ambivalence, in effect, unmet needs. And the 24 Social Priority Trees determine your sense of what kind of needs they are.

As for the photo, I doubt you've resisted looking at the next drawing. This said, even with that fourth filter—Character Type—removed, can you be sure you know what's left to see? Here, I mean scientifically certain. Not just a guess. A certainty.

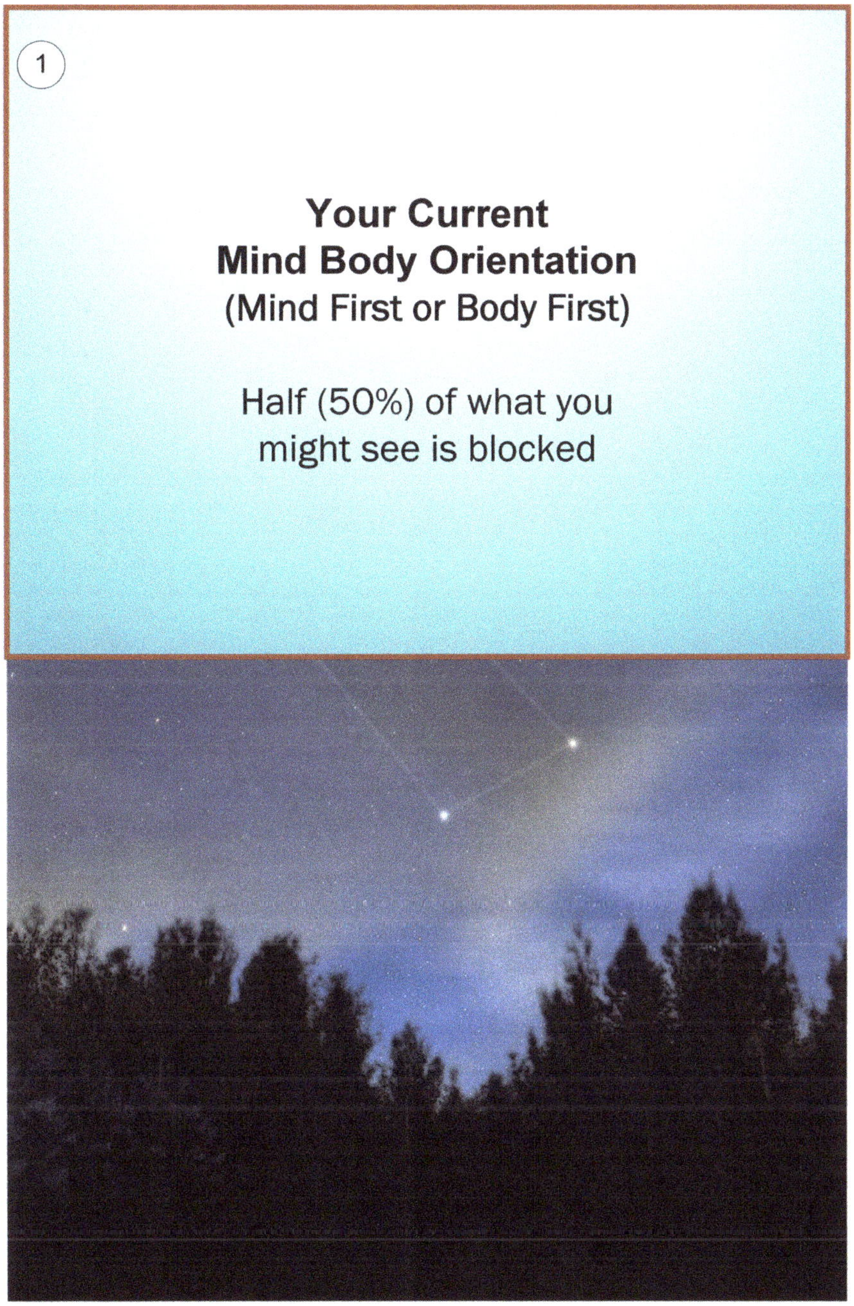

So what do you think? Obviously you can make an educated guess. But can you be sure you know what's left to see behind that fifth and final filter?

Realize, what I've just asked you to do—to guess—is what all existing diagnostic manuals do. Nothing in them is measurably clear, certain, or scientifically defined. Now think back to where you began a moment ago when all you saw was a small, dark space. Trying to guess what was in this space is a lot like how all diagnostic efforts begin. Even given sufficient information, we normally recognize very little.

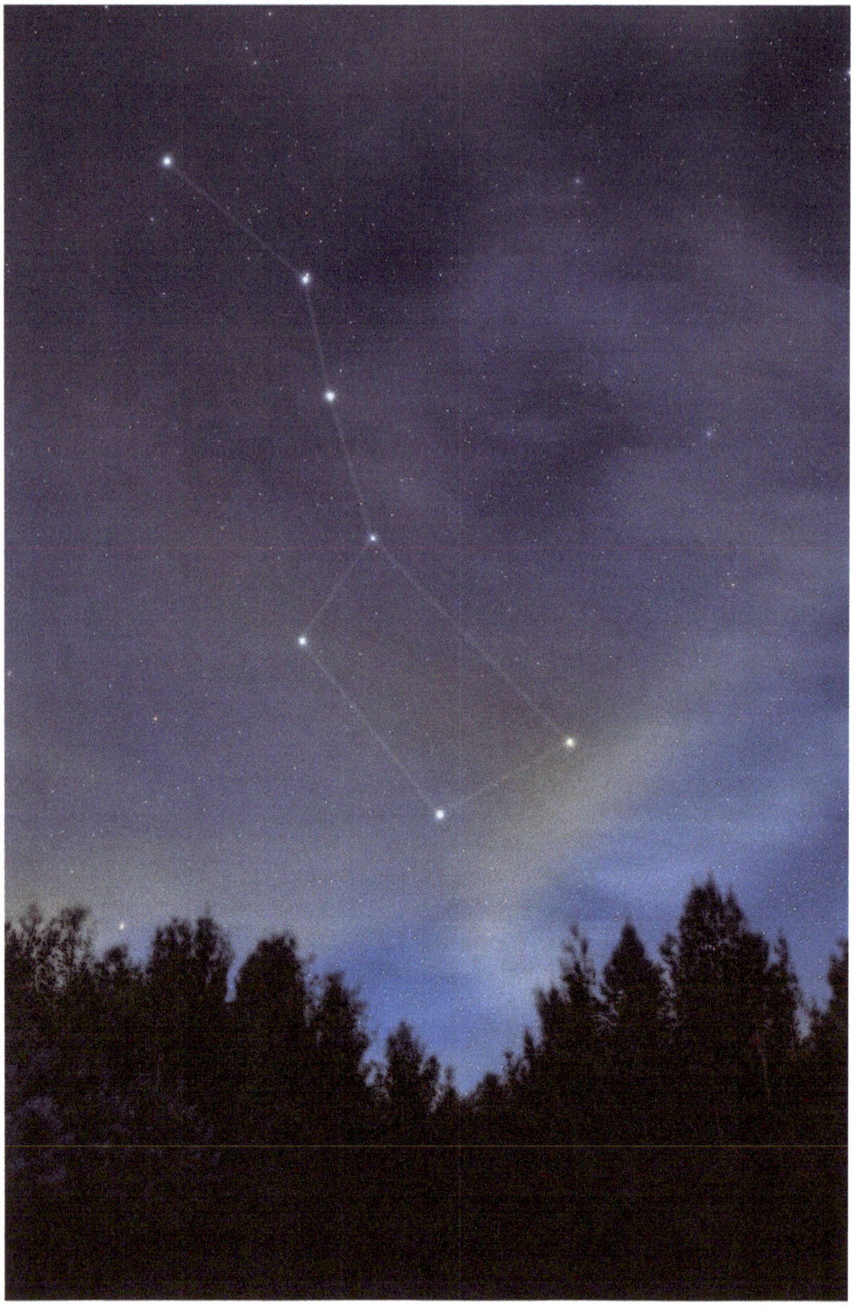

My point?

Shouldn't diagnostic efforts lead to clear and certain scientific outcomes?

What I am claiming is that a diagnostic manual based on a measurable personality theory will allow you to do this. With it, you could feel just as certain as you now feel about what is in this photograph. Can you see it? Of course, you can. It's The Big Dipper. No chance you feel unsure now.

Imagine diagnosing with this much certainty—every single time.

A Brief Look at Those Five "Fractal" Filters

Now let's briefly talk about what those five filters represent. The big idea this time? That despite the claims that personality is just a set of qualities which describe who we are, it's not. Rather, personality refers to a sequence of five nested filters, each of which reduces our ability to experience life. Here each filter acts like a layer of colored cellophane placed in front of a video-set light. And with each additional layer, less light gets through—and more and more colors get filtered out.

Do you realize what I'm saying here? Not only do these filters make us see life less vividly. Some of them hide or distort our needs beyond recognition. Keep in mind, consciousness is the ability to visualize and sense these needs from a personal perspective. And personality is what prevents—or allows—these needs to manifest in our minds. Together with wounds then, personality drastically reduces our ability to recognize any and all needs.

The thing is, given the mind's limited ability to process information, in one sense, this is likely a good thing. Seeing all of our needs and the needs of those we love in one big gulp would surely overwhelm us. Then again, not seeing these needs can and often does lead to far worse outcomes.

Fortunately, we humans have a workable alternative here. We can learn to recognize the meta-patterns of these needs. Like candle flame patterns they remain visible even under very low light.

Meaning what?

Think about it. How many candle flames must a five-year-old see in order to then recognize any and all future examples? Normally, only one. Usually, a single example is all a child needs to see to become visually able to identify candle flame patterns for life. This is not to say there's no more to learn. Most people, if asked, can't draw the entire candle-flame fractal pattern. The outer shape? Yes. Easy-peasy. But the temperature-based tipping-points within this flame? Probably not.

Those tear-drop-shaped rings of vertical temperature change are tipping-point based. Candle-flame temperatures don't just increase. They increase incrementally, in differently-colored layers. Can you picture what those colors are and how many rings candles have? Are you feeling curious? If so, then you're doing well.

Whenever you feel curious, this meta-pattern tells you, you are personally aware of a need. And since you can't meet a need you can't see, feeling curious is the key to becoming an excellent diagnostician.

Have You Ever Opened a Russian Nesting Doll?

On the next page, we're going to briefly explore a drawing I expect will look at least mildly familiar. This drawing—a cross-section of a group of 10 Russian Nesting Dolls—represents Emergence Personality Theory's 10 nested layers of personality. I have, in my office, a hand-made set of 10 dolls which I had made for me, in Russia, some years back. I vividly recall sending the money for this set, then worrying I'd been scammed when months later, it still hadn't arrived.

Personality as the Ten Russian Nesting Dolls

(according to Emergence Personality Theory)

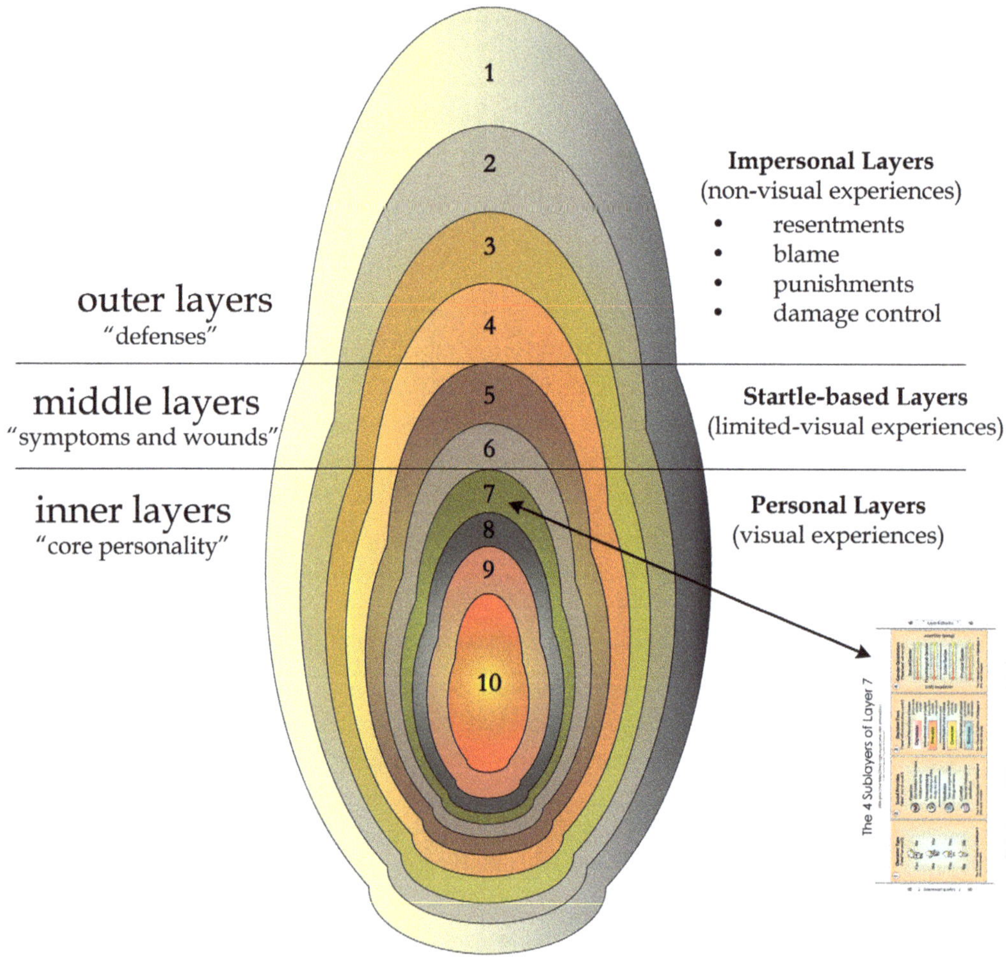

Stories aside, the point of all this is that people have been using nesting dolls—and onions—to describe personality for some time now. For one thing, despite what it may seem like from seeing cross-sections of these things, to move from one layer to another in them, you cannot skip any layers.

Can you picture what doing this looks like? To move from one doll to another in an actual set of nesting dolls, you must open—and set aside—each prior doll, one at a time, in a fixed order. This is why nesting dolls, and onions, have so often been used to describe personality.

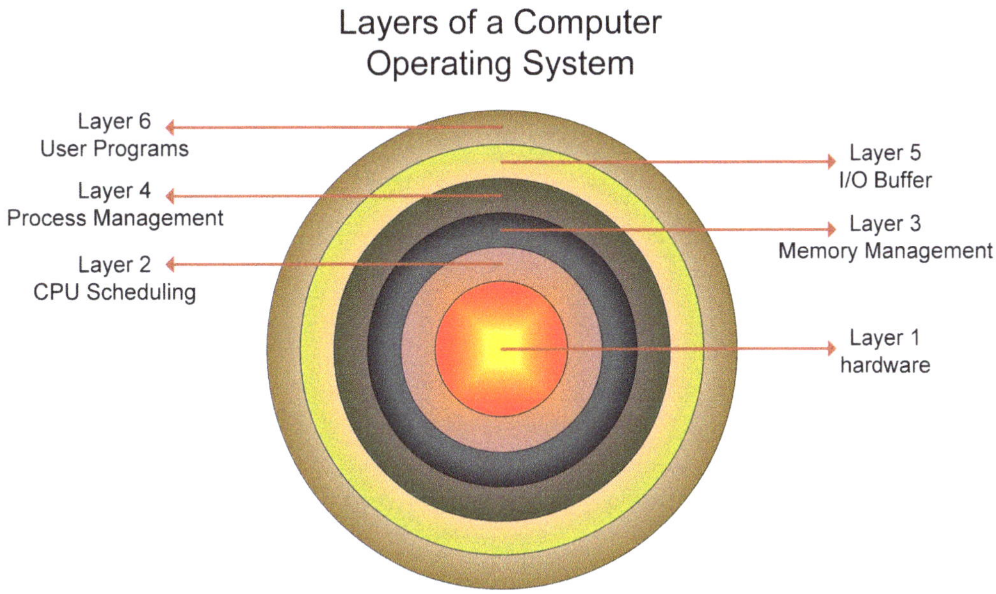

This nesting visually and physically reveals the way the different parts of the mind are organized and interact. How did I come to discover the particulars of this organization when no one before me had? I, for some time in my late thirties, worked as a computer whiz-kid for a major corporation. At the time, PCs were just becoming part of this company's information services infrastructure. Back then, no colleges offered degrees involving personal computers. This meant, much of what I learned about computers I had to teach myself.

Part of what I learned was that all computers have what amounts to a personality. A Mac has one type. A PC, another. And Linux, yet another. Computer professionals call these personalities, "operating systems." Fascinated, I taught myself how computer programmers design these operating systems.

Obviously, each of them gets designed by human beings. I posited that because of this, the designs of the minds of these human designers had to be reflected in the way they designed the minds of these computers. I then reverse-engineered those computer operating systems and in doing so, discovered the underlying structure of the human mind. The result is what you see in the 10 Russian Nesting Dolls drawing. All computer operating systems are designed in nested layers. I reasoned that human personalities must be similarly designed. And they are.

What is particularly important to see here is how this nesting affects the way our minds function. For example, locate Layer 9 in the 10 Nesting Dolls cross-section drawing. Now picture moving from Layer 9 to Layer 7. If these layers are nested, then you cannot jump from Layer 9 to Layer 7. To move from 9 to 7, you must move from Layer 9, through Layer 8, to get to Layer 7.

What does this tell us about how personality functions?

It turns out, understanding the way nested layers work holds the key to it all.

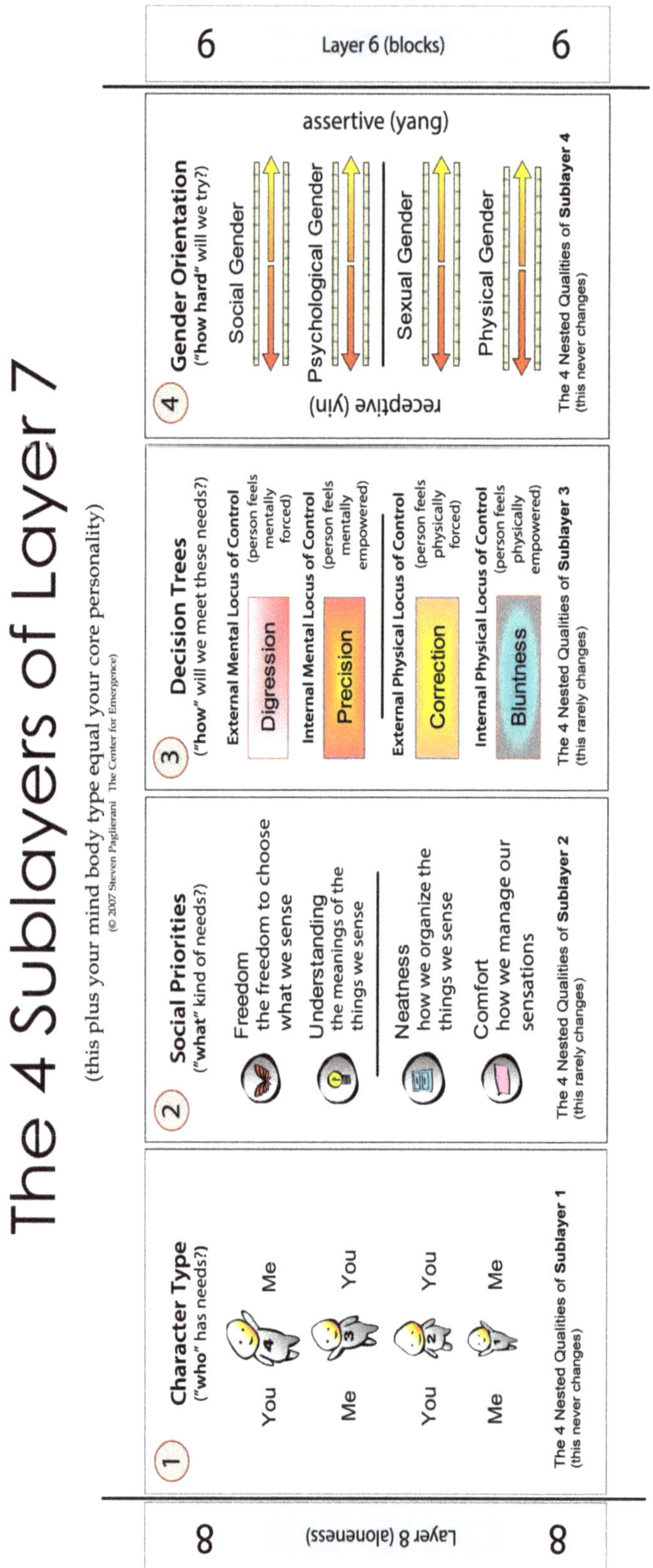

The Core Personality as The Four Nested Sublayers of Layer 7

Did you notice, in the Ten Nesting Dolls drawing a page or so back, the small upright rectangle in the lower right? What you see here is a much larger, more readable version of that rectangle. In it, you'll find the basics of the four ***sublayers*** of Layer 7. Please keep in mind, these four sublayers nest between Layer 6 and Layer 8.

Now imagine you are currently in Layer 10 and want to move your mental attention up and out into the real world. Can you see that to do this, you'd need to move through all ten layers, starting with Layer 10? This would, of course, include going through all 4 sublayers of Layer 7. Admittedly, this is a lot to picture. So please do remember to use the drawings as you try.

Collectively, those ten layers, in that order, are how the mind stores and organizes its content. It's also how the mind filters and focuses in on our life experiences. This means we can learn a lot about human nature just by exploring this one drawing. For one thing, since each layer stores a different kind of content, we can focus in on only one kind of content at a time.

What kind of content do we process and focus in on in Layer 7?

Any and all human experiences of pure need.

What do I mean by "pure need?"

"Pure need" is the uncomplicated urges newborn babies feel. As adults, this term refers to the unpleasant feelings we feel whenever we feel lost and can't understand something important in life. Technically, this can be any experience wherein we feel we need something but haven't a clue what this something is—as well as the kinds of feelings which no amount of logic or facts can resolve.

Realize, these needy feelings do not arise in us as thoughts, or decisions, or as urges to do specific behaviors. Rather they emerge in our minds as a sequence of 4 kinds of urges. Here the first urge we feel after leaving Layer 8 is our "Character Type" urge. This urge is what we'll look at next.

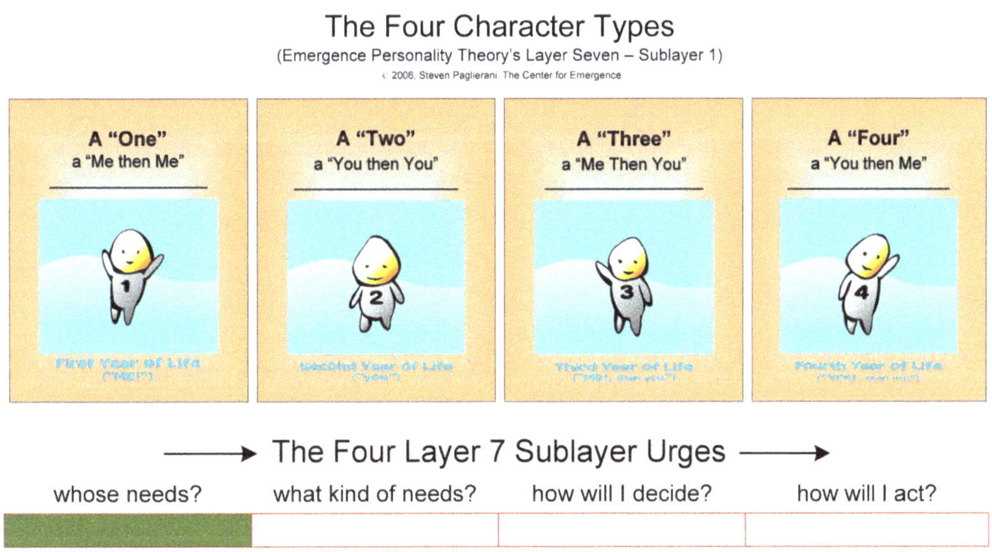

Character State / Type Urges: the 1st Sublayer of Layer 7

When does our Character Type develop in us? Between birth and four years old.

Where do the numbers come from? These numbers, One through Four, refer to the year in which this particular pattern of urges most resembles that year's normal.

What does our Character Type do? Very simply, it's a sequence of two urges. These urges are the first thing we feel each time we feel ambivalent about something.

In these times, our Character Type automatically decides for us "*where these needs exist—in us or in others.*" Our personality then defaults to one of two possible Character States—either the Me state, or the You state.

Either we believe we are sensing our own needs. Here, we are said to be in a Me state. Or we believe we are sensing someone else's needs. So we are said to be in a You state.

In effect, Character Type is an urge we feel in certain situations—those times in which we feel we must decide between our needs and the needs of someone else. Arriving at a bookstore entrance where there is only one door and two people trying to go in. Coming up to an interstate toll booth plaza where you must merge into one lane.

In these times, your Character Type instantly tries to resolve the situation. It does this by urging us to accept an answer to the question, "Whose needs are the legitimate needs here, mine or the other person's?"

Realize, we never actually hear this question being asked. This process happens unconsciously. How? Our Character Type simply hides the needs it thinks are not legitimate, in effect, filtering that choice out.

Character Type - The Primary and Secondary States

Please note, all four Character Types (Character Types One, Two, Three, and Four) do this filtering twice for each need. The first time is called, the primary urge state; the second, the secondary urge state. Know the time between these two outcomes can be anywhere from minutes to weeks or years. In a case where you and a friend are going back and forth as to which movie to go to, it can occur in minutes. In a case where you've always thought your parents screwed you up? Sometimes, it can take years. And sometimes, you never reach the secondary state.

How many possible ways can a Character Type filter out needs?

Since there are only two possible Character States, there must be exactly four possible Character Type filters.

"Whose needs are the legitimate needs here, mine or the other person's?"

First possibility? I'm a Character Type **One**. The needs are mine (I'm in a Me state), then mine again (I checked and I'm still in a Me State).

Second possibility? I'm a Character Type **Two**. The needs are yours (I'm in a You state), then yours again (I checked and I'm still in a You state).

Third possibility? I'm a Character Type **Three**. The needs are mine (I'm in a Me state), then they're yours (I checked and now I'm in a You State).

Fourth possibility? I'm a Character Type **Four**. The needs are yours (I'm in a You state), then they're mine (I checked and now I'm in a Me state).

Realize, each of these four possibilities is entirely tipping-point based. Like coin tosses, each time we feel the urge to decide whose needs the needs are, our personality hides one of the two possible Character states.

Equally important, consider how I've said our personality arrives at this "choice." We never see where this answer comes from. Rather we simply feel urges to focus on whichever needs remain visible to us.

Know that all four of Layer 7's sublayer urges function this way. They hide all but one possible outcome. This is not to say we then automatically choose how we respond to these urges. Here, we can feel choices. We can choose to respond based on our urges. Or we can employ logic, or culture, or situational restrictions.

How The 4 Character Types Hide Urges

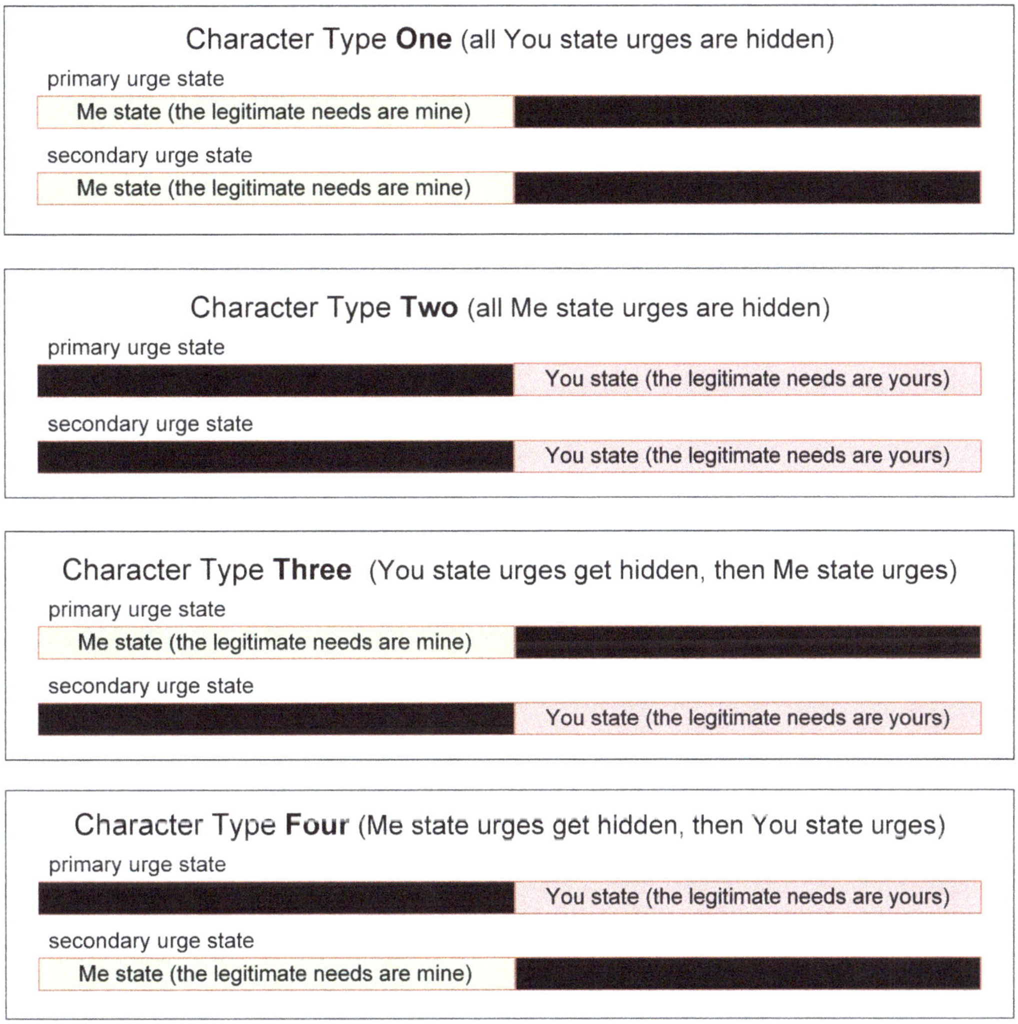

My point is, how we respond can and often does include conscious choices as to how we behave. But the urges behind these choices are largely predetermined by our personalities.

This points to yet another mistaken idea diagnosticians get told is true. They get taught to assume that most of what human beings do, they do for logical reasons. What is true? That we largely get pushed into doing things based on responding to the needs which don't get filtered out. And since our personalities hide all but one possible source of these needs, it's our personality—and not logic or reason, that provokes much of what occurs in our minds.

What about facts and logic? Where do they come in?

After the fact, they function as the justifications and rationalizations for how we ultimately responded.

Realize, there are infinite nuances at play here. The patterns in personality are as complex as candle flame patterns. This said, should you be interested in exploring these ideas further, please know I've done this in depth in my 2011 book, ***Unraveling Human Nature***. At the same time, know that what I've written here builds on what I wrote there, adding quite a bit of new and useful explanation.

As for logic and reasons, obviously we do use these things to explain why we do what we do. But attributing our behaviors to logic alone assumes we are unaffected by our inner natures. So much for "therapies" which claim better logic makes us healthier people. Then again, it does make us function like healthy robots.

Here then is the first of the four sublayers of Layer 7—Character Type. This is the part of personality which instantly hides the urges you are programmed to ignore. And the urges that are left are what you will feel you need to respond to.

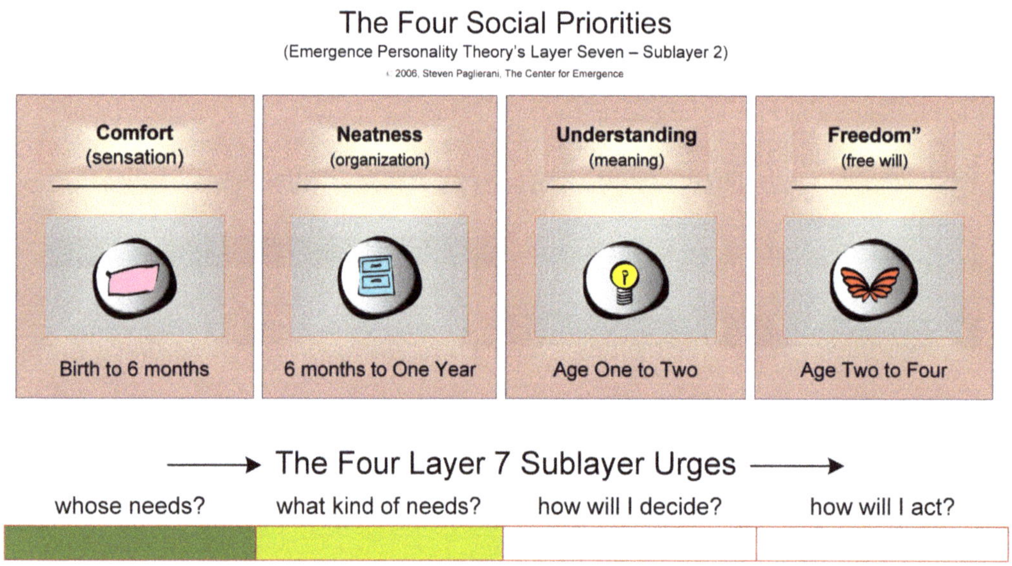

Social Priorities Urges: the 2nd Sublayer of Layer 7

Obviously, you can't address an urge if you don't know what it is. And so far, all that's happened is you've felt urges as to *whose* needs you're feeling—where to look. This in no way tells you what kind of needs these needs are. And this is where the second of Layer 7's sublayer urges—your Social Priorities—come into play.

These four qualities are the four ways human beings categorize needs. By age four, all human beings will have, for the rest of their lives, permanently prioritized these four categories of urges. Realize, by "prioritized," I'm referring to the order in which each of these priorities gets unhidden. In other words, like Character Type, our personality filters out all but one of the possibilities at a time.

The thing is, unlike Character Type—where all possible urges come from the two Character State urges (the Me state and the You state), with Social Priorities, there are four possible States—Comfort, Neatness, Understanding, and Freedom.

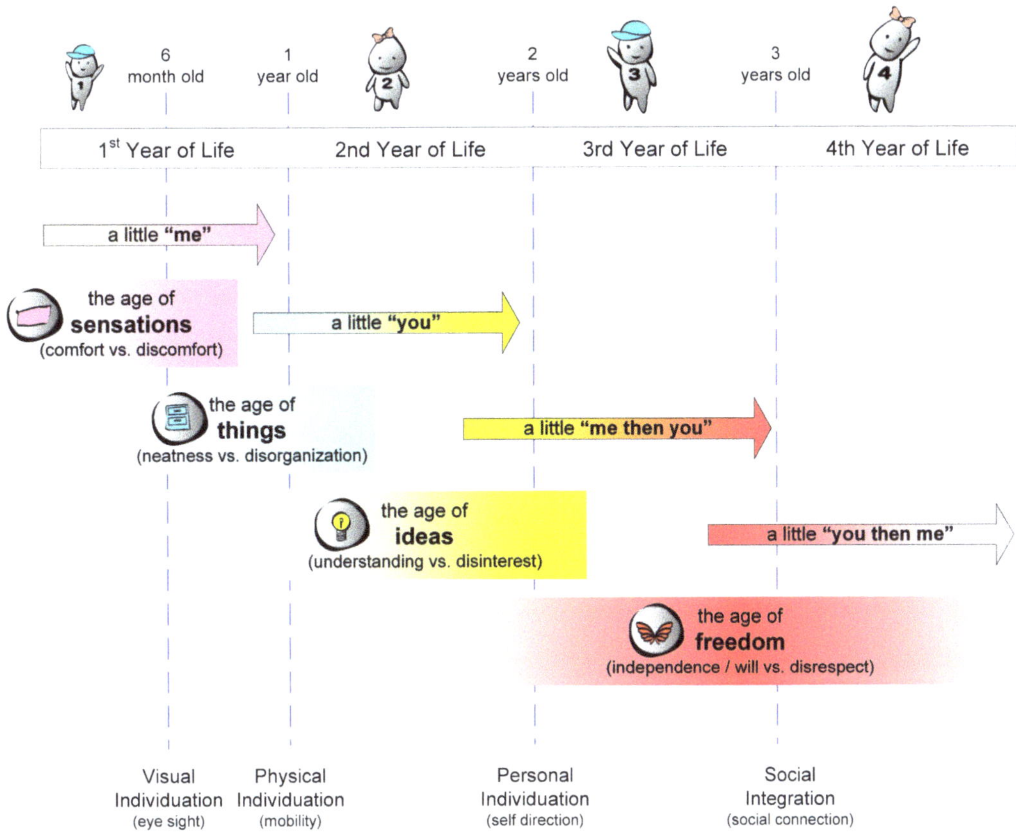

What you see in this drawing then is the developmental origins of these four urges.

First, between birth and about six months old, we look to master our urges for *Comfort*. Here we work on mastering our five senses.

Next, from roughly age six months to about one year—we look to master our urges for *Neatness*—the ability to arrange the things we've learned to sense.

Then—from about age one to age two—we look to master our urges for *Understanding*. Here we begin to assign word meanings to the things we've learned to arrange.

And lastly—from about age two to age four—we look to master our urges for *Freedom*. Freedom is "the ability to forget about the first three kinds of urges." We do this so we can be free to socialize with others. Or not, if we choose to be alone.

Identifying Regressions Based on Social Priorities

Something I've previously mentioned is that our core personality is entirely comprised of a nested set of just five unconscious urges. What I may have failed to mention though is that all of these urges arise in us developmentally. This is to say, each and every one of these urges is tied to a certain time in human development.

Knowing what these times are can be especially helpful to diagnosticians.

The 4 Social Priority-Based Regressions

(the Trauma Determines the Depth of the Regression)

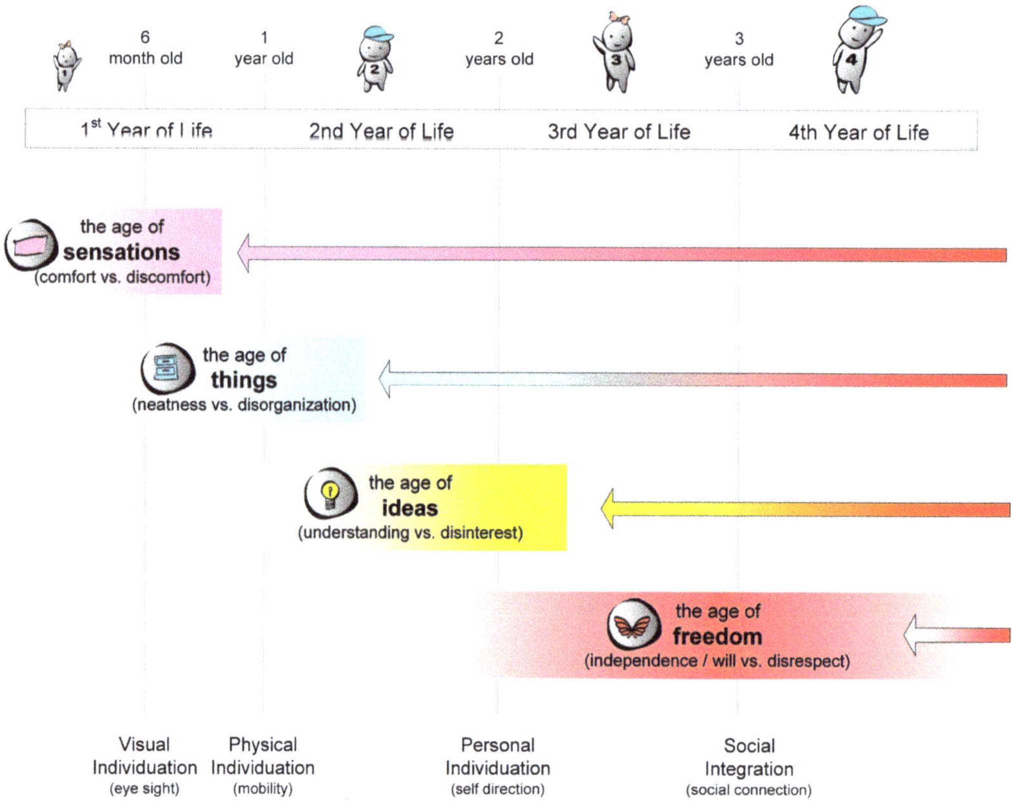

Indeed, if you wish to properly process your patient's regressions and transferences, you must be able to connect these urges to the ages in which they first developed. For this reason and more, all diagnosticians should be fairly expert in recognizing the developmental indicators present during these regressions. However, here again, what I'm presenting is merely a brief introduction to these aspects of personality. For an in-depth discussion of the 4 Social Priorities, please consult my 2011 book, ***Unraveling Human Nature***.

What I will offer here is a series of drawings which visually represent aspects of this second sublayer. For instance, in the drawing on the next page is an example of a completed Social Priorities test.

All Social Priority tests employ just 6, tipping-point based questions.

Social Priority Questions	Choices
Which is harder, being hungry or being ignorant?	(C or U)
Which is harder, losing your day off or losing a day's pay?	(F or N)
Which is worse, a cluttered closet or a dull movie?	(N or U)
Which is harder, to be restricted or to be overtired?	(F or C)
Which is worse, tasteless food or tattered clothes?	(C or N)
Which is harder, being outsmarted or taking orders?	(U or F)

Because they are tipping-point based, 6 questions is all it takes to identify this order.

Please note, however, that there are conditions which must be met for these tests to be valid. Again, if you're curious, see that previous book.

In this example, the four circled letters on the far right reveal this person's Social Priorities. ***The Upper Pair***—**U**nderstanding (meaning), then **F**reedom (free will). ***The Lower Pair***—**N**eatness (organization), then **C**omfort (sensation).

Why divide these four urges into two pairs?

The Upper Pair indicates people's normal response to their Character Type urges.

The Lower Pair, ***with an inverted order***, is how people respond to these urges when they're under significant stress.

In this example, that inverted pair would be C, N—rather than N,C.

So say this person is a Character Type Two (a You, then You). To describe this person's normal CT & SP urges, a diagnostician would say this person "Gives Understanding Freely." And under significant stress? Their urges would become "to Urgently Give Comfort Neatly."

Now consider what this tells us about this person.

Comfort is normally this person's lowest priority. Thus if you knew this and you were diagnosing them—and if you saw them focusing on Comfort-based things like over-eating or over-sleeping—you'd know they were experiencing significant stress.

Please realize, I am treating you here like you've been trained in all this. I apologize for any stress I may be causing you to feel.

My goal here is only to give you a brief example of how knowing these things can be used to set a baseline from which to diagnose.

How would you use this information to diagnose this person?

You would evaluate this person's current stress levels in various life situations.

How? By asking about things like "how are you sleeping?"

And if they say, "a lot more than usual?" Then you have two pieces of evidence for this person being under a lot of stress. This would not be true for a person whose Social Priorities are **C**omfort, **F**reedom, **U**nderstanding, **N**eatness (CFUN). Here Neatness, then Understanding, would be their lower pair. Inverted, this would mean that when this person is stressed out, they would have trouble sleeping and lie awake (C)—likely trying to organize what they need to do the next day (N).

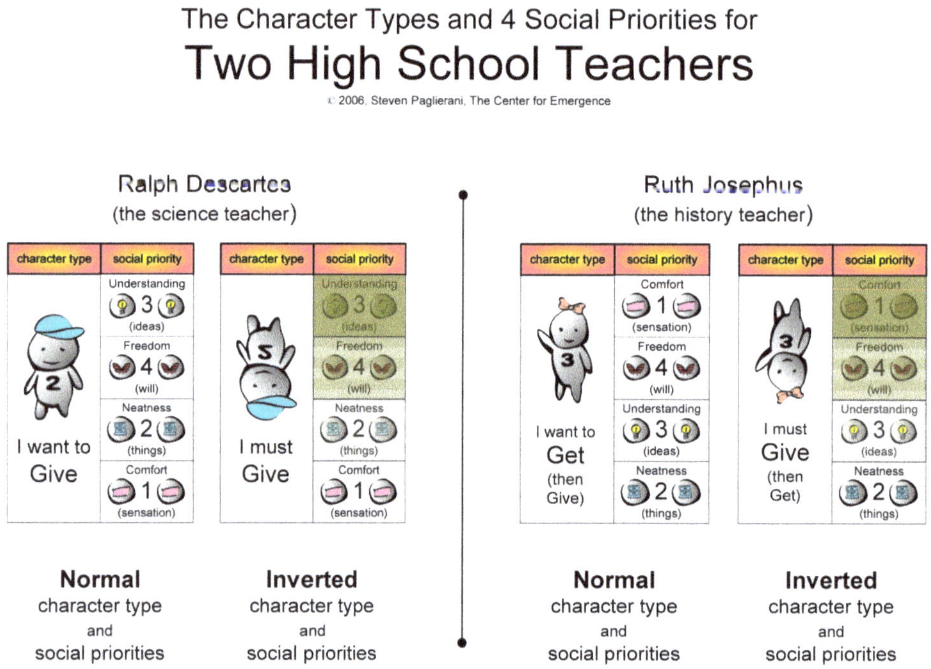

Finally, as I've likely used too many words and have given you no picture, here's a drawing which may help you to see how all this works. In this drawing, you'll find the normal and inverted states for two people—Ralph Descartes, a science teacher who is a Two (You then You) with Understanding, Freedom, Neatness, and Comfort (2UFNC)—and Ruth Josephus, a history teacher who is a Three (Me then You) with Comfort, Freedom, Understanding, and Neatness (3CFUN).

Can you see how each of their Character Types, and the order of their Social Priorities, change based on how much stress they are feeling? Normal vs Inverted. Not hard to see.

One final set of pictures may give you an even better sense of all this. You'll find them on the next page. In these two drawings, I've used water to represent the mind filtering things out. What's under water is what's being filtered out—and what's above water is what is visible. And in the first drawing, you'll find Ralph's variations; in the second, Ruth's.

Both drawings show four states, each of which represents how the person's levels of stress are affecting their Character Type and Social Priorities.

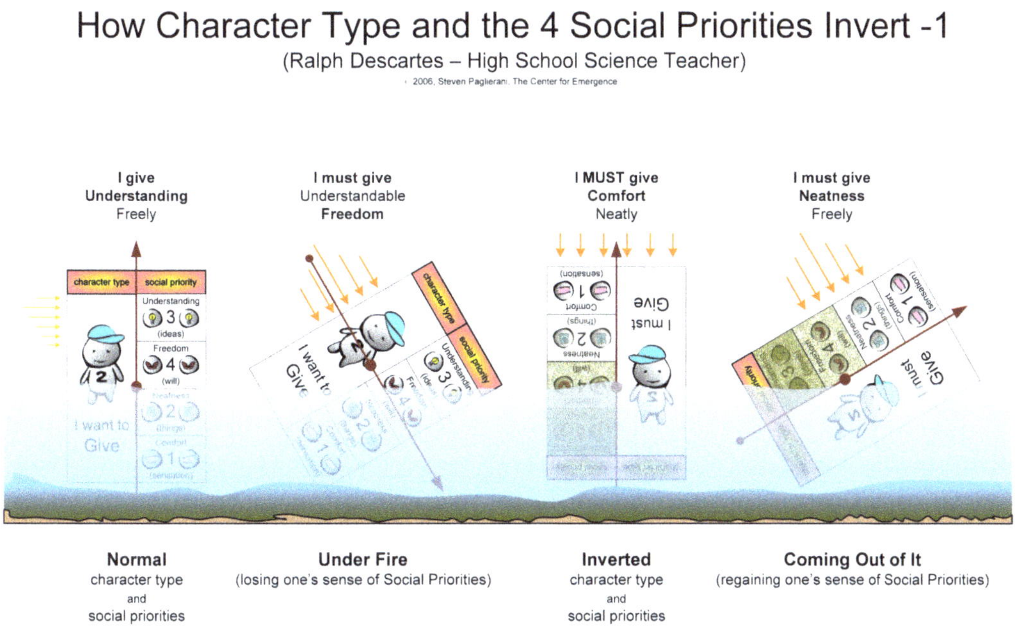

Note the way the four states in both examples include an arrow pointing towards normal. Pay particular attention to the words above each example, as these words typify what these changes feel like.

Now read through the words above all four groups, in order, from left to right.

The changes you observe should tell you a heck of a lot about how stress affects people's Character Type and Social Priority urges.

Baseline readings for personality must be taken in the Normal state.

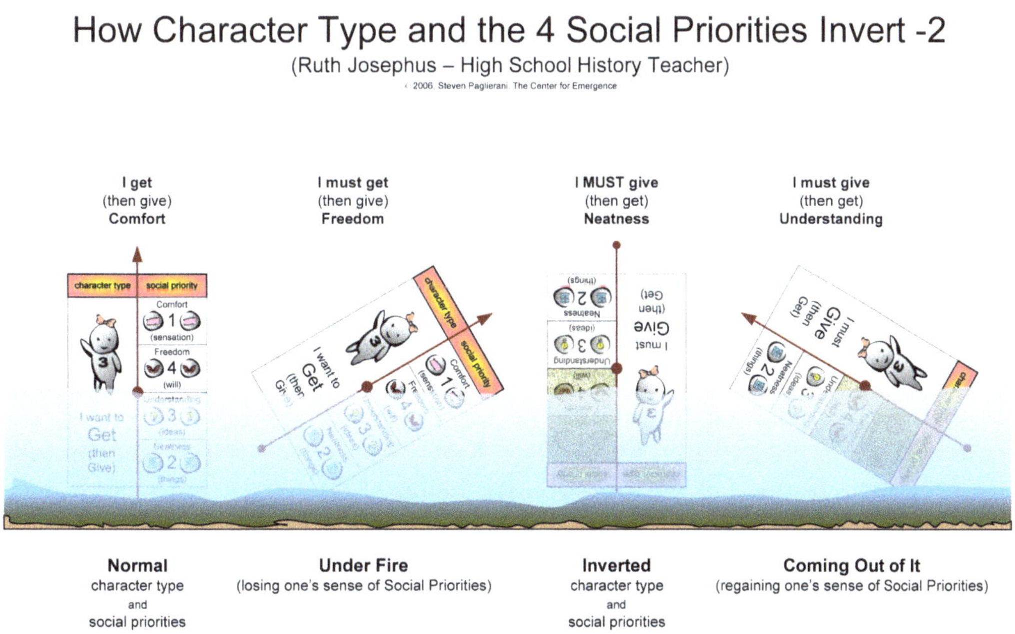

Finally take some time to contrast and compare the differences between these two people. Twos and Threes experience urges quite differently. For example, contrast and compare both people's Inverted states.

Ralph feels he "MUST give Comfort Neatly."

Ruth feels she "MUST give (then get) Neatness in an Understandable way."

Now take a moment to consider how differently these words could explain, ***and predict***, each person's behavior.

Can you imagine feeling like either of these things?

What are you like under stress?

Now do your best to take in what I am about to say.

None of these words refer to behavior. They only refer to urges.

This is what I've been trying to get across to you. A patient's urges are the true measure of their personality. Their behavior is something else. Now consider this. What is the main thing current diagnostic manuals use to diagnose?

Behavior.

Good luck with that.

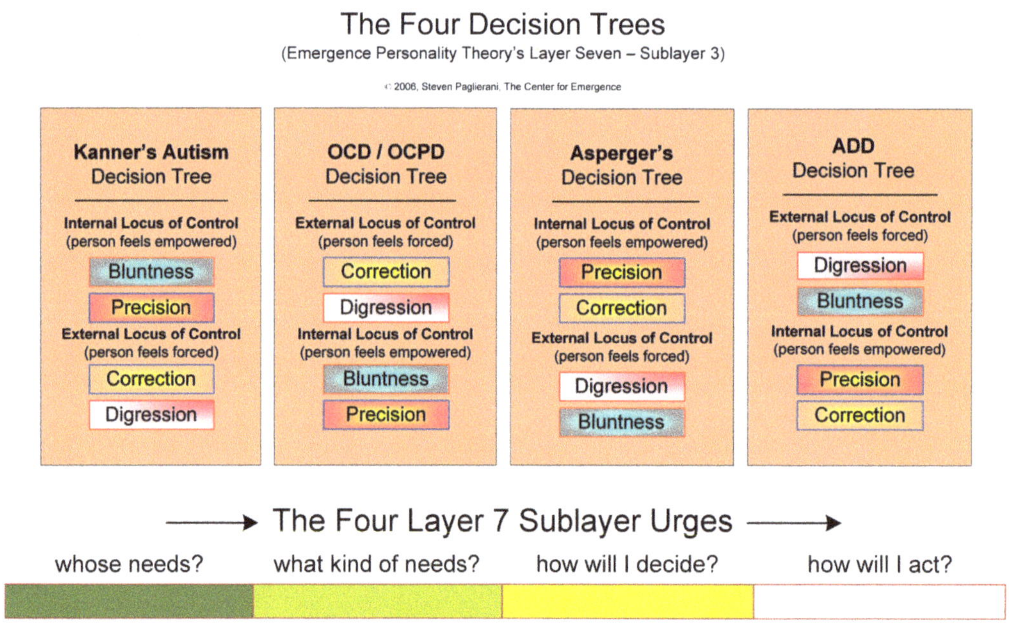

Decision Tree Urges: the 3rd Sublayer of Layer 7

OK. At this point, all but one choice for ***who has needs*** and for ***what kinds of needs these needs are*** has been filtered out. Now you have to decide "***how you will decide,***" how to respond to the urges you are feeling. And yes, this is an odd way to say this. Words describing urges often sound odd. We normally voice urges as the urge to do "such and such," but rarely consider that "such and such" is the *response* to an urge, not the urge. What then is an urge? This is what we are going to explore.

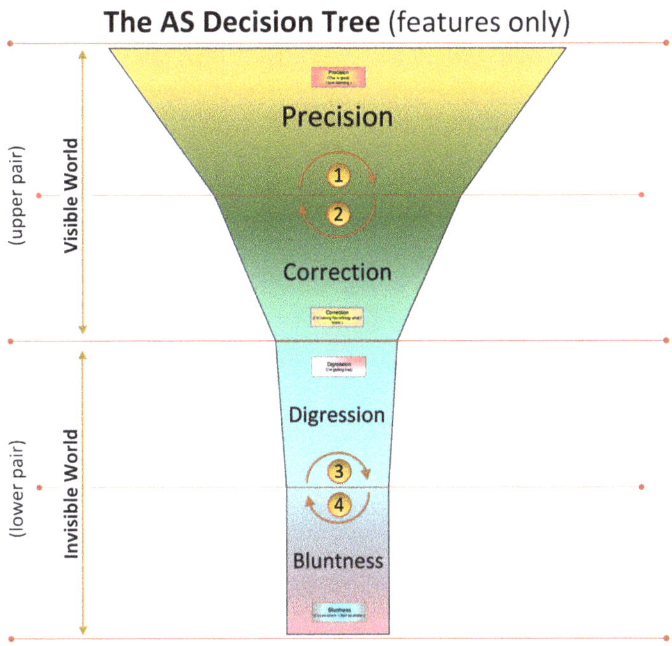

We'll begin with a look at Ralph—the High School science teacher's—Decision Tree. Imagine you're him and you're in his Normal urge state. Ralph is a Character Type Two with Understanding Freedom as the Upper Pair of his Social Priorities (2UF). So Ralph's Normal urges are to Give (he's a Two) **U**nderstanding **F**reely (UF - his upper pair of social priorities).

I am also a Two with UF as my Upper Pair (2UF). Thus I now feel the need to give you a clear and precise Understanding as to what Decision Trees are. But with Freedom as my second social Priority, I don't want to force you to accept these ideas. I'd actually love it if you felt Free to ask me for my evidence.

What do Decision Tree urges add to this already complex picture?

In my case, the words "*clear*" and "*precise*" indicate that.

Precision is the first thing I consider when making decisions. No surprise, I research everything I'm thinking of buying for weeks before I buy. And if you look up at the small drawing of the Four Decision trees at the top of this page, you'll see why. For now, please ignore the title—The AS (Asperger's) Decision Tree.

Recall, Ralph has the same Decision Tree as I do—the AS tree. Can you locate the Precision urge at the top of this Decision Tree? Does the title mean he is, or that I am, on the Autism Spectrum? After all, it says "Asperger's."

In Ralph's case, no, it does not mean that. Hence the qualifier at the end of the title—features only). Why then does this title refer to something current diagnostic manuals claim is diagnosable? And how can I, a man with Asperger's, have the same Decision Tree? This is what we're going to look at next.

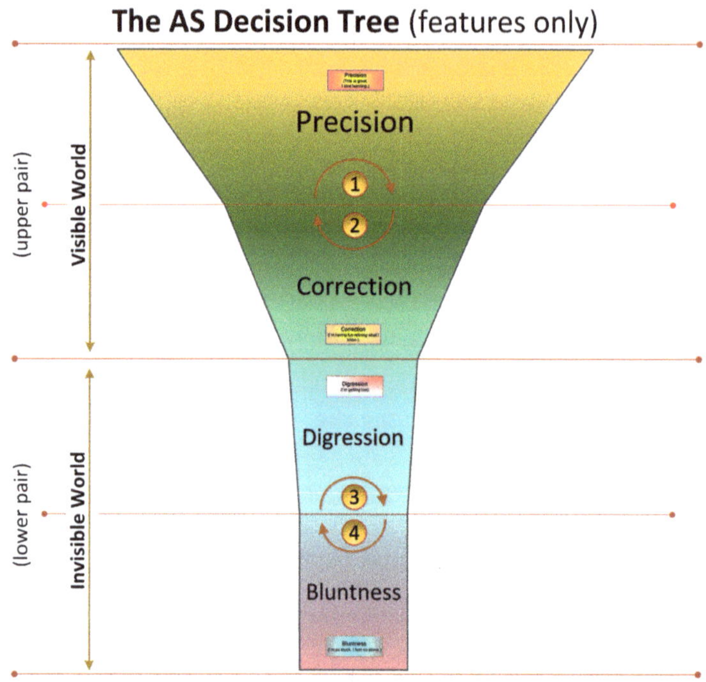

How Can Ralph and I Have the Same Decision Tree?

Begin with this drawing. It's Ralph's yet again. Can you see his four Decision Tree urges? All Decision Trees list these same urges in one of four possible orders. Ralph's tree lists them as Precision, Correction, Digression, and Bluntness (PCDB). This particular ordering is known as the AS (Asperger's) Decision Tree. As I previously pointed out, this funnel indicates Ralph has the features only. How then can I have the same Decision Tree? I have the same ordering. Let's look.

Decision Trees as a Factor in Majority vs Minority Personalities

The thing I'm about to tell you is one of the more important ideas in this book. The idea? That there is just one baseline from which to diagnose. The standard variation of this baseline is called, "The Majority Personalities." These personalities all exist in the upper part of bell of the Bell-Shaped Curve. There are then four less common variations of this same baseline. Each of these "minority" personalities lie 2 to 3 deviations from that norm. Nonetheless, they are all baselines as well. And all five of these variations measure the same five urges—Mind Body Orientation urges, Character Type urges, Social Priority urges, Decision Tree urges, and Gender Identity urges. Know that three of these measures are identical in both Majority and Minority personalities. And the other two, the Social Priority and Decision Tree measures, then differ only in how weak or strong these urges are.

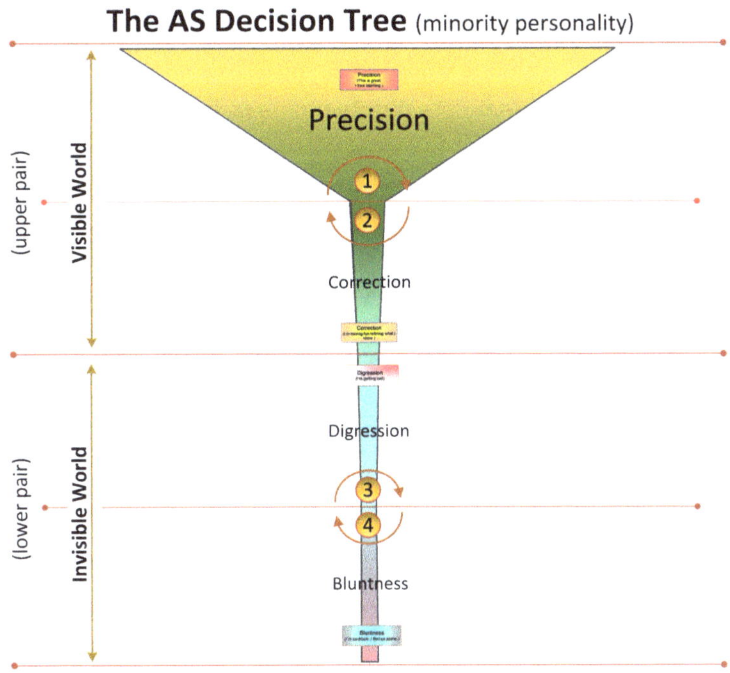

Realize, this difference should be easy to see in these two drawings. Contrast and compare Ralph's Decision Tree (prior page) to mine (on this page). Both drawings share the same main title—the AS Decision tree—and the same Decision Tree urges. But Ralph's says, "features only," whereas mine says, "minority personality."

Did you just catch the diagnostic significance of these two drawings? *Full-blown* Asperger's vs *features of* Asperger's. Again, you see drawings which clearly describe diagnostic criteria. As before, in no way do I intend this to be a comprehensive discussion. Rather, I only wish to point to something you'll learn later in this book.

Now look closely at how the shapes of these two funnels differ. Obviously, the one on the left looks like a normal funnel. Whereas the one on the right is shaped oddly. Can you guess what this shape tells you about me? If you picture yourself pouring something like wet beach-sand into these two funnels, you'll see it. How would wet beach-sand flow differently through these two funnels?

Obviously, it would flow through Ralph's funnel more easily and smoothly. And the sand in my funnel? It would go in fine. But then it would slow down—and might even jam up. This is true despite the fact that both funnels list the same four urges, in the same order—Precision, Correction, Digression, and Bluntness (PCDB).

Please keep this in mind. Same order. Only the funnel shapes differ. My skinny funnel? It indicates I have a Minority Personality. Ralph's fat funnel? It indicates he has a Majority Personality, which includes the features of AS. Could you possibly not recognize this difference? No more than you could not recognize a candle flame.

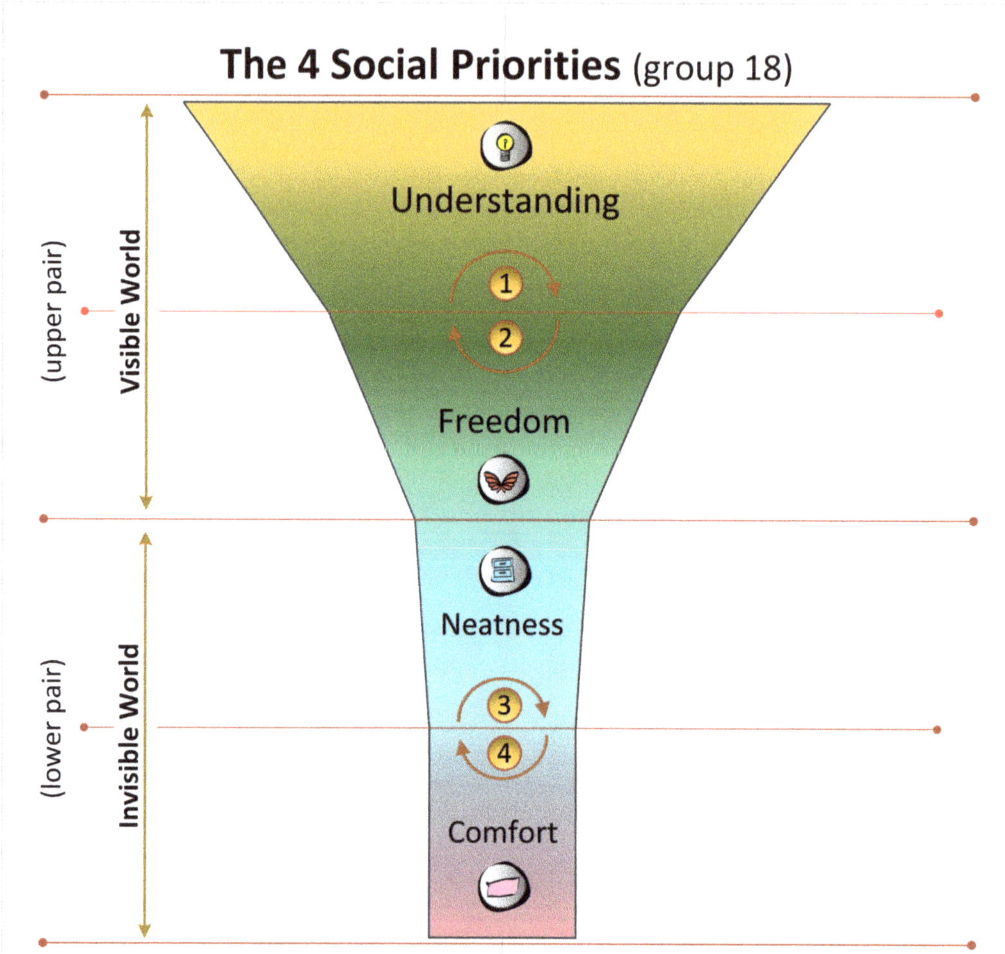

Majority vs Minority Personalities: Part 1 - the Social Priorities

Now contrast and compare the Social Priority Tree drawings at the tops of these two pages. Even a quick glance at the one on this page should tell you, this person has a Majority Personality. Whereas according to the drawing on the next page, that person has a Minority Personality. Are you beginning to see that like my previous drawings, even a quick glance makes diagnostic differences easy to see?

Now do take a breath and go slow. What I'm about to say is extremely important. Why? Because to properly diagnose, you must keep in mind, there are actually five variations of this baseline. One occupies the upper portion of the bell. The other four lie 2 to 3 deviations away. And together, these five "normal" baselines allow diagnostician's to easily discern between what is diagnosable and what is not.

Why the need for this? Because being in a minority group does not make someone broken. These folks shouldn't get a diagnosis just because they are in a statistical minority. Moreover, three measures of personality look and function exactly the same in all human beings. The only difference here is how two of the five measures are distributed in the funnels of Majority and Minority Personalities.

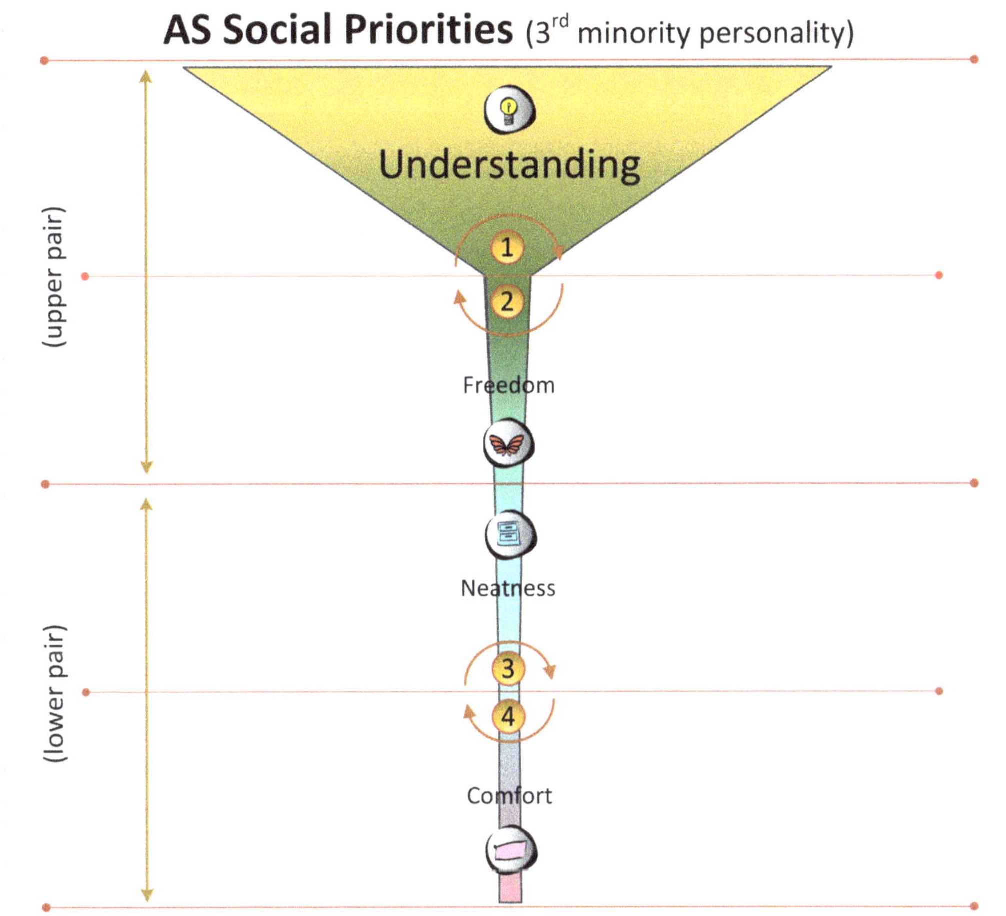

Now imagine pouring wet sand into the funnel on the previous page. Based on that funnel's shape, sand would flow through this funnel smoothly and easily. This flow tells you how this person's urges flow through their mind and body. This smooth easy flow indicates this person has a Majority Personality.

Now imagine doing the same for the funnel on this page. This time, the funnel neck abruptly narrows. So we know, this person has a Minority Personality. Wet sand in this funnel would likely slow down and get stuck. And being these are "social" urges—and being this person would only notice the topmost urge—this person would experience an extremely narrowed focus in social situations.

Can you see it? Both funnels have the same urges in the same order. Only the distribution is different. Now recall, the Social Priority Tree on the left is Ralph's and the one on the right is mine. At least, it was mine most of my life. After discovering these patterns some two plus decades ago, I became able to see these limitations in myself. So I taught myself how to switch between these two funnels. In truth, currently, the shape of my funnel is usually much closer to the funnel on the left than to the one on the right. More on how this is possible in a bit.

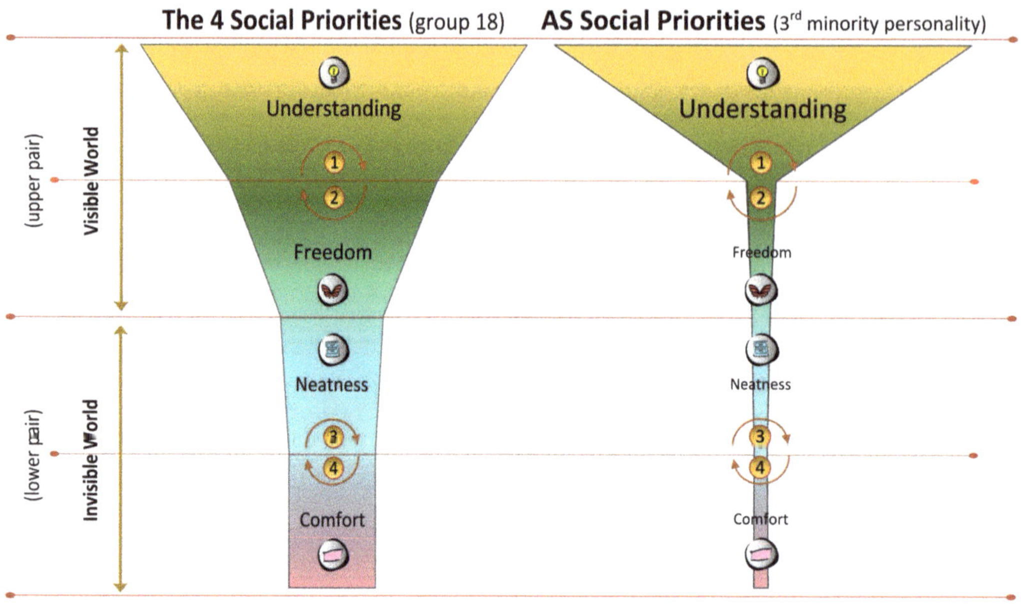

Majority vs Minority Personalities: part 2 -the 4 Decision Trees

Are you feeling overwhelmed? If so, know there's nothing wrong with you. What the heck does all this stuff mean? Oh, boy. Where do I even begin?

Start by looking at the pair of Social Priority funnels on this page. Then look over at the two Decision Tree funnels on the next page.

Now realize—in both drawings—both left funnels represent a person with a Majority Personality (group 18). Whereas both right funnels represent a person with a Minority Personality (AS).

Based on these drawings, hopefully you can see what's the same—and what's different. The same?

The person with a Majority Personality and the person with the Minority Personality share all the *same qualities*, in the *same order*. The only difference? How the urges move through the wide funnel neck vs the narrow one.

The size of this neck predicts how many urges will get through—or filtered out.

Now try picturing something being poured into these funnels. For instance, consider how differently wet sand would flow through the two **Social Priority** funnels in the drawing on this page. As I said, the funnel on the left is one of the 24 common Majority Personalities (group 18). Whereas the funnel on the right is one of the four Minority Personalities—the one people with Asperger's have.

Can you see how that second funnel accurately reflects and predicts how people with Asperger's experience life? All that matters to folks with this funnel is that they feel free to discuss (2nd priority) what they're currently interested in (1st priority). Why? Because these urges are "Social" Priority urges. So socially sharing the meanings of the things they're interested in is all that matters to them.

What if the people they're talking to have no interest in these things?

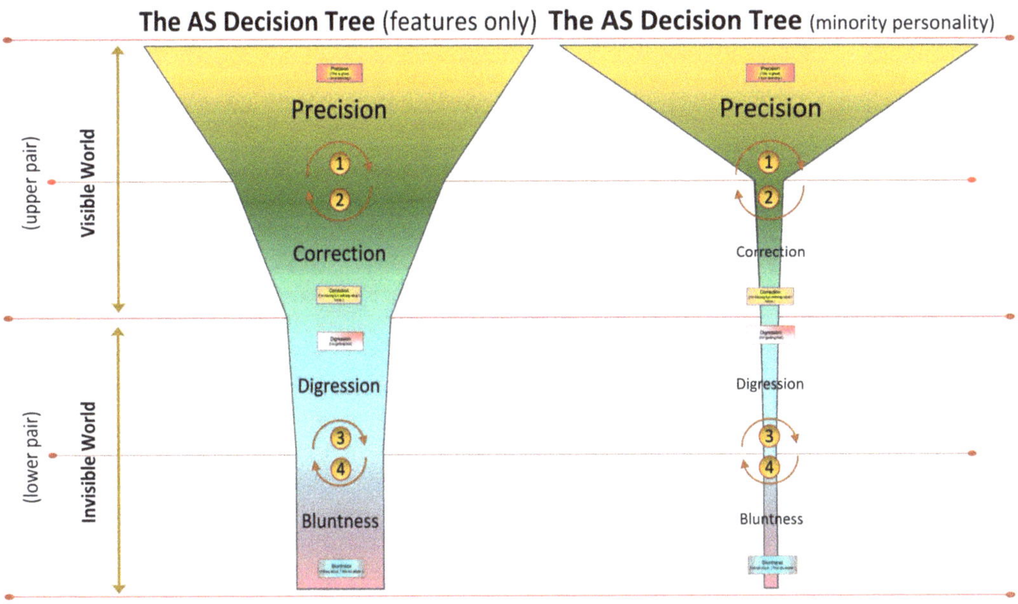

Clearly, folks with AS hardly notice. Not because they don't care about hurting people. Rather, because the urges they can sense eclipse (and so hide) the other three urges. It doesn't occur to them to try to see if you're interested or not. Lacking the other urges, they remain blind to how they're affecting other people. And with Comfort last, they never notice when they're making people uncomfortable.

Now add to this mix the AS (Asperger's) **Decision Tree**. What does this tree tell you about these people? That they feel compelled to share their Understandings (1st Social urge), Precisely (1st Decision urge). Perfectly. And should they misspeak? Then they feel compelled to immediately offer a Correction. Indeed, these corrections can often occur mid-sentence, derailing the entire conversation.

Now recall, I have this Minority Personality. So I can personally attest to what this is like. For example, say I've just told you I did something last Thursday. If I realize it occurred last Wednesday, then mid-sentence, I'll feel compelled to correct what I said. I actually feel like I have no choice. Small Freedom (my second Social urge) to avoid offering a Correction (my second Decision Tree urge) points to this.

It's taken me years to learn that to most folks, these corrections don't matter.

Back to my Social Priorities. Consider how that lack of Freedom urges has affected other social interactions. People like me can literally trap people in conversations they have no interest in, never even realizing this has happened. Nor do people with this Minority Personality realize that what they're telling you may have little to do with what you were talking about. No urges for Neatness? No sense of how what we say to you does or does not follow what you've said.

Finally, with Comfort urges located at the bottom of the funnel, we have no way to gauge the discomfort you're feeling. Keep in mind, this is not because we do not care about you. Rather it's because our Social Priority and Decision Trees filter out these urges, rendering them—and you—invisible to us.

The KA Social Priority Grouping (1 - 6)

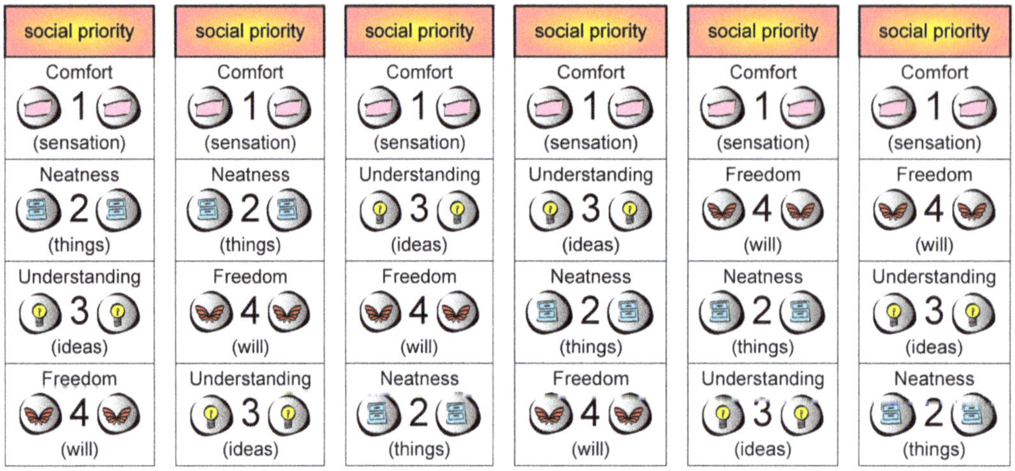

Determining a Person's Diagnostic Baseline

In what follows, I'm going to briefly show you how to use these things to determine a patient's diagnostic baseline. After all, you can't hope to diagnose properly if you can't differentiate between what is diagnosable and what is not. And yes, I realize, it's quite controversial to claim there are five variations of the "normal" baseline. But this claim is no different than saying we should treat people in other minority groups (skin, culture, religion) as being equal to people in majority groups—and that being "statistically normal" (meaning "in the *majority*") should in no way be seen as proof a person is a good person, let alone healthy.

How do you determine which baseline to use? It all comes down to knowing your patient's Social Priorities. For now, assume you've tested your patient and that you know their Social Priorities are just like mine—UFNC. Obviously, the next thing you need to do is to interpret this data.

The following is a brief, albeit densely complex, overview. Please try to keep breathing and refer back to the diagrams as you read through this.

To begin with, as you know by now, there are 4 Social Priority urges. **Comfort** (urges to respond to sensory information). **Neatness** (urges to organize information). **Understanding** (urges to assign meanings to information). And **Freedom** (urges to be free to socialize, and talk about this information, at any time and in any place). All four categories of urges appear and develop—in all human beings—during the first four years of life. The order of these four urges also gets fixed for life in this time as well.

How many possible orders can these 4 things end up in? Twenty four in all. How did I arrive at this? From the permutation of four things taken four at a time. Based on the highest priority, this can then be broken down into four groups of six. The first six are at the top of this page. The next six are on the next page. And if you then turn the page, you'll see the third and fourth groupings there. The groupings?

The OCD Social Priority Grouping (7 - 12)

social priority	social priority	social priority	social priority	social priority	social priority
Neatness 2 (things)	Neatness 2 (things)	Neatness 2 (things)	Neatness 2 (things)	Neatness 2 (things)	Neatness 2 (things)
Understanding 3 (ideas)	Understanding 3 (ideas)	Freedom 4 (will)	Freedom 4 (will)	Comfort 1 (sensation)	Comfort 1 (sensation)
Freedom 4 (will)	Comfort 1 (sensation)	Comfort 1 (sensation)	Understanding 3 (ideas)	Understanding 3 (ideas)	Freedom 4 (will)
Comfort 1 (sensation)	Freedom 4 (will)	Understanding 3 (ideas)	Comfort 1 (sensation)	Freedom 4 (will)	Understanding 3 (ideas)

- In the first grouping (groups 1-6), the highest priority is **Comfort**.
- In the second grouping (groups 7-12), the highest priority is **Neatness**.
- In the third grouping (groups 13-18), the highest priority is **Understanding**.
- In the fourth grouping (groups 19-24), the highest priority is **Freedom**.

Know the sixth group in each of these four groupings (group 6, 12, 18, 24) either indicates a person with a Minority Personality—or a person with the *features* of a Minority Personality. What determines which it is? Not the order. It's the shape of the neck in the funnel. Does it suddenly narrow and stay that way, or gradually get smaller? Suddenly narrow. Minority Personality. Gradually? Then features only.

From this, each grouping is then associated with a different Minority Personality.

- Groups 1 - 6 are the **KA Grouping**—and Group 6 is either a person with the KA Minority Personality or a person with the features of KA.
- Groups 7 - 12 are the **OCD Grouping**—and Group 12 is either a person with the OCD Minority Personality or a person with the features of OCD.
- Groups 13 - 18 are the **AS Grouping**—and Group 18 is either a person with the AS Minority Personality or a person with the features of AS.
- Groups 19 - 24 are the **ADD Grouping**—and Group 24 is either a person with the ADD Minority Personality or a person with the features of ADD.

Am I implying all human beings in some way act like people with a Minority Personality? In some ways, yes, I am. But only people with groups 6, 12, 18, or 24 can say this is them. This is similar to how we all have two eyes and a nose. While no two people have identical eyes or noses, we sometimes say, "He has an English nose." Also notable is the idea that the first group in each grouping (1, 7, 13, 19) is most opposite from this grouping's Minority group, while also being oddly similar to the Minority group in the previous grouping. Group 7, NUFC, is a first group. It's the reverse of Group 12—NCFU, but similar to Minority Group 6—CFUN.

The AS Social Priority Grouping (13 - 18)

social priority	social priority	social priority	social priority	social priority	social priority
Understanding 3 (ideas)	Understanding 3 (ideas)	Understanding 3 (ideas)	Understanding 3 (ideas)	Understanding 3 (ideas)	Understanding 3 (ideas)
Comfort 1 (sensation)	Comfort 1 (sensation)	Neatness 2 (things)	Neatness 2 (things)	Freedom 4 (will)	Freedom 4 (will)
Neatness 2 (things)	Freedom 4 (will)	Freedom 4 (will)	Comfort 1 (sensation)	Comfort 1 (sensation)	Neatness 2 (things)
Freedom 4 (will)	Neatness 2 (things)	Comfort 1 (sensation)	Freedom 4 (will)	Neatness 2 (things)	Comfort 1 (sensation)

The ADD Social Priority Grouping (19 - 24)

social priority	social priority	social priority	social priority	social priority	social priority
Freedom 4 (will)	Freedom 4 (will)	Freedom 4 (will)	Freedom 4 (will)	Freedom 4 (will)	Freedom 4 (will)
Comfort 1 (sensation)	Comfort 1 (sensation)	Neatness 2 (things)	Neatness 2 (things)	Understanding 3 (ideas)	Understanding 3 (ideas)
Neatness 2 (things)	Understanding 3 (ideas)	Understanding 3 (ideas)	Comfort 1 (sensation)	Comfort 1 (sensation)	Neatness 2 (things)
Understanding 3 (ideas)	Neatness 2 (things)	Comfort 1 (sensation)	Understanding 3 (ideas)	Neatness 2 (things)	Comfort 1 (sensation)

Are you ready to scream? Is this too complex? I can so empathize. Imagine what I went through to realize all this? I suspect this is why no one has previously discovered any of it. If I hadn't made these drawings, I wouldn't have either. After all, as I've been telling you for some time now, making the drawings holds the key.

Finally, try to do what I did with the KA and OCD groupings on the previous two pages. This time, compare Group 19 (a first group) with last Groups 18 and 24. Can you find them? If a person has the priorities in Group 18, then depending on the shape of their funnel, they either have the *features* of, or *full-blown* AS. And if a person has last Group 24, then depending on the shape of their funnel, they either have the *features* of, or *full-blown* ADD.

Finally, if you're familiar with how the Periodic Table of the Elements works, then you may suspect that stacking these four tables on top of one another functions similarly to that table. And it does. More on this in a future chapter.

the Twenty-Four Social Priorities

Least like either the features of— or a full-blown— Minority Personality

KA Grouping (groups 1 - 6)

social priority	social priority	social priority	social priority	social priority	social priority
Comfort 1 (sensation)	Comfort 1 (sensation)	Comfort 1 (sensation)	Comfort 1 (sensation)	Comfort 1 (sensation)	Comfort 1 (sensation)
Neatness 2 (things)	Neatness 2 (things)	Understanding 3 (ideas)	Understanding 3 (ideas)	Freedom 4 (will)	Freedom 4 (will)
Understanding 3 (ideas)	Freedom 4 (will)	Freedom 4 (will)	Neatness 2 (things)	Neatness 2 (things)	Understanding 3 (ideas)
Freedom 4 (will)	Understanding 3 (ideas)	Neatness 2 (things)	Freedom 4 (will)	Understanding 3 (ideas)	Neatness 2 (things)

OCD Grouping (groups 7 -12)

social priority	social priority	social priority	social priority	social priority	social priority
Neatness 2 (things)	Neatness 2 (things)	Neatness 2 (things)	Neatness 2 (things)	Neatness 2 (things)	Neatness 2 (things)
Understanding 3 (ideas)	Understanding 3 (ideas)	Freedom 4 (will)	Freedom 4 (will)	Comfort 1 (sensation)	Comfort 1 (sensation)
Freedom 4 (will)	Comfort 1 (sensation)	Comfort 1 (sensation)	Understanding 3 (ideas)	Understanding 3 (ideas)	Freedom 4 (will)
Comfort 1 (sensation)	Freedom 4 (will)	Understanding 3 (ideas)	Comfort 1 (sensation)	Freedom 4 (will)	Understanding 3 (ideas)

AS Grouping (groups 13 -18)

social priority	social priority	social priority	social priority	social priority	social priority
Understanding 3 (ideas)	Understanding 3 (ideas)	Understanding 3 (ideas)	Understanding 3 (ideas)	Understanding 3 (ideas)	Understanding 3 (ideas)
Comfort 1 (sensation)	Comfort 1 (sensation)	Neatness 2 (things)	Neatness 2 (things)	Freedom 4 (will)	Freedom 4 (will)
Neatness 2 (things)	Freedom 4 (will)	Freedom 4 (will)	Comfort 1 (sensation)	Comfort 1 (sensation)	Neatness 2 (things)
Freedom 4 (will)	Neatness 2 (things)	Comfort 1 (sensation)	Freedom 4 (will)	Neatness 2 (things)	Comfort 1 (sensation)

ADD Grouping (groups 19 - 24)

social priority	social priority	social priority	social priority	social priority	social priority
Freedom 4 (will)	Freedom 4 (will)	Freedom 4 (will)	Freedom 4 (will)	Freedom 4 (will)	Freedom 4 (will)
Comfort 1 (sensation)	Comfort 1 (sensation)	Neatness 2 (things)	Neatness 2 (things)	Understanding 3 (ideas)	Understanding 3 (ideas)
Neatness 2 (things)	Understanding 3 (ideas)	Understanding 3 (ideas)	Comfort 1 (sensation)	Comfort 1 (sensation)	Neatness 2 (things)
Understanding 3 (ideas)	Neatness 2 (things)	Comfort 1 (sensation)	Understanding 3 (ideas)	Neatness 2 (things)	Comfort 1 (sensation)

Either features of— or a full-blown— Minority Personality

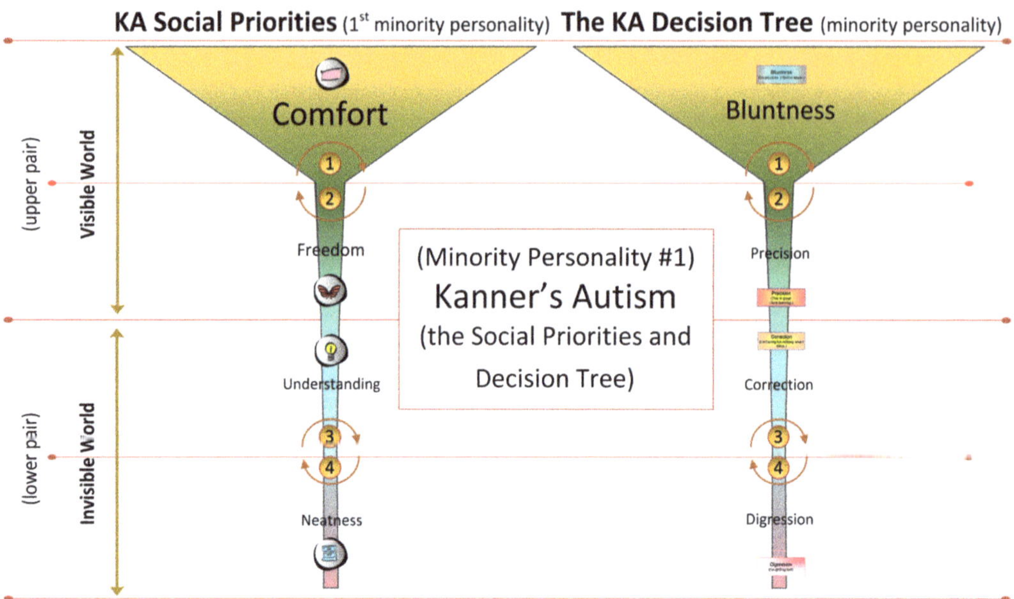

Rant Warning: Unprofessional Words Ahead

Know that what I'm about to say is a complete and utter digression. Based on this book's title, you've no doubt noticed, I can, at times, be patently unprofessional. Translation. I am often honest, authentic, blunt, impolite, angry, and crude. In other words, even in a book as important to me as this one is, I will not hide behind my profession—especially when it involves calling out people who mistreat suffering people.

To see why I'm saying this, notice the pairs of funnels at the tops of these two pages. Each pair of funnels is a person with a full-blown Minority Personality. Each person's Social Priorities are on the left—and their Decision Trees are on the right. Now let me ask you. Do these two people—the person on this page and the one on the next—look the same to you? Please, look closely.

The most recent diagnostic manuals claim they are the same. They also claim both of these people are diagnosably broken and should get the same diagnosis. To see if you agree, let's contrast and compare these two people. Please ignore the drawing titles for now. Focus only on the drawings themselves.

Begin by noticing the necks of all four funnels. They narrow *abruptly,* then stay that way—unlike the funnels of people with Majority Personalities, where the funnel necks *gradually* narrow. This narrowness tells you these urges rarely, if ever, affect the person's life. In effect, these narrow necks all but filter out the lower three urges.

Now notice the titles of these two pairs of funnels. The pair of funnels on this page represent a person with the 1st Minority Personality—KA. The pair of funnels on the next page represent a person with the 3rd Minority Personality—AS. This narrowness is reflected in the personalities of these two people. Both are missing a lot of information. Both have a Minority Personality.

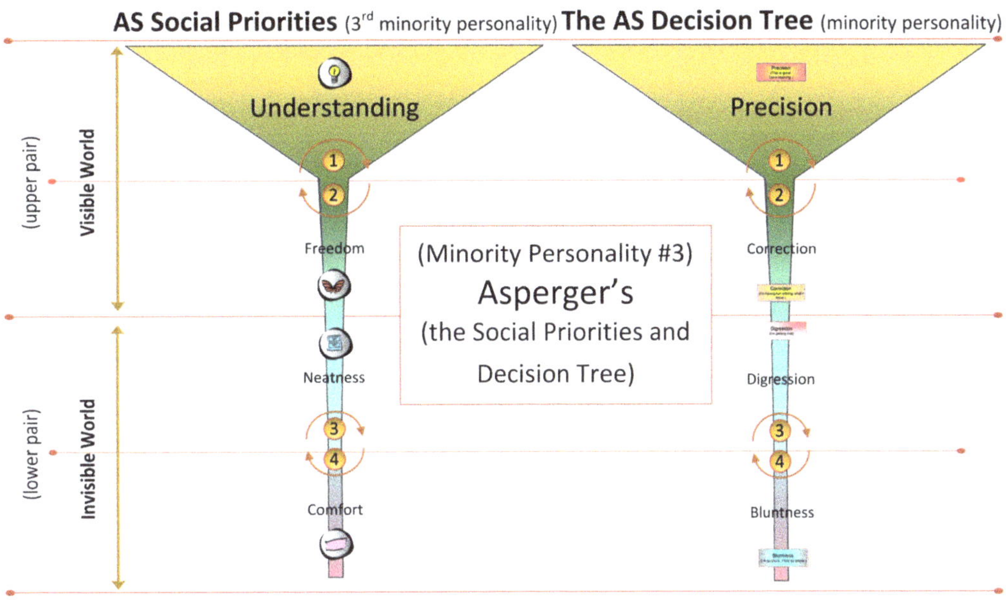

Does it look to you like these two people are missing the same information though? From the shapes of the funnels, it could seem like they are. Look closely now at what's inside the funnels. Obviously, they're not the same. Thus despite how diagnostic manuals love to reduce people to numbers and meaningless words, these two people are human beings. So let's take the time to take a closer look.

What Makes Minority Personalities Measurably Different?

In a moment, I'm hopefully going to offer you a clear explanation for my soon-to-begin rant. First I need to explain how Minority and Majority Personalities differ. To begin with, Emergence Personality Theory employs five real world measures.

- **Mind Body Orientation** (the speed at which the person sends and receives information, in particular, information involving needs)
- **Character Type** (the person's sense of who has the needs they've just sensed)
- **Social Priorities** (the person's sense of what kind of needs these needs are)
- **Decision Tree** (the person's sense of how to best decide to meet these needs)
- **Gender Identity** (the person's sense of how to execute these decisions)

People with Majority and Minority Personalities differ only in how their Social Priority and Decision Tree funnels change size. Internally, the ordering of the qualities within these two measures can be the same for both types of personalities. The difference then? How the upper-most quality in these two measures does or does not eclipse the other three qualities. This is the only difference. In funnel drawings, this difference is represented by the way the funnel necks get narrow.

In Majority Personalities, necks narrow gradually. So there's a lot of change.

In Minority Personalities, necks narrow abruptly, then don't change much at all.

Finally, Here Comes the Rant

Despite copious numbers of people protesting the change, the authors of the current diagnostic manual chose to lump together people with Leo Kanner's autism and people with Hans Asperger's autism. Why do this? Because the majority (not all) of these authors are cold-hearted, self-righteous assholes—"professional" know-it-alls who rarely see the need to treat suffering human beings with respect.

Do you recall what I told you, in the Introduction, about how psychiatrists in the US and Europe have different licensing requirements? Most (not all) of these manual's authors have no training whatsoever in personality or therapy.

Despite this lack of education and experience, these authors chose to ignore the objections of thousands of people, most of whom were actually professionally educated and experienced. Fuck human nature and well-grounded advice, and who cares about the feelings of suffering people. Let's pretend we've discovered some previously hidden, unifying pattern in the symptoms of these poor souls.

Do I think these two groups of people should be lumped together?

To answer this, I need to offer more than blatantly unprofessional words. I need to offer scientifically-sound proof.

Hopefully, the following descriptions will suffice.

Again, please forgive any curse words that I may blurt onto the page.

Can We Scientifically Define "Autism?"

No endeavor can claim to be proper science without first defining its terms. In the old science, dictionary-style lists of qualities can suffice. Often, these lists so overlap that it becomes logically impossible to differentiate between similar things. Sadly, no diagnostic manual has even managed to do this well.

To wit, no diagnostic manual has defined any of its terms. Rather, each diagnosis consists of a simple list of undefined words. These words are then assumed to be understood by all trained professionals. But as I've already shown you, were you to ask 100 professionals what the symptoms of depression are, most would wrongly mention, "sadness."

Sadness is a kind of perceived change. Depression is the lack of perceived change.

Contrast this with the science which underpins this book—"Constellated Science." My 2016 book, "The Science of Discovery," formally explains—in depth—what it is and why it's different. Specifically, in Constellated Science, terms must be defined using pairs of complementary opposites. Why? Because to truly know the nature of a thing, we must know "what this thing is **and** what it is not"; it's ***sine qua non***. By defining our terms this way, we discover the actual nature of a thing, specifically, it's relationships to other, similar things. These relationships—how similar things connect and interact—are what a good science looks to discover. This is especially true for complex things like human nature. Take KA and AS. This simple drawing does exactly this. KA is defined as "significant internal *physical* distractions." AS is defined as "significant internal *mental* distractions."

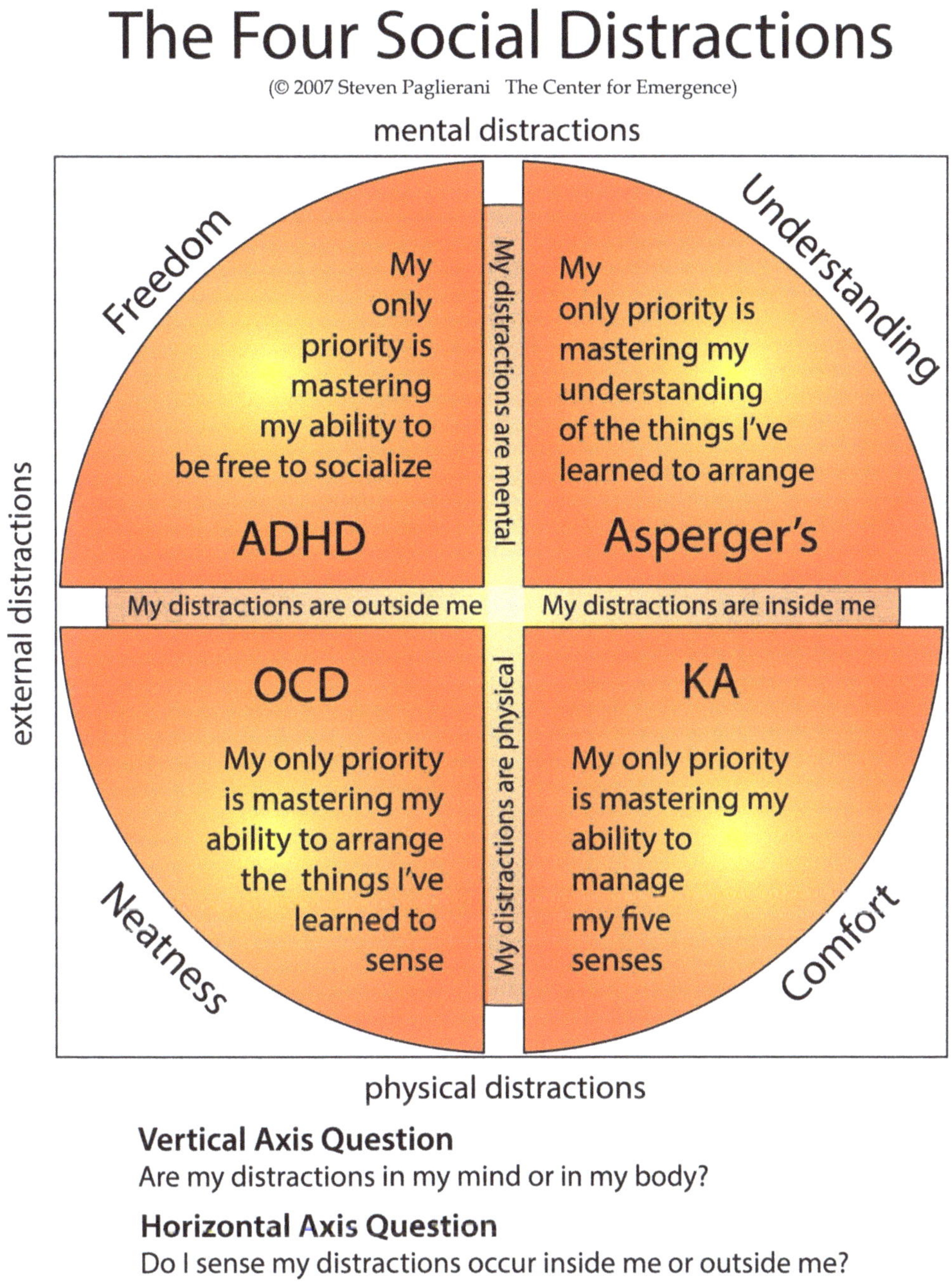

So can Leo Kanner's Autism (significant internal *physical* distractions) and Hans Asperger's Autism (significant internal *mental* distractions) be the same thing? No more than a single person can have both AS (significant internal mental distractions) and ADD (significant external mental distractions). But because the word "distraction" is used in the term, ADD, I've seen many people get both diagnoses. Assholes. Who writes these manuals anyway? Assholes. That's who.

What Does the Word "Autism" Actually Refer To?

Something I now feel the need to address is why I am using the word "autism." Shouldn't I eschew this word in favor of the formal titles of the four Minority Personalities? I'm using this word here because this was the way I originally referenced these four personalities. Over time, "The Four Autism's" became "The Four Distractions," which then became "The Four Minority Personalities."

I'll leave the story of how these changes came to happen for another time. Suffice to say, I was quite surprised when I realized how these four things are the same and how they are different. Their sameness? It all goes back to the word, "autism," clearly a baggage-ridden, ill-defined term. In a moment, I'll offer an excerpt from an article I wrote back then, when I was still using the word "autism."

Know that when I wrote that article, I was just finishing the first version of my personality theory. So when I read this article today, I, like many writers, feel compelled to go back and update it. The thing is, while I voice my ideas, including some terms, differently today, the ideas themselves remain unchanged—especially the idea that treating people on the Autism Spectrum as "diagnosably broken" is just plain ignorant, cruel, and wrong.

In truth, people on the spectrum are folks who have extreme versions of one of the four ways we socially master life—[1] we master our sensations, [2] we master the ability to sense things, [3] we master the ability to assign meanings to the things we sense, and [4] we master the ability to free ourselves from the ongoing need to master these three skills. Moreover, this idea—that folks with a Minority Personality have an extreme focus on only one of these four social skills—remains true no matter what causes people to be like this and no matter what we call it.

This means the best way to see people on the spectrum is as folks with Minority Personalities. And the best way to integrate them into society is for all of us to learn how we are the same and how we are different. Sadly, as long as we continue to define "normal" as the characteristics of the statistically largest group, we'll continue to see people on the spectrum as broken and in need of being taught to act more like normal people. This is truly ironic. By forcing them to imitate some fake normal—instead of being themselves—we cause much of their social oddness. In truth, this is just about the cruelest thing you could ever do to a person—on or off the spectrum. Tell a person they can never be themselves. Rather, they must master the ability to pretend to be like "normal people." And yes, folks on the spectrum do not easily fit into the molds society casts for us all. But all of these folks, including me, are human beings first. Only then do we become a person on "the spectrum."

Does this sound more compassionate than the usual medical drivel? Are you chomping at the bit to tell me how misguided I am? Either way, please remember my point. The most caring thing you can ever do for someone you love is to take the time to get to know them. So if you love someone on the spectrum, care enough to look past the labels. Then get to know this person as the beautiful being he or she was born to be. Hopefully, my article will point you in that direction.

(excerpted from an article I originally posted in 2004, on theEmergenceSite.com)

Autism, OCD, Asperger's, and ADD as Normal Responses to Life

Let me say this right up front: My skill at presenting the theory you'll find here is still in the early stages. Even so, what I'm about to tell you is the result of more than nine years of observations and explorations, involving many hundreds of people. What am I about to tell you? That Autism, OCD / OCPD, Asperger's Syndrome, and ADD are the same condition contracted at different ages; more so, that the age of onset determines what will distract the person. Equally important, because these ideas come from the theories and practice of a personality theorist (me), they reveal an even deeper truth. This truth is that all symptoms, including these four groups of clustered distractions, are ***normal life responses experienced at abnormal times and in abnormal ways.***

Meaning what? That all symptoms are a compulsive repetition of what was once a normal, natural response to life.

This means symptoms are like the sound of a stuck phonograph record which "compulsively" replays a small section of what may in fact be beautiful music. Even the most beautiful music endlessly replayed will feel terribly annoying or worse. All symptoms, then, including the symptoms of these four conditions, are simply a "compulsive" replaying of what was once a normal human response to life.

Now let's take this idea a step further. Given you can blamelessly explore peoples' symptoms (including the symptoms of these four conditions), what will you find? You'll find that all symptoms reveal, not the source of a condition, but rather the onset of the condition; not the "cause" of an illness, but rather the literal life stage on which a particular symptom, or cluster of symptoms, was once a normal, natural, healthy response to the person's life events. What do you gain by looking at symptoms in this light? For one thing, better focused interventions. For another, less suffering during the healing process. For another, more natural compassion and blamelessness.

Here, then, are the two ideas I will explore in this article: [1] the connections between the four conditions I've previously named: the connections between Autism, OCD / OCPD, Asperger's Syndrome and ADD, and [2] that using symptoms to find the literal life stage and onset of illness can be a far more potent, compassionate, and potentially healing approach than using symptoms to project and infer a pathological cause.

What is Autism?

What is "autism?

According to current diagnostic manuals, autism is "a social impairment wherein a person suffers from a pervasive category of socially disconnecting distractions."

The principle symptom?

A profound inability to connect to socially normal people.

The principle behavior? Compulsively focusing on things other than personal relationships at the expense of personal relationships.

Using this definition then, all four of the conditions I've listed here can be considered a variety of autism.

Is this link—a common definition—enough though? Not really. However, this common definition does function as a good starting point for understanding these four conditions. Before offering specifics, allow me, first, to comment on the word "autism" itself—many people, when they hear the word autism, cringe. Why? Because for them, the word "autism" carries a deeply shaming charge.

Originally, the word "autism" referred to Leo Kanner's Autism—the isolated, rocking, wordless, removed, head-banging autism. So if you feel angry at me for suggesting that your recently-diagnosed-with-ADD, little boy or girl has a form of autism, I can understand. As I said, the word has a lot of baggage, so much so that most people cannot even tolerate the thought that anyone they love has "autism."

Why even use this word then? First, because it is still the best way to describe to medical people what folks with these four conditions have in common. These folks all suffer from a significant social impairment, a personality deficit which causes them to repeatedly fail to make or maintain normal social connections to others.

Certainly the word "autism" conveys this impairment well.

Second, because the aversion people feel to this word so mirrors the aversion people feel to those who have these conditions. In a sense, the word "autism" conveys much of the meaning of this condition, even to those who don't understand it.

Third, because facing this aversion head-on with blamelessness, honesty, and compassion is the only way we will even learn to offer genuinely helpful assistance to those with autism—as well as be able to connect to them as fellow human beings.

Fourth, since we all have some degree of the symptoms present in these four conditions, learning to understand these four conditions can forever change how we understand ourselves and each other. At the same time, it can teach us how to improve the way we live, learn, love, grow, and connect to one another.

Does this sound like something worthwhile?

Does a bear do his stuff in the woods?

We All Suffer From Some Degree of Autism

Am I saying we all suffer from some degree of autism? Yes. I am saying this. Unless, of course, your social skills lie beyond those of human beings. Hopefully, by the time I'm done here, I'll have helped you to see this idea through loving eyes. Why say this though? Why say we all suffer from some degree of autism? Because I believe it is only through seeing the four "autisms" in ourselves that we can ever hope to help the more severely autistic among us. At the same time, doing this will allow us to learn to see our differing learning styles and social abilities as "diversity" rather than disease. (from ***The Autism Spectrum: the Four Ways We Feel Compelled to Master Our World, 2004, https://theEmergenceSite.com***.)

~

For anyone wishing to read the rest of this "novelette-length" article, you'll find it listed in the menu of theEmergenceSite.com. There, along with this article, you'll also find articles documenting the story of how I came to make these discoveries. It also lists articles with better ways to help. The thing is, I have to admit, as I read those words back, I felt pained by how many medical terms I used back then.

I did, however, notice I'd just begun using the term "minority personality" twenty years ago. Not capitalized, let alone well defined. But I was using it just the same. Why mention this? It tells you something important. It tells you nothing, other than a few terms, has had to be revised or deleted. Rather, all this book adds is twenty plus years of scientific support to back up what I originally wrote.

This said, I realize the way I shun most medical language, in a book on diagnosis, must seem strange to some of you. Then again, if you've managed to read this far, I'm sure you realize, I am indeed one rather strange man. Right now I'm more concerned with whether any of this is making sense to you. And are you beginning to see what makes Majority and Minority Personalities different? The sameness?

- Both types of personalities share the same set of five measurable qualities.
- The kinds of outcomes for three of these measures are identical in both groups.
- Except for how the funnels are shaped, the kinds of outcomes for the other two are identical as well.

The only oppositeness? How the shapes of these two measures cause certain social qualities to get distributed then filtered out.

In people with Majority Personalities, the distributions in the funnels change gradually, predictably, and socially. Less gets filtered out. So these folks have more information with which to manage their lives.

In people with Minority Personalities, one quality in their Social Priorities and one in their Decision Trees eclipses the other three kinds of urges. And lacking this social data, most people with Majority Personalities assume these folks just don't try hard enough, or are too broken to care.

Need further proof?

Speak to some of the professionals I've trained. Better yet, speak to the people whose lives they and I have changed. Even better, do your own research into why these two things are not the same—beginning with reading for yourself what the original authors of these two autisms wrote. If you do, know it's wise to avoid those over-cooked-string-bean descriptions in college texts. Rather, please read Leo Kanner and Hans Asperger in their own words. I'm confident even a cursory read of their work will show, these two autisms cannot possibly be the same thing. As the Map of the Four Minority Personalities drawing shows,

Leo Kanner's autism focuses mostly on *physical* struggles.

Hans Asperger's autism focuses mostly on *mental* struggles.

The Spectrum of Distraction

KA (group 6)	OCD (group 12)
What distracts me? "too many sensations"	What distracts me? "too many things"
If extreme, I have Kanner's Autism	If extreme, I have OCD / OCPD
Focus of my compulsion? Regulating my sensory input by self imposed repetition (sensory rituals)	**Focus of my compulsion?** Regulating how I sense things by repetitive rearranging (material rituals)
How? Predictable sensory repetitions (e.g. compulsive head banging, rocking, squeeze machine, etc.)	**How?** Predictable object repetitions (compulsive touching and / or sorting of objects)
The Goal: predictable repetition of my sensations avoids discomfort (find the rules for arranging me)	**The Goal:** predictable repetition of how I sense things avoids discomfort (find the rules for arranging things)
Feeling compelled by nature to Organize **my sensations**	Feeling compelled by oneself to Organize **the things I sense** **with** my sensations

birth — age → 6 months — 12 months

birth	"comfort"	6 months	"neatness"	12 months

The Spectrum of Distraction

AS (group 18)	ADD (group 24)
What distracts me? "too many ideas"	What distracts me? "too many rules"
If extreme, I have Asperger's Syndrome	If extreme, I have ADD
Focus of my compulsion? Regulating how I understand ideas by repetitive mental sorting (mental rituals)	**Focus of my compulsion?** Regulating how others make me think or feel (avoidance rituals)
How? Predictable intellectual repetitions (compulsive sorting of and / or learning about ideas)	**How?** Predictable absence of repetitions (compulsive rule breaking, never being forced)
The Goal: predictable repetition of how I arrange ideas avoids discomfort (find the rules for arranging ideas)	**The Goal:** predictable absence of repetition avoids discomfort (avoid rules / never feel forced)
Feeling compelled by oneself to Organize **what I think about** the things I sense with my sensations	Feeling compelled by others to Organize **what others think about** the things I sense with my sensations

12 months — 22 months — 48 months (age →)

"understanding" | **"freedom"**

Personality is Not *Behavior*. It's What Does Not Get Filtered Out.

What you've just read in this chapter is but a first look at the five baselines from which to diagnose. These baselines all stem from an understanding of, and ability to distinguish between, Majority and Minority Personalities. Neither category, in and of itself, indicates a diagnosable condition. Rather, both serve only as necessary starting points from which to diagnose.

Finally, before we move on to the next chapter, I need to offer you a few "big picture" ideas. My hope is that these ideas will further ground what I've just tried to present to you.

One. Human suffering never comes from brokenness. Brokenness is a view from the outside with no real understanding of who the person is inside. Regardless of who and what we appear to be, on the inside, we are all the same. All human suffering comes from the same place. It comes from feeling alone and unseen.

Two. Know this is true even for people with serious mental illnesses. Feeling alone and unseen is what transforms their serious mental illnesses into serious suffering. And the distortions in their external behaviors? They simply have fewer ways to remedy their aloneness. Over time then, this so exceeds their ability to learn better ways that they give up. They then sink into who the medical world claims they are.

Three. How can I claim all prior personality theories are patently lacking in scientific rigor? For the same reasons I see dictionary-style definitions as total bullshit. For one thing, most of these qualities refer to human behavior. So while I admit, human behavior does often reflect the personality of the doer, the reverse is often not true. Behavior often does not reflect a person's true personality.

What then is ***personality***? According to Emergence Personality Theory, it's the result of a person's life experiences, ***after they've traveled through a rather complex set of filters***. These filters are all nonlinear and fractal. So there are an infinite number of ways they affect the person's ability to see life. Moreover, each of them, in some way, reduces a person's ability to see other, better choices.

Now add to this infinite complexity the even more complex possibilities of everyday life. No one can account for how external influences like situation and culture confound any attempts to say behavior is an adequate measure of personality. This difference in how the funnels change shape was what we explored in funnels throughout this chapter. There I contrasted and compared how the Social Priority and Decision Tree funnels of people with a Majority Personality (group 18) differ from people with a Minority Personality (AS).

Again, the differences all come down to how the filtering occurs in these two measures. In Minority Personalities, this filtering is more severe. "Severe" means a harder life. But a harder life often leads to a better life—given a person receives, as I have, the love, care and teaching they deserve.

Diagnosticians can learn to love and care more—and become better teachers.

I hope this book is, in some way, already making this happen for you.

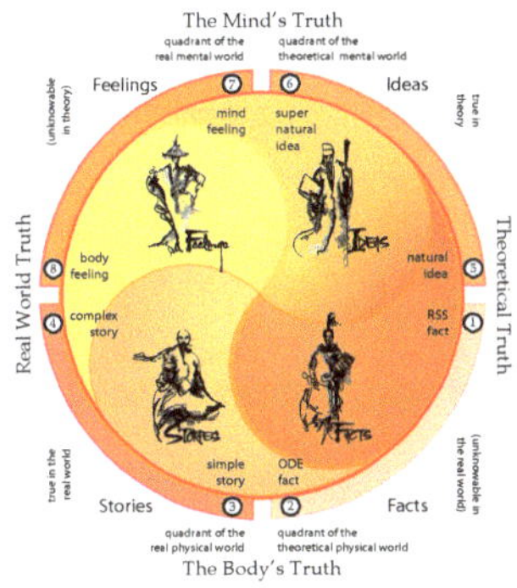

Chapter 4

Classifying "Disorders"
(what can we learn about . . . ?)

Can We Stop Treating People Like They're Broken?

As I begin to write this chapter, I am again feeling overwhelmed. After all, I am just one person. How can I possibly classify an entire volume of disorders. The thing is, I have a good hunch about where I need to focus in this chapter. I need to focus on the word "disorder." My hope is that by doing this, we'll begin to create a template for a more kind, caring diagnostic system.

Before I do that—and being we are at the half-way mark in this book—I want to briefly recap what we've done so far. Specifically, I'm going to divide this second half of the book from the first. I also want to check-in with you to see what has and has not made sense. To do this, I'll be offering you a checklist of those ideas so you can inventory them for yourself.

And if you find you've still got questions?

Then I suggest you go back and review those parts before reading this chapter.

Perhaps you and a colleague can review the difficult parts together.

I, myself, never attempt to learn anything without having partners in the learning process. This includes how I'm writing this book. Each time I finish a draft chapter, I send copies to all those I supervise, asking for their thoughts and questions.

Where will we actually begin this chapter then? With yet another funnel drawing. This time, it will be a drawing of the "Diagnostic Sequence." This funnel is the outline master diagnosticians should follow. Obviously, we have a lot to discuss.

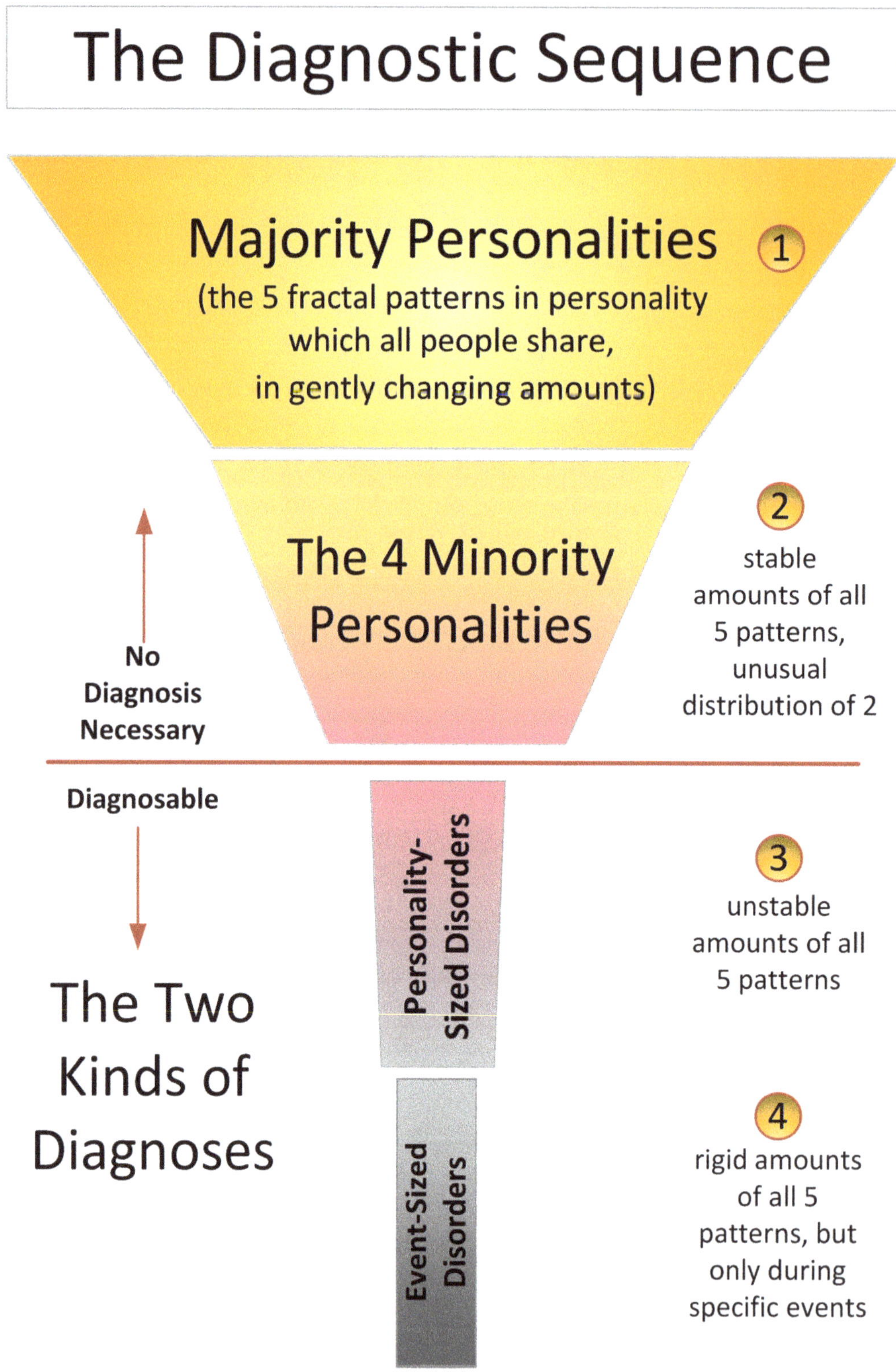
The Diagnostic Sequence
Majority Personalities
1
(the 5 fractal patterns in personality which all people share, in gently changing amounts)
The 4 Minority Personalities
2
stable amounts of all 5 patterns, unusual distribution of 2
No Diagnosis Necessary
Diagnosable
Personality-Sized Disorders
3
unstable amounts of all 5 patterns
Event-Sized Disorders
4
rigid amounts of all 5 patterns, but only during specific events
The Two Kinds of Diagnoses

The Diagnostic Sequence (the Next Three Chapter's Topics)

Obviously, there is much to explain in this drawing. It describes the four steps diagnosticians must take each time they evaluate their patients. Already, even before explaining a single thing—and just based on this drawing, I am introducing a number of significant changes to what all prior diagnosticians have been taught they must do.

The short list?

- All people, diagnosable or not, share some variation of the same five patterns which define human personality. The diagnostician must begin all diagnostic processes by determining at least a provisional sense of the first three of these five patterns. These results will then be used to set the baseline for a provisional diagnosis. However, regardless of how severe the patient's symptoms are, at this point, no diagnosis should be given. To properly diagnose, you must first know "who this person is."
- Next, the diagnostician must refine this provisional baseline, by determining whether the patient has a Majority or Minority Personality. Patients cannot be properly evaluated without first doing this, as this is what determines how you will voice your diagnostic questions. Literally, there are five ways these questions can be voiced. In most cases, they will be voiced in the Majority Personality voice. For now, please set aside any questions you may have about how to do this as I will address this in a future chapter.

No Diagnosis Necessary

Diagnosable

- Having determined a solid provisional diagnostic baseline, data is then gathered to determine whether the patient's symptoms indicate a possible diagnosis or not. Here, the diagnostician must take care to not prematurely assign meanings to any observable symptoms. The goal here is to determine the scope of these symptoms within the person's life. Have there been symptoms for most of the person's life and can these symptoms be seen in all walks of life? If yes, then consider assessing for a Personality-sized Disorder.
- Given there is not solid evidence for a Personality-sized Disorder, assess for one or more Event-sized Disorders. Realize, all people have Event-sized Disorders, including people with Personality-sized Disorders. However, to properly assess for Event-sized Disorders in people with Personality-sized Disorders, the full scope of this disorder must first be clearly defined.

Recall, I introduced you to the basics of Event-sized Disorders in Chapter 2. There we spoke about the relationship between wounds, regression, and transference. Then in Chapter 3, I described the basics of Majority and Minority Personalities.

In this chapter, I plan on introducing you to Personality-sized Disorders. Hopefully, by chapter's end, you'll have internalized the diagnostic "big picture." Even more, I hope this four step sequence will eventually ground and guide all of your diagnostic assessments. Granted, it will take some time, effort, and experience. But as I said in the Reader's Guide, I believe in you. Now let's begin.

There Are Two Kinds of Disorder—One Kind Is *Not* Diagnosable

All people have a personality—a constellation of five nested categories of urges. Together they describe and define our nature. Because these urges pressure us to focus only on certain things, in essence, they render other things invisible to us. What remains visible to us is then what we commonly refer to as, "personality."

Based on how much of each urge remains visible, we are then said to have either a Majority or a Minority Personality. In Majority Personalities, all urges take up some amount of recognizable space. In Minority Personalities, certain urges take up little to no space—they become invisible. Please notice, up to this point, nothing has been considered a diagnosable disorder, this despite the fact that we each live far from perfectly organized lives.

This contradicts what diagnostic manuals have led us to believe—that any significant deviations from a "norm" should be considered diagnosable. In truth, most of our differences are just that—mere differences. What's the main distinction between these ordinary aspects of personality and diagnosable conditions then?

Two things.

One—The speed of the onset of the signs of the disorder—knowably gradual or unpredictably abrupt.

Two—The presence, or lack, of a recognizably ordinary context in which this disorder occurs.

- Disorder which *is not* diagnosable includes all disorder which [1] has a knowably gradual onset and [2] a recognizably ordinary context.
- Disorder which *is* diagnosable includes all disorder which has [1] an abrupt onset and [2] which lacks a recognizable context.
- An already existing diagnosis is not a context.

∞

Now consider how being able to properly diagnose rests entirely on having the ability to differentiate between these two kinds of disorder—normal and diagnosable. Here, the differences all amount to the timing of, and context in which, the disorder occurs. Clearly, no human behaviors occur in anything resembling perfect order. Disorganization in the hair on our heads is the norm when we wake up. Disorganization in the sequences of thoughts in our minds is normal as well.

This reminds me of a referral I got from a couple I saw early in my career. The couple asked me to see their then 15-year-old daughter, but offered a caveat. They told me she had a birth defect, something having to do with her hair. And they made such a big deal of telling me this that on the morning I was to first meet her, I felt extremely anxious.

I so didn't want my reaction to hurt this girl.

At the time I had yet to discover any of what I now know about human nature. So I did what any normal caring human being might have done in that situation. I tried to steel myself against having any kind of negative reactions. Of course, when she came in and sat down, she chose to sit in the chair closest to mine. And having been damned by the parents to a horrible curiosity, I tried to not look—while simultaneously trying to see what it was they had warned me about.

The truth? I couldn't see anything like what they'd mentioned to me. But they'd put so much effort into warning me that I must have seemed like a crazy man to that girl. But finally, after what seemed like an eternity but was actually more like ten minutes, I welled up with tears and said to her, "I'm so sorry I'm acting strange. Your parents told me something about your hair being odd. But I can't see anything at all."

At this point, she too teared up. I've assumed, all these years, that no one had ever cared enough—or been brave enough—to speak to her like a human being. I knew even then that she'd likely suffered from this unfounded characterization all her life. But to this day, I have no idea what the parents found wrong with her, let alone why they sent her to see me.

In the months that followed, I found her to be a sweet, quiet, perfectly normal teenaged girl. Yet somehow, those parents saw the way her hair grew as being pathologically disorganized. Are you feeling confused by what they might have been seeing? Are you having a hard time imagining what it could have been? If so, realize, this is the point for my having told you this story.

To me, most differences between human beings are either similarly hard to see or hard to see why they matter. Conversely, almost all diagnosable disorders are impossibly hard to see. Like the urges in our personalities, the actual disorders will forever remain invisible. In a way then, this is what makes our jobs as diagnosticians challenging.

We must focus entirely on finding acceptable external evidence, which then points to there being invisible, internal diagnosable disorders.

Hopefully, as you begin this process, you will remember to see the human being first. Only then should you begin to look for disorder of any kind. Know this is true even in cases where a patient is so disordered as to be dangerously incoherent. Granted, you must also know how to make this process safe for the both of you.

Sometimes, this can require more than one of you to be present. This said, and despite the way existing diagnostic manuals see all notably disordered behaviors as brokenness, human beings are not broken machines to be fixed. Even the worst narcissist has feelings and a heart. Thus we should never mistake "the need to help while remaining safe" for a need to punish and correct.

Our own humanity as clinicians depends on our doing this.

Diagnosable Disorders Come in Two Sizes—Event & Personality

All human beings have in them an infinitely complex, in theory, countable constellation of Event-sized disorders. Each of these Event-sized disorders originated from the person getting startled during a single event. Here, the word "event" in "Event-sized Disorder," in part, refers to that original event. More specifically though, it refers to a three-to-five second, slice of ***context*** from that event.

The word "event" also refers to what happens to us ***after*** that three-to-five seconds. Each startle programs us—from then on—to respond to this context, by feeling the same pattern of urges we felt just before we got startled. Keep in mind, we not only can get startled during an actual, "out there," life event. We can also get startled by events which occur only in our minds. Either way, from then on—we react to a specific three-to-five second triggering pattern. This triggering pattern is whatever happened in that small slice of the original ***context***. Anytime we experience that small slice of the original ***context***, we involuntarily react to it with the same pattern of urges we felt during the original event. And this idea—***context***, not cause—is the key to understanding and diagnosing Event-sized Disorders.

In these events, our minds record only two things—that small slice of the original context, and the urges we felt in response to it. We do not record how we behaved, nor any of the rest of the context. This is why we can relive this event even in times which in no way resemble the original event. This also explains why we often cannot accurately recall how we've behaved, no matter how hard we try.

We will also never again respond to this context as we once did ***before*** we got startled. Once programmed, we respond to this small slice of context as if we are responding to the entire context of the original event. Realize, what I'm saying here is that afterwards, we respond to that small slice of context, "out of context." Now take a few moments to consider the importance of what I've just said.

This idea is surely in the top three in importance in this entire book.

The idea? That getting startled programs us to involuntarily and automatically pay special attention to a small slice of context. Notably, this three-to-five seconds of context has become "context independent." No matter when we relive it, we react to it the same way. This means, we can relive it in any number of dissimilar events. And when we do, we'll respond to it as if we're reliving the entire wounding event.

The problem here is that we will inevitably relive this three-to-five seconds of context in any number of completely unrelated events. This is why most psychotherapies never properly identify most wounds. Most wounds will never recur within the full, original context. But any event which contains this small slice of context will trigger those urges, even when the rest of the context of an event is nothing like that original event. This is what's happening in the Blood Draw drawing on the next page. Most people, reading the title, will assume the injury involves blood and needles. The timing of the startle tells a different story though. How much of this story made it into the small slice of context? Only section number 5.

The woman bumping his arm and the sound of the glass breaking on the floor.

A Blood Draw Injury

I enter a medical office waiting room. I see seats and I choose one. I get called to the desk, take a pad and fill out the forms. I bring the pad and pen back and sit down.	I get called to the desk and am given a plastic vial, then told to go give a urine sample. I return the vial to the person at the desk, then get told to go to the blood draw station.	I sit in the blood draw chair and a young woman in a white gown comes in. She has brown hair and eyes, and says, "Good morning."	The young woman rolls up my left sleeve, then puts a tan rubber tourniquet on my arm. I hear her say, "Make a fist."	She then inserts a needle into my arm. I'm fine. But then she bumps the vial of blood, knocking it onto the floor. As it hits the floor, I hear the glass breaking and get startled.	She blankly looks at the floor, says "I'm so sorry," then begins to clean up. She then finishes with me and again says, "I'm so sorry." I feel blank inside, then get up and leave.	I get up, walk down a hall, then leave and go to my car. I feel blank inside, then drive away.
1	2	3	4	5	6	7

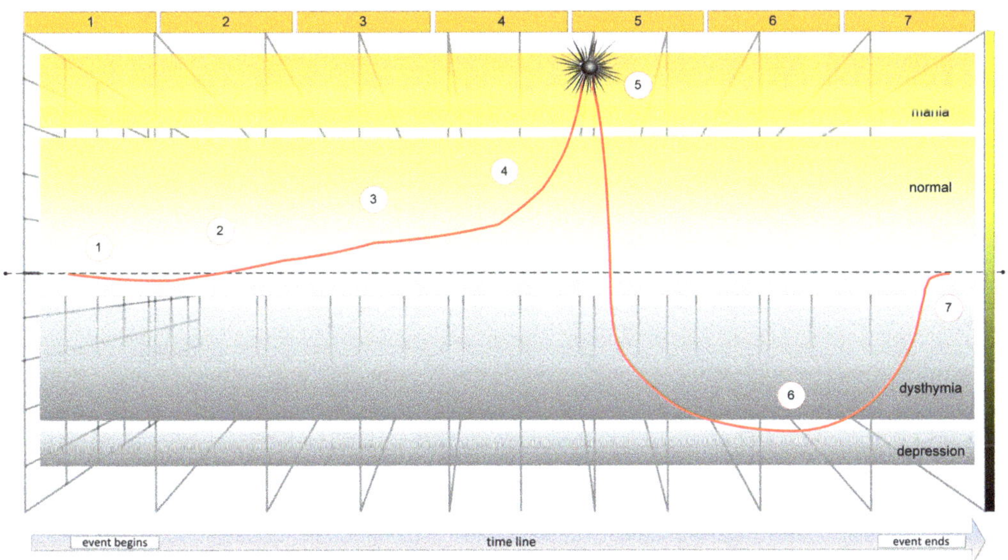

What did not make it into the triggering slice of context?

Every detail after the startle. Also, every detail before the startle, except for what happened in the three to five seconds right before it. This includes feeling the needle go in. Notably here, the man says, "I'm fine." It also includes the woman saying "sorry" several times. None of that made it into the triggering slice.

How many dissimilar events could this slice of context affect? Can you guess?

Any event in which a woman ***bumped*** his left arm would be one part of the slice of context. The ***sound*** of the glass vial hitting the floor and breaking would be another. More significantly though, if someone bumped his left arm then dropped something, he would never hear them say, "sorry." So no matter how many times they apologized for bumping into him, he would feel like they didn't care.

How many situations could include him getting bumped where someone dropped something, then said a "sorry" he didn't hear?

I can't begin to imagine how many situations this could effect. And each time this happened, he'd relive the urges he felt when he was in that blood-draw chair, including what he'd felt while he had a needle in his arm. Other than those urges though, that three-to-five second slice of context would include very few things. Being bumped on his left arm while he was seated would be one. Hearing the sound of something falling, and then the sound of breaking glass on the floor would be another.

What it would not include—and indeed, what he would likely be unable to picture—would be things like hearing someone say "sorry" for what had just happened. Why? Because without exception, startles cause people's minds to suddenly go blank. This means, anything which happened right after the startle would have occurred while his mind was offline. Thus he would never experience these things.

Now consider what would happen to this man if his therapist asked him what happened? He'd likely be able to recall much of the event before the startle—slices 1 through 4. He'd also likely be able to recall leaving the building (slice 7). But if the blood got on his pants in slice 6, would he know how this happened? Logically he might? But would he be able to picture this happening? Probably not.

Primary Causes of the "Disorder" in Event-Sized Disorders

There are two things I'd like to point out yet again.

Both are primary causes of the disorder in these Event-sized Disorders.

The first involves the urges people feel when they relive one of these events.

The second involves these peoples' abilities to process these events.

The first? When people get triggered, they relive the same kinds of urges they experienced in the ***original*** event—***and nothing else***. And yes, the intensity of these urges may and often does progressively increase over time. But the kinds of urges themselves remain the same.

The second? The idea that when people relive these urges, their understanding of what's happening to them remains the same as well. If the person is now 26, but they were age 6 in the original event—they will temporarily lose access to any and all knowledge and abilities they acquired after age 6.

Realize, both of these things occur because of the regression/transference feedback loops we looked at in Chapter 2. No one, no matter how healthy, can escape this fate. This contradicts what many therapists claim—that having better logic, and being taught better ways to behave, can prevent this. In truth, nothing can prevent the onset of regressions, even in healed wounds.

Taken together, these two things explain why people can "know better," yet still behave as if they do not. They also explain why even otherwise healthy adults posit all manner of chaotic and wrongheaded explanations for what is happening to them, each time they relive one of these events. Realize, these well-meant but wrongheaded explanations account for much of the resulting disorder. But as I said, even better explanations cannot prevent regressions.

Secondary Causes of the "Disorder" in Event-Sized Disorders

What do I mean by "secondary causes?"

Specifically, the way people's expectations exacerbate this disorder even more.

Over time, wounded people come to see these bad outcomes as inevitable. Moreover, because no conventional therapy addresses, let alone knows to look for, the actual source of this disorder—those three-to-five second triggers—both therapists and patients alike turn to logic to try to make sense of these events.

Admittedly, better logic can tell you what better behaviors would look like. But since no human being has unlimited will power, these efforts to behave like proper adults inevitably fail. And yes, there are times where these will-powered efforts can prevent harm. But ultimately, the therapy must either locate those three-to-five second triggers and deal with them—or these efforts will continue to fail.

As for the expectations which cause this disorder to worsen, to be blunt, they're as complicated as a hurricane. The main problem? Even when these events turn out well, people still feel like they have turned out badly. How is this possible? Because over time, people's expectations of where and when the pain will occur continue to broaden and generalize. Eventually then, these expectations become so embedded in them that even when nothing hurtful happens, they still feel the hurt.

Does this make sense to you? These expectations of pain ARE painful. And over time, repeatedly feeling this pain just makes these expectations worsen. Ironically, much of this worsening comes from failures experienced in conventional therapies. And these failures are unavoidable, as no amount of logic, caring talk therapy, or newfound will power can alter these urges or expectations.

Then there's what happens to people each time one of those three-to-five second triggers sets off a regression transference feedback loop. These loops so distort and exaggerate people's symptoms that from their point of view, the wound itself seems to keep getting worse. This makes identifying the original wounding events logically impossible. The pain of the reliving is many times worse than the pain of the original event. And with each failed effort, the mental and physical disorder which surrounds these relived events gets worse as well.

Realize, in large part, it's the primary disorder that fuels these expectations. From the wounded person's perspective, the pain always does occur. In large part, this happens because being startled always causes the mind to suddenly go blank.

So even when the outcomes of these events improve, this blankness keeps people from seeing these improvements.

Add to this that because these triggers are but a small slice of context taken out of context, they eventually affect any number of completely unrelated areas of life. This is why even the most seemingly insignificant wound can wreak havoc on people's ability to make sense of why they act so poorly in those parts of their lives. And because most therapies focus on fixing this dysfunction (the disorder) rather than on healing it, in the end, people just continue to accumulate failures.

Now consider how using logic affects our ability to find the wounds themselves. All logic generalizes a series of real world events into ideas. There are no exceptions. This means the more logic you use, the more you generalize the problems beyond the original scope of the event. Over time, these broad mental generalizations then poison many completely unrelated events—things we would normally not get triggered by as we have no wounds there.

For example, I've previously mentioned that before I was a therapist, I worked in computer technology.

I hated working for that company and several times tried to apply for computer jobs in other companies.

After several job interviews, all of which failed, I came to believe these failures were in me—that I just must be horrible at doing interviews.

In one case, I interviewed for a job—and when they called me back to take a computer skills exam, I felt encouraged. I'd easily passed this test and assumed I'd get the job. But then, two weeks passed and they hadn't called me back. So I called them to see if they'd hired someone else. Realize, I made this call at a time before cell phones were common. So I'd called on my lunch break, from a phone booth.

In that call, I asked if they'd given the job to someone. They said they had.

Impulsively and completely out of character for me, I then asked why I hadn't gotten the job. I then heard something which made me feel sure I'd been right about the problem being me.

The HR person I was speaking to told me, "You aren't fit to work with people."

Those were his exact words.

I can picture myself outside that phone booth, in a suit, standing there sobbing. Strangely, it was this failure which led to me applying for work as a counselor. I'd never before considered this career change and had no idea if I'd like doing it. Within a little over a month though, I'd received two job offers.

Both jobs involved working as a counselor for teens. One job was in a residential, 18-month program for troubled teens. As I write these words, I can picture the boy who had been tasked with showing me around.

To this day, I feel I missed out on something I would have loved there.

The other position was as the family therapist in an inpatient rehab for addicted teens. Keep in mind, I'd never worked as a counselor before. Ever. Nor did I have a degree or any sort of training. Yet somehow, I got that job.

Strangely, I was later told by the woman who hired me that this job normally required a master's degree and ten years experience. Back then, due to my failures, my self-worth was lower than whale shit. So most of what she told me that day didn't get in. With one exception. She told me in that same conversation—something I couldn't write off even back then.

She told me that when I interviewed, that there had been no job opening.

She then added, they'd created that job for me.

Why?

Because, she said, I had interviewed so well.

How Do Personality-sized Disorders Differ?

Finally we come to the other major category of disorders, the ones I'm calling, "personality-sized." How do these disorders differ from Event-sized Disorders?

For one thing, unlike Event-sized Disorders—which result from being startled, Personality-sized Disorders have nothing to do with getting startled. Nothing at all.

This explains why the disorder caused by Personality-sized Disorders isn't limited to a specific kind of event.

In effect, this disorder is literally "personality sized." This means it can and does occur in any and all areas of the person's life. So any and all life events can, and often will, be affected by this disorder in unpredictable ways and times.

The result?

This person's life events will never have a predictable, stable, reliable *context*.

For these people, the *context* for everything in their life IS this disorder.

What does this mean?

Depending on the specific condition, the meaning will vary. We'll begin to address this question in a moment. But to put it bluntly, again, it's complicated.

What can help is to keep coming back to the following statement which describes the principle difference between these two classes of disorders.

Please review this statement whenever you feel confused about how these two classes of disorders differ. After all, the amount of words you've already had to endure in this chapter has been tedious, I'm sure. With few pictures to guide you, I know understanding what I've said has to have been hard.

The statement which can help? Just this.

The principle difference between these two categories of disorders is the degree to which they cause disorder in human relationships.

Event-sized Disorders create ***time-limited***, ***event-based disorder*** and only in situations where people relive the small-slice of context from a startling event. Moreover, this kind of disorder can and often does occur, even in otherwise healthy people's lives—where the word, "healthy," means they can, for the most part, create and sustain well-organized relationships.

With Personality-sized Disorders, however, ***there are no knowable limits to the disorder they create in relationships.***

Neither time, nor place, nor relationship, are in any way limiting factors. In truth, the disorder in Personality-sized Disorders is so unpredictable that even with their best efforts, these folks cannot sustain even marginally healthy relationships.

Not ever.

Again, realize, I'm using the word "healthy" here as a reference to the ability to create and sustain reasonably well-organized relationships.

Notably, even "reasonably well-organized relationships" can at times appear to be seriously disorganized. Some would even fall into a category most diagnosticians and therapists would label "abusive." Realize, all I'm saying here is that these reasonably well-organized, abusive relationships do not fall into the Personality-sized Disorders category.

Why not?

Mainly, for just one reason.

These relationships are well-organized.

Now realize how the presence of this degree of organization tells us something important about how these two classes of disorders differ. It means the disorder present in well-organized, abusive relationships is not due to one or both people having Personality-sized Disorders. Rather, this abuse results from the presence of a special class of Event-sized Disorders. Here, an example would be domestic abuse cases wherein spouses and or children are being seriously mistreated.

Any therapist or diagnostician who has worked with people in this category can attest to there being well-organized patterns of abuse. More important, these well-organized patterns of abuse are always followed by well-organized patterns of healthy behaviors. This sequence then continues until the next incident involving the well-organized patterns of abuse, which is then followed by the next period of well-organized healthy behaviors.

Is this idea sinking in yet?

Admittedly, we've a lot to discuss.

This includes me explaining how I could possibly say these abusive relationships contain periods of health.

Indeed, most diagnosticians and clinicians will likely balk at what I've just said.

If this is you, I certainly can understand.

The thing to keep in mind here however is how I am defining the word, "disorder."

"Disorder" is "a clinically significant lack of organization in either specific events or in an entire personality."

In other words, disorder is either "event-sized" or "personality-sized."

The disorder in domestic violence cases is event-sized.

It gets triggered by, and occurs, only in specific events.

Granted, clinically, these cases are always heartbreaking, as they're among the most difficult to treat. I've personally tried—and failed—to make a difference in a number of these cases. I've also succeeded in a small number of these cases as well. This said, I never assume success or even expect to succeed.

Why?

Because as I've just said, the Event-sized Disorder present in these relationships is a special kind. This is what we'll look at next.

The Two Kinds of Event-sized Disorders: Simple and Complex

Simple Event-sized Disorders exist within, and are limited to, an individual person. Here, when this person gets triggered, any other people present do not get triggered. And yes, obviously, these other people do get affected, often in painful ways. At the same time, they can also clearly see, the disorder is originating in the triggered person, and not in themselves.

Complex Event-sized Disorders, on the other hand, exist within and between two or more people. Here, both people have an Event-sized Disorder and their triggers exactly complement those in the other person. This kind of complexity is always present in cases of domestic violence where neither person has a Personality-sized Disorder. Thus this category does not apply to—and is literally too difficult to diagnose—in cases which involve Personality-sized Disorders.

Why?

Because the context of Personality-sized Disorders is personality-sized. Thus the onset of any violence is never limited to specific kinds of events.

Realize, this exclusion includes cases where one or both people have a chronically active Substance Use Disorder. You cannot reliably diagnose a Complex Event-sized Disorder in these cases. After all, you wouldn't try to understand, let alone try to predict, tomorrow's weather during a hurricane. And the craziness present in cases involving chronically-active Substance Use Disorders is definitely hurricane-sized.

Nothing in these people's relationships is safely away from the shitstorm.

The point?

Before considering a Complex Event-sized Disorder, diagnosticians must first rule out the presence of a Personality-sized Disorder.

Fortunately, doing this is easier than it at first may appear.

The lives of people with Complex Event-sized Disorders always include—and intertwine with—broad swaths of life which are otherwise well-organized.

Here, the presence of this well-organized "order" is sufficient to rule out a Personality-sized Disorder.

Please keep this diagnostic measure in mind as we begin our look at the kinds of Personality-sized Disorders. And for those who may have previously noticed the many instances of things coming in fours in earlier chapters, it won't surprise you to know that overall, there are four kinds of diagnosable disorders.

Two of them are event-sized, the two kinds I just mentioned. And two of them are personality-sized.

This latter pair is what we are about to look at next.

There Are Two Kinds of Personality-sized Disorders

The first thing to know—and something to keep in mind here—is that all Personality-sized Disorders are ***permanent.***

For reasons I will enumerate as we go forward, ***they cannot be healed.***

This is not to say people with these disorders cannot learn to better manage their lives. With proper help, many can and often do.

The thing is, in this book, I only use the word "healing" to refer to "permanent, positive changes made to Event-sized Disorders." These changes permanently alter the paths that regression-transference feedback loops take. By doing this, "healing" restores the wounded person's visual access to the parts of life which being startled previously blocked from view. This restored visual ability then leads to people developing better organized, less disordered lives—including in, but not limited to, these particular kinds of life events.

What about cases where a person with a Personality-sized Disorder markedly improves? Don't these improvements point to something having been healed as well?

In many cases, yes, something can have been healed. But these observed improvements cannot, and should not, be attributed to them having healed anything in their Personality-sized Disorder. Rather these changes should be attributed to them having healed one or more Event-sized Disorders.

Even here, helping people with Personality-sized Disorders to heal Event-sized Disorders can be incredibly difficult. In most cases, treatment goals should take this into account. This said, in rare cases, healing can happen, given the therapeutic relationship is sufficiently developed. But few therapists can tolerate this level of disorder in their patient/therapist relationships.

This brings us to the idea that there are actually two kinds of Personality-sized Disorders.

The main difference between them?

The degree to which a ***sustainable***, healthy order can be restored in relationships.

In the first class of Personality-sized Disorders, this cannot occur, not ever.

In the second class, with sufficient help, this can happen.

Obviously, we have a lot to discuss.

The Two Kinds of Personality-sized Disorders: Fixed and Transitional

Let's begin with what they both have in common.

Both types of Personality-sized Disorders result from ***chronically*** painful experiences during the first year of life.

Please pay particular attention to the word "chronically." As used here, it means these disorders do not result from being startled. A startle is acute.

"No startle" means none of these disorders are event-sized. Rather they always involve, and result from, extended periods of neglect or abuse. Moreover, these periods of neglect or abuse always occur during specific, measurable, developmental periods—and these periods always occur during the first year of life.

Diagnostically, the specifics of these developmental periods then form the basis for the entire diagnostic differential. This means, all diagnosticians must be well-versed in first-year-of-life, developmental sequences. In particular, they must know the way each step in this sequence affects the next. Moreover, since all diagnosis must begin with ruling out Personality-sized Disorders, all diagnosticians—even those who rarely if ever work with people with Personality-sized Disorders, must be highly skilled in identifying deficits in these specific developmental steps.

Know we will look at this process in some detail in the next chapter, when we explore the evidence-gathering process. For now, consider how using specific, early childhood features of personality could and should form the basis for diagnosing any and all Personality-sized Disorders.

My evidence? Consider for a moment the difference between a diagnostic differential based mainly on the existence of symptoms, versus one based on identifying specific developmental deficits. The same symptoms can easily occur in very different people—as well as in any and all types of life situations.

In truth, many of the flaws in existing diagnostic manuals are rooted in symptoms alone being used to tell different diagnoses apart. This flaw is particularly egregious when diagnosticians attempt to rule out personality disorders. The types of symptoms these folks present with can occur in almost all human beings. Even the severity can be similar, given a person experiences sufficient trauma.

The same can be said for using behavior alone as a diagnostic gauge. All of us can act crazy at times. We all have Event-sized Disorders, each of which can lead to displays of context-limited doses of behavioral insanities. In truth, even once-perfectly normal developmental behaviors can be seen as pathological when they occur in adults. Where is the line between a normal adult who is regressing to an earlier developmental stage and an adult who is in need of more serious help? Without referencing personality and child-development, there is no scientific line.

How is a differential based on the presence and absence of clearly defined developmental deficits different from one based entirely on symptoms and behavior? This is like asking how a McDonald's burger differs from world-class restaurant filet mignon. Only by basing diagnosis on personality and child development can we hope to define both the origins of, and the measurable evidence for, the existence of a diagnosis. Equally important, only when we have a proper, science-based diagnosis can we then hope to develop a proper treatment protocol.

Realize, nowhere does this matter more than when trying to discern the difference between a Fixed versus a Transitional Personality-sized Disorder. Know that in the next chapter, we'll contrast and compare examples of the underlying differences between Fixed and Transitional Personality-sized Disorders. Here, we'll explore an example of the Fixed type—the origin of, and prognosis for, Borderline Personality Disorders. We'll then contrast and compare this origin and prognosis to that of a Transitional example, one which has frequently been mistaken for a Fixed disorder—the origin of and prognosis for Substance Use Disorders.

Realize, the word "transitional," as used here, holds the key to understanding what makes these two classes of disorders differ. People with Fixed Personality-sized Disorders cannot sustain well-organized, healthy relationships—not even just functionally. People with Transitional Personality-sized Disorders, however, can ***functionally*** transition from having a Personality-sized Disorder to living as if they do not have one. In effect, they can come to sustain well-organized, healthy relationships just as well as people who do not have a Personality-sized disorder.

Now take a moment to think about what I've just said.

When this happens, and it doesn't always happen, they, in almost every way, function as if they no longer have a Personality-sized Disorder. And for all intents and purposes, this is true. The thing is, even in people with Transitional Personality-sized Disorders, the disorder itself never actually goes away. Rather, it lingers in the background. And given the person experiences a sufficiently painful event, it can resurface at any time.

This pattern will be easily recognizable to anyone who is personally or professionally familiar with Substance Use Disorders. In these cases, being in an extended period of recovery can restore much of a person's normal functioning. The thing is, this restored functioning does not and cannot guarantee a relapse will never occur. Conversely, being in an extended period of relapse does not preclude the person's return once again to a healthy life.

The Two Kinds of Bipolar Information (affective vs schizophrenic)

Back in Chapter 1, we briefly looked at the Single Moment Square (Information times Meaning). I've placed a variation of this drawing on the next page. This square contains a number of single moment plots which represent the kinds of experiences people with Bipolar or Schizophrenia diagnoses experience. And were you to connect the dots within each of these two vertical stripes, you'd find these two diagnoses vary only based on the placement of those two lines.

Does this make sense yet? It should not. I'm making a big claim here.

I'm claiming that a Bipolar diagnosis and a Schizophrenia diagnosis differ only in the kinds of Information present in the person—and not in the way the Meanings of events change over Time. More specifically, I'm claiming both diagnoses are actually bipolar diagnoses, and that both flip between a manic phase and a depressed phase—moreover, that there are two kinds of Mania and two kinds of Depression.

Have I just confused you again? If so, I can understand. People with these two diagnoses can present with very dissimilar symptoms. Recall though that all truly scientific definitions must be based on at least one pair of perfect opposites. Bipolar and Schizophrenia, as defined in this book, are two variations of just such a pair.

Now to see why I'm saying this, look closely at the arrangements of dots in this drawing's two vertical stripes. Notice there are no Information dots between these two stripes. Now notice how each stripe has no Information dots between the upper and lower portions of each of these stripes. This distribution is what creates

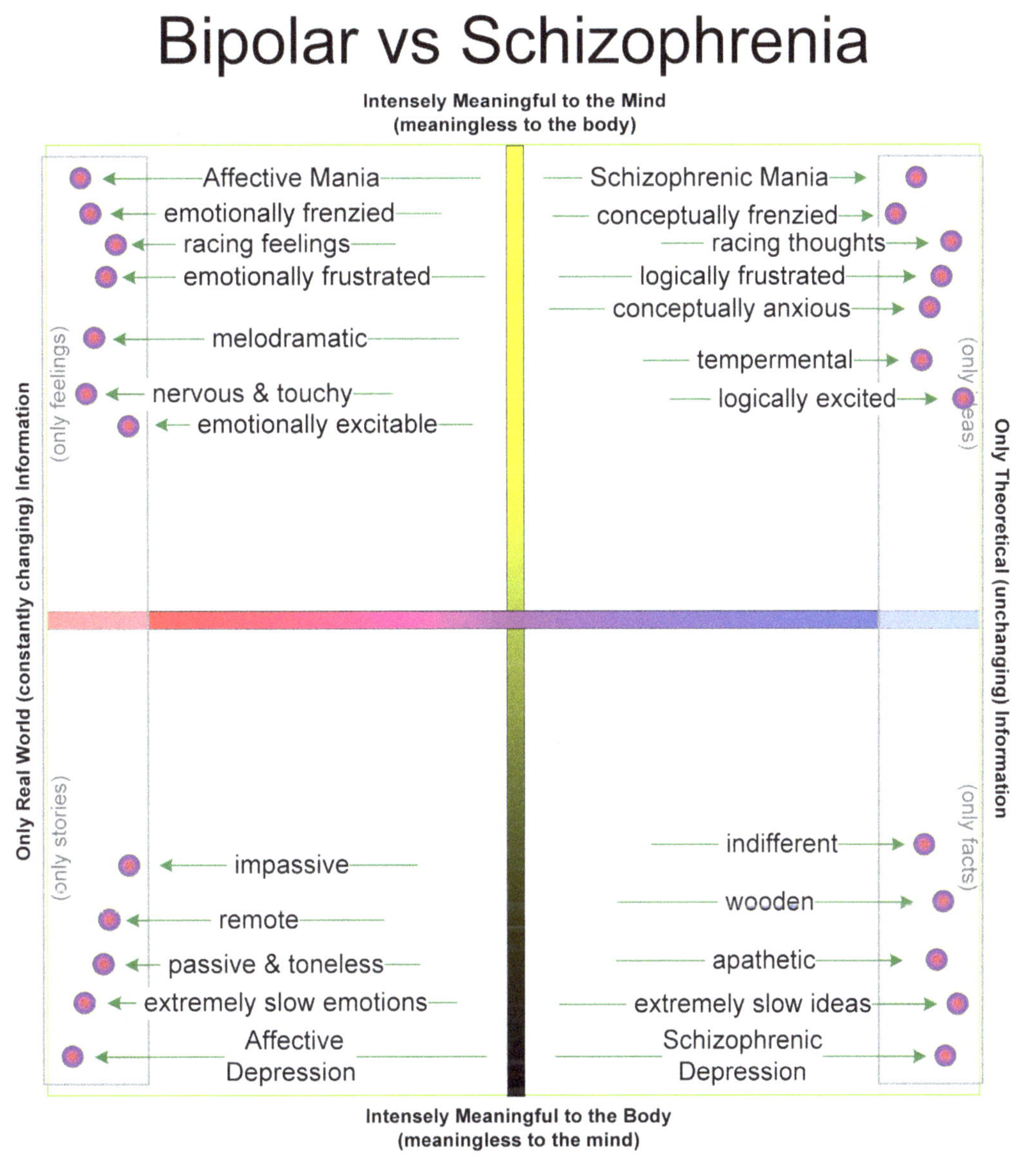

the basis for calling these conditions, "bipolar." In effect, these patterns of dots are distributed into two vertical, polarized stripes of bipolar information—the dots in the two gray zones. And within each gray zone, this Information is limited to two of the four corners of this Single Moment Square.

Keep in mind, together, these dots represent the limits to the kinds of Information people with these two Personality-sized Disorders can experience. What's missing—the other kinds of Information—is what creates the Personality-sized Disorder. Take a moment to let this sink in. It's a good portion of what is necessary to create a science-based diagnostic system. Obviously, we have a lot to discuss. Fortunately, we'll have drawings containing shaped-lines to help us.

The Front View of the Cube

(how Meaning changes over Time)

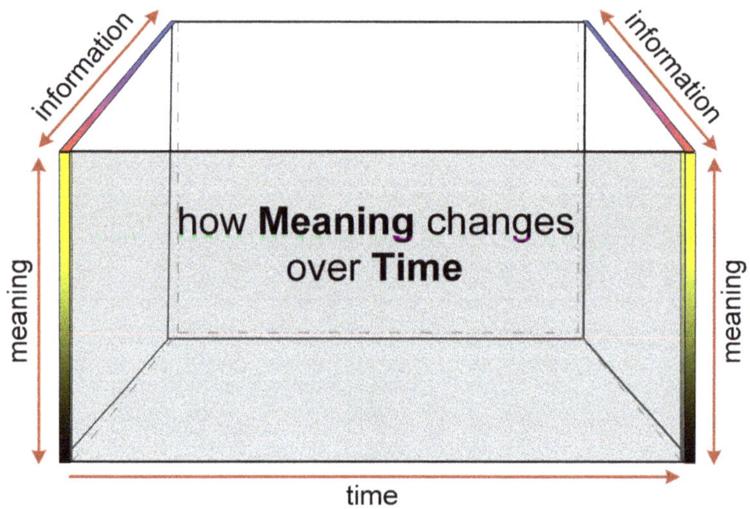

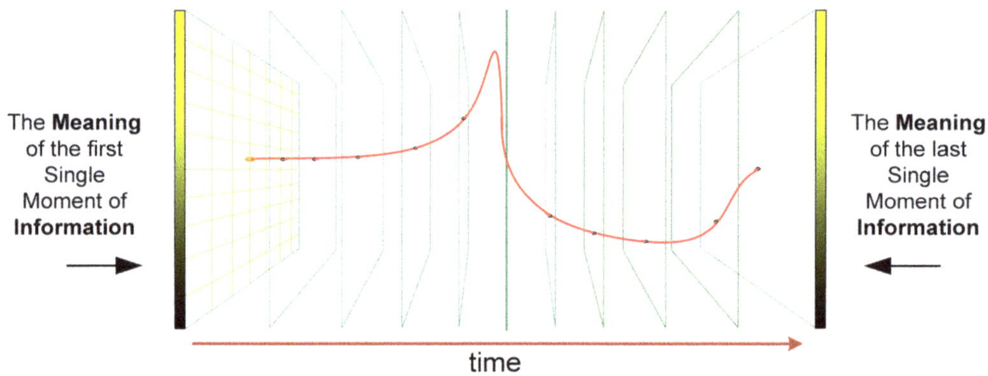

Meaning Over Time Line

(as viewed from the **front** of the cube)

Picturing the Diagnostic Lines in Three-Dimensional Space

By now, the line in this drawing should be somewhat familiar. It's the Meaning-over-Time line which people experience when they get wounded. This line plots how the Meaning of these painful events changes *within the event,* over Time. And the shape of this line is fractal, meaning, we can learn to recognize it similarly to how we learn to recognize a candle flame. Think about it. Candle flames change constantly, minute to minute. They also never change the same way twice. Yet despite these constantly evolving visual changes, young children can effortlessly learn to recognize them as candle flames. And know this for life. These lines are the same.

The Top View of the Cube

(how Information changes over Time)

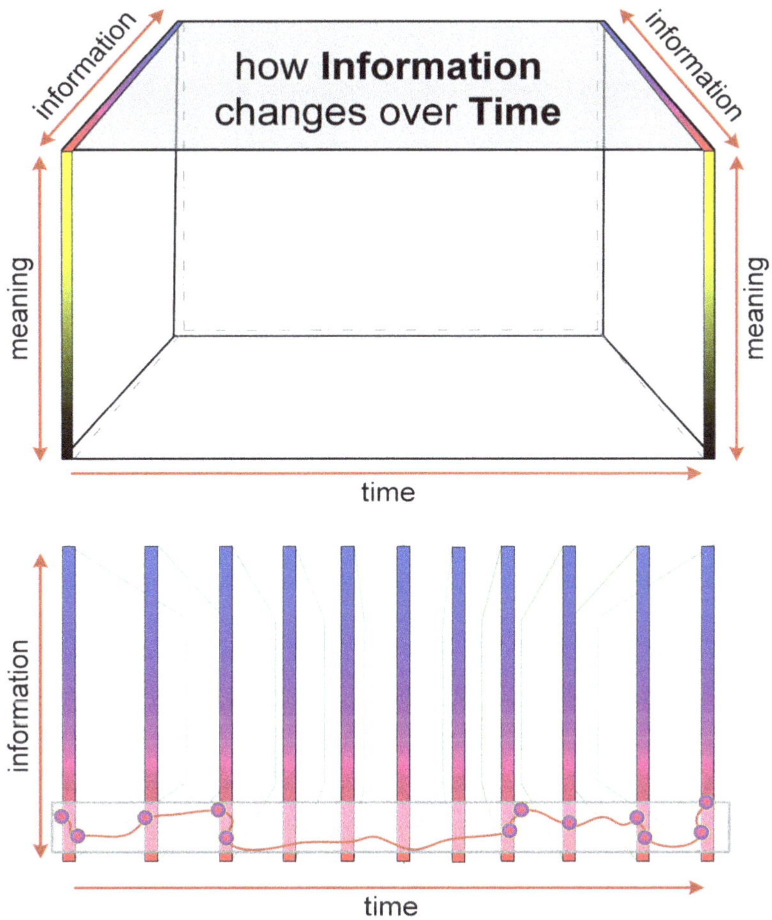

Information Over Time Line

(as viewed from the **top** of the cube)

Now imagine you turn this cube down, so the top is in front. This is how the Meaning-over-Time line on the previous page would look if we looked at this line from above. This "from above" view is what the Information in that Meaning-over-Time line looks like. Here, we see that all of the Information in this wounding event exists within a thin stripe of extremely Real World (changing) Information.

We also see that there is no Theoretical (unchanging) Information present, nor any normal mixes of the two kinds of Information.

Is this hard to imagine? Then do your best to try to picture this line, inside that 3-D rectangular cube shaped box. Can you flip it up and down between views?

The End Views of the Cube

(how Information exists in a single moment)

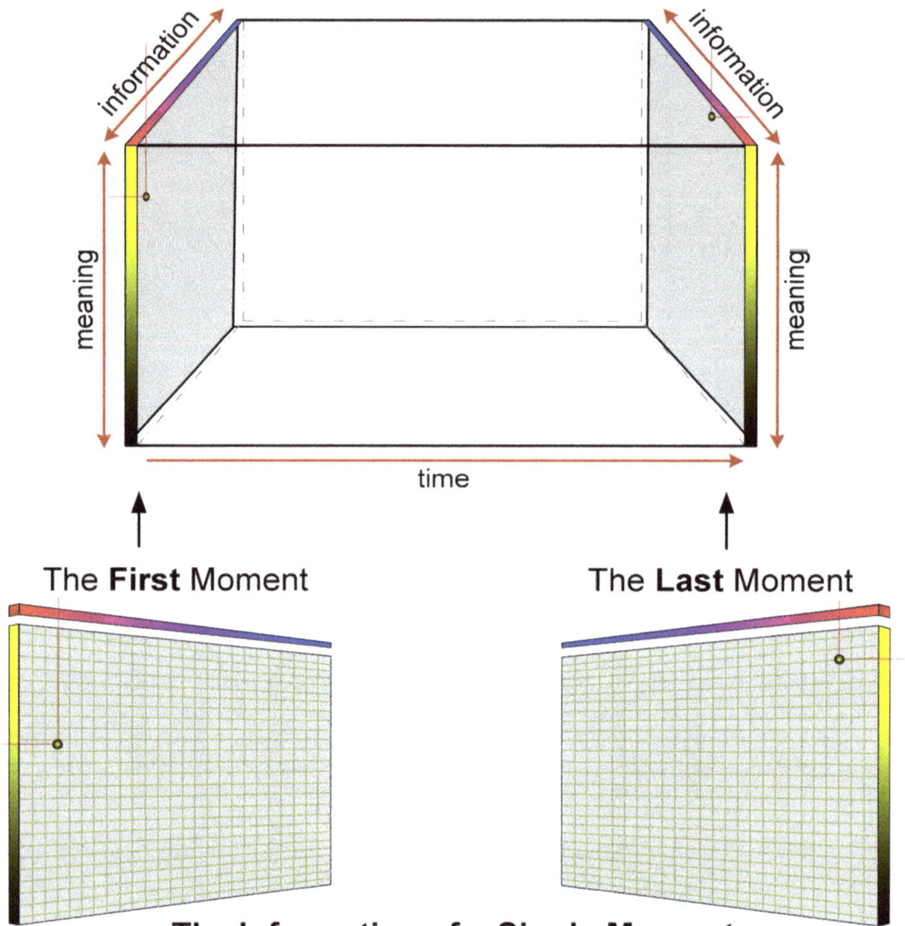

The Information of a Single Moment
(as viewed from the **ends** of the cube)

Finally, here are the two ends of this 3-D rectangular space. Each end represents a plot of a single moment, specifically, the first and last moments of this event. Visually, this assumes these two plots exist on a hard-to-see-through slide. So viewed from outside of the cube, only the very ends of this line are visible.

Know I myself hope, before this book ends, to become able to visually represent the full lines through translucent ends. As of today, I don't know how. For now, hopefully, these end points will suffice for you to be able to picture this 3-D space. Also, please note, before we proceed, I first need to offer you a few caveats about some of the terms I used a few pages back, in the Bipolar vs Schizophrenia drawing.

The Two Bipolar - Information Lines

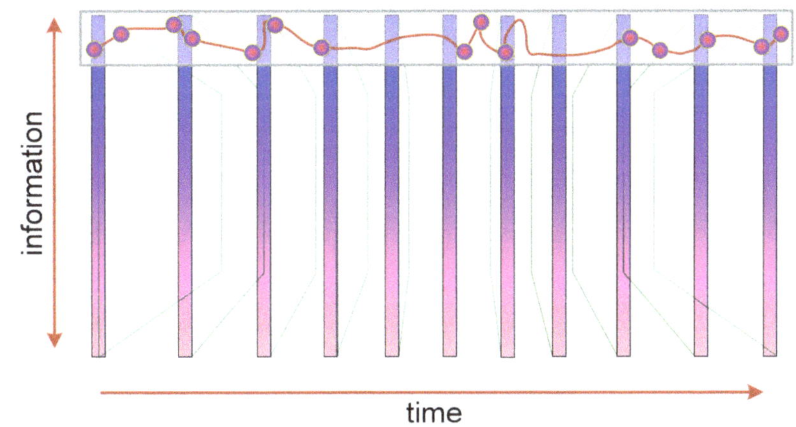

Schizophrenic Bipolar (information line)
(as viewed from the **top** of the cube)

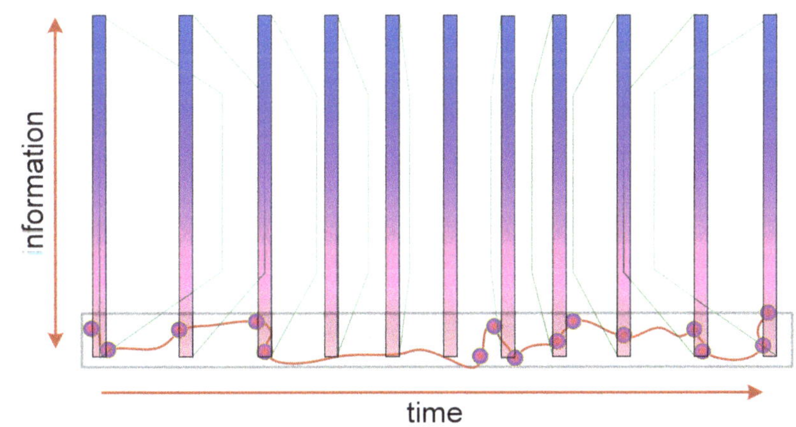

Affective Bipolar (information line)
(as viewed from the **top** of the cube)

Clearly, without recognizable lines, at this point, those terms remain vague and unscientific. In truth, despite that drawing's title using the words "Bipolar" and "Schizophrenia," a more accurate way to classify these two conditions would refer to both of them as "bipolar disorders." As I've previously told you, in this book, I'm trying to build a bridge between existing language and what would be more accurate and accessible terms. Were I to do that here, I'd call these two Personality-sized Disorders, "Affective Bipolar" and "Schizophrenic Bipolar." To see why, contrast and compare these two Information over Time Lines. Pay particular attention to all the places where there are no dots in both of these drawings.

Affective Bipolar

(Information & Meaning Lines)

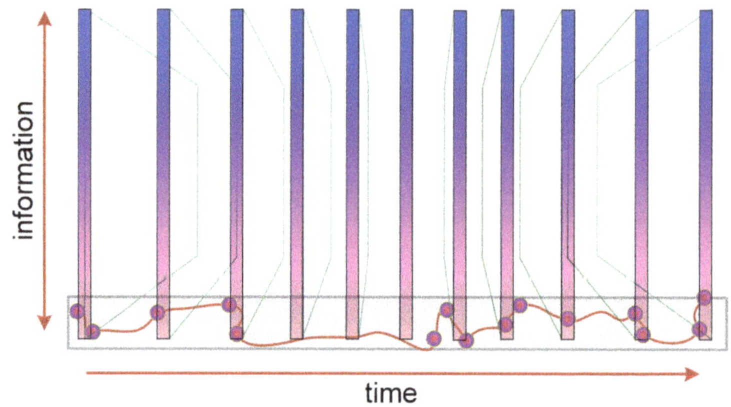

Affective Bipolar (information line)

(as viewed from the **top** of the cube)

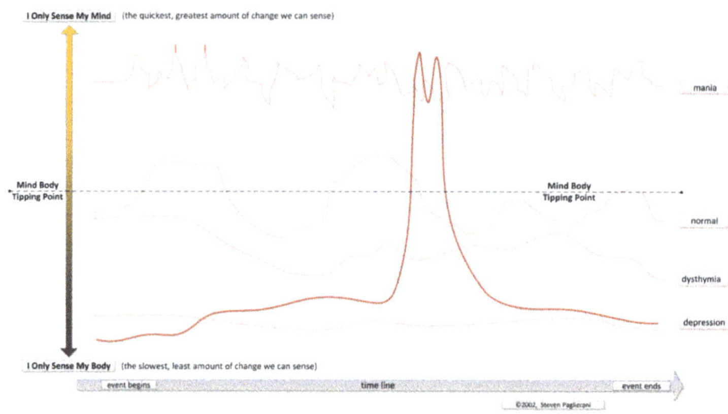

Affective Bipolar (meaning line)

(as viewed from the **front** of the cube)

Know we'll return to variations of that Bipolar vs Schizophrenia Single Moment drawing many times before this chapter ends. For one thing, I need to explain how that drawing connects to the line drawings I've used in previous chapters. Specifically, I need to show you how it connects to the Four States of Mind and the Four Kinds of Change. For instance, one of the Four States of Mind uses a single line shape to define the word "depression." So how can there be two kinds of depression, when there is only one depression line?

Start with the terms I've used in that drawing. In this book, the word "catatonia" will be called "Schizophrenic Depression." This refers to "an unmoving body of deadened ideas." As opposed to "Bipolar Depression," which refers to "an unmoving

Schizophrenic Bipolar

(Information & Meaning Lines)

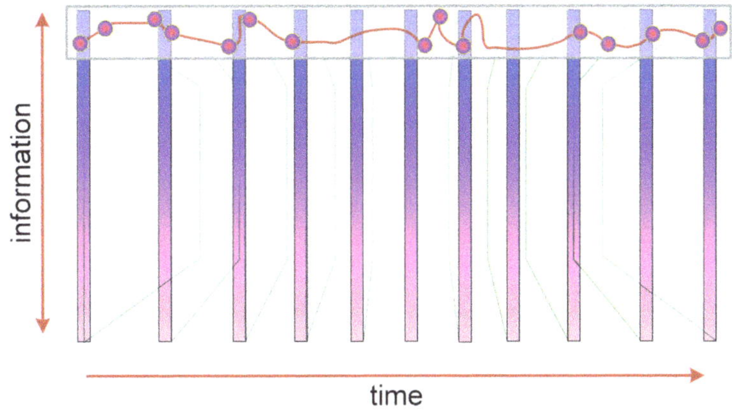

Schizophrenic Bipolar (information line)

(as viewed from the **top** of the cube)

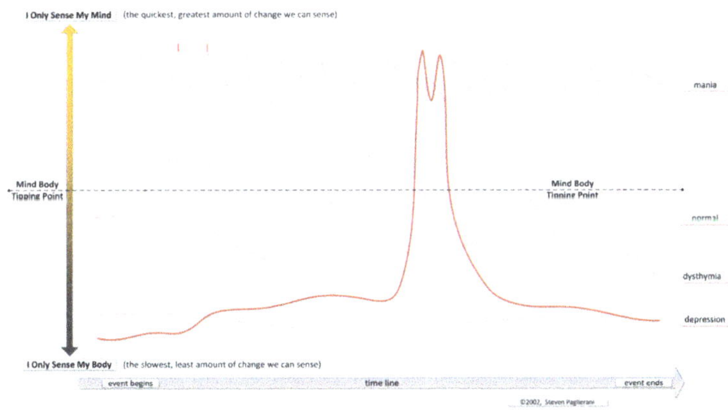

Schizophrenic Bipolar (meaning line)

(as viewed from the **front** of the cube)

flood of deadened feeling." This means, they both use the same State of Mind, Meaning Line shape—*but with different Information*.

What does it feel like to be experiencing these two kinds of depression?

Here's the five-cent tour.

Schizophrenic Depression feels like endlessly staring at an undifferentiated mass of ideas. This mass of ideas is standing stock-still, and you are blankly staring at the words. You don't understand them. But you just don't care.

Bipolar Depression feels like endlessly staring into an undifferentiated mass of feelings. This mass of feelings is close-to-imperceptibly moving and you are blankly staring into it. You don't understand this either. But you also don't care.

Schizoaffective Bipolar - Types 1 & 2

(Information Lines)

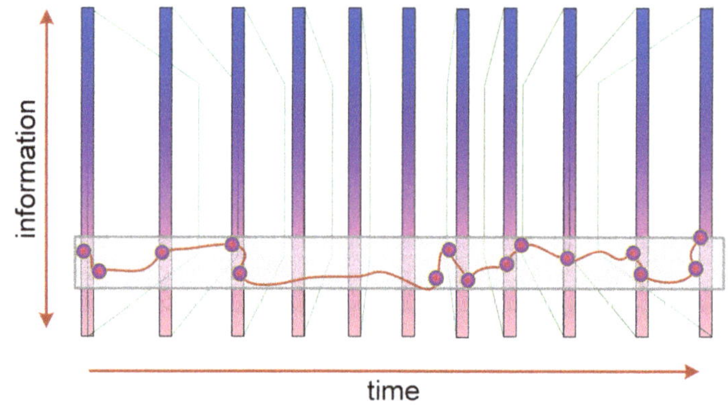

Schizoaffective Bipolar Type 1
(information line)
(as viewed from the **top** of the cube)

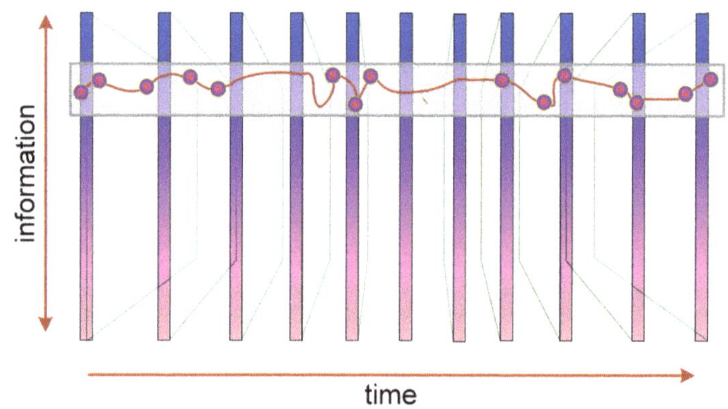

Schizoaffective Bipolar Type 2
(information line)
(as viewed from the **top** of the cube)

The point?

Clinically-significant amounts of "not caring" (diagnosable depression) come in two flavors—as in not caring about your feelings (affective), and as not caring about your ideas (schizophrenic). And if you now look at the drawing on this page, you'll see I've expanded on this theme. This time, you'll see the Information in the two Schizoaffective Bipolars. Again, these two Bipolars differ based on the kinds of Information the person can experience. Schizoaffective Bipolar Type 1 is a less extreme version of Affective Bipolar. Schizoaffective Bipolar Type 2 is a less extreme version of Schizophrenic Bipolar.

Here again you see this same theme—feelings vs ideas.

Schizoaffective Borderline - Types 1 & 2

(Information Lines)

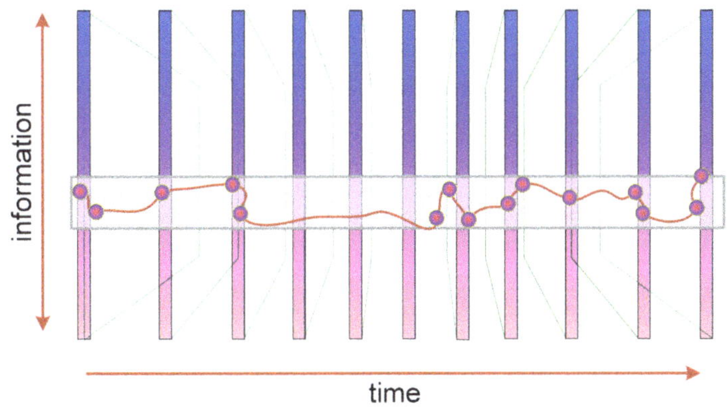

Schizoaffective Borderline Type 1
(information line)
(as viewed from the **top** of the cube)

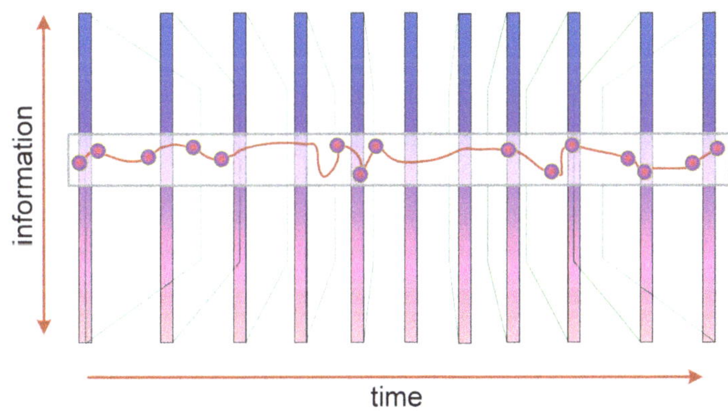

Schizoaffective Borderline Type 2
(information line)
(as viewed from the **top** of the cube)

Continuing with this pattern, we now come to a more intelligent description of Borderline Personality Disorder. The Information lines for this condition are in the drawing on this page. Here the term "borderline" refers to the fact that these two narrowed ranges of Information border on either side of the Information midline. And the terms, Type 1 and Type 2, refer to which side of this border they are on.

Type 1 is towards the affective side, mainly, disordered feelings.

Type 2 is toward the schizophrenic side, mainly, disordered ideas.

Keep in mind, the placement of the Information dots, within the grayed-out stripes in each of six of these conditions, can vary widely. But these dots cannot exist outside of these stripes.

This means a principal feature in the nature of all six of these Personality-sized Disorders is the narrow range within which the person can experience Information. Realize, this explains the difficulty these folks have with organizing interpersonal relationships. Vast swaths of the life experience necessary to manage relationships are missing from their view. Indeed, this aspect of Personality-sized Disorders already has a name—***anosognosia,*** a neurological condition which impairs people's awareness of their mental health symptoms.

People with anosognosia may have no awareness of their condition—or an inaccurate perception of it. Either way, in each case, what is missing is a large amount of the Information necessary to understand specific parts of human relationships. This condition is said to commonly affect people with certain mental health conditions. No coincidence, schizophrenia and bipolar disorder are the main two.

Now consider how those six Information-line maps explain these interpersonal deficits. To begin with, as I've said, all people experience Event-sized Disorders. When they do, they too experience a severely limited amount of Information. Here, the Information which people can access during these events gets limited to what the person experienced during the critical period in the original wounding event.

This means, all people can at times look like they have a Personality-sized Disorder. However, when this reliving ends, people who do not have a Personality-sized Disorder regain access to a normal amount of Information. Whereas people with a Personality-sized Disorder often never had access to this Information in the first place. Even in normal times, they're unaware of huge swaths of Information.

Now consider how this affects a diagnostician's ability to diagnose. All diagnosis must begin with ruling out Personality-sized Disorders. The problem is, Event-sized Disorders blind even "normal" people to all but a small bit of Information. So in these moments, all people effectively become as severely disordered as—and so, can look just like—people with a Personality-sized disorder.

This is why diagnosticians should never try to diagnose a Personality-sized Disorder when a patient is reliving an Event-sized Disorder. Diagnostically, it becomes impossible to determine which diagnosis to give. In these times, the interactions are simply too complex to pull apart. Here, observation is the key.

Therapists trying to help such people should also keep this in mind. Often, much of what the therapist says will have no meaning to people with these disorders. You cannot experience Meaning without having relevant Information. M=IT. And people with a Personality-sized Disorder can lack access to even basic Information. This means, their ability to tolerate talk therapies—even when they're not reliving an Event-sized Disorder—is severely impaired. Why? For one thing, they simply cannot make sense of, let alone believe, that the source of their suffering may exist within themselves. This leads them to logically assume, it is other people who are causing their problems. Can you imagine how this belief affects their ability to have personal relationships? They think their suffering is always someone else's fault.

As for why this happens, I'll explain why in the next chapter.

What About All The Other Kinds of "Personality" Disorders?

Existing diagnostic manuals list quite a few "personality disorders." There have been as many as 13 types. As of today (September 28, 2023), the current manual lists 10. Realize, the titles of each of these disorders simply derive from what is seen as the main class of symptoms present. And this is where the train runs off the track.

The list?

- Antisocial Personality Disorder
- Avoidant Personality Disorder
- Borderline Personality Disorder
- Dependent Personality Disorder
- Histrionic Personality Disorder
- Narcissistic Personality Disorder
- Obsessive-Compulsive Personality Disorder
- Paranoid Personality Disorder
- Schizoid Personality Disorder
- Schizotypal Personality Disorder

My take on all this? For the most part, it's all unscientific bullshit. Why? Each of these diagnoses is based entirely on specific symptoms and behaviors. Setting aside the idea that these authors never scientifically define these symptoms and behaviors, how do you differentiate between these diagnoses—when all these people can present with any and all of these symptoms and behaviors?

Think about it. As defined in these manuals, a person with Schizoid Personality Disorder can appear to be just as avoidant, sensitive, and shy as a person with Avoidant Personality Disorder. A person with Dependent Personality Disorder and a person with Borderline Personality Disorder can both appear to be just as dependent, clingy, and needy when they feel they've been abandoned. A person with Histrionic Personality Disorder and a person with Borderline Personality Disorder can both seem to be just as attention seeking and excessively emotional. And all of these people, at times, will appear to be just as narcissistic and lacking in empathy towards others—as a person with Narcissistic Personality Disorder.

This brings us to what are surely some of the most important questions in this book. Why is it so hard to define Personality-sized Disorders? Is it because all of these features so badly overlap? If so, how can those authors have managed to overlook such a serious flaw? And what makes it impossible to heal these disorders?

These questions are some of what we're about to explore.

The First Year of Life - Undifferentiated Information

In the past dozen or so pages, I've mentioned several things all Personality-sized Disorders share.

First, all Personality-sized Disorders are ***permanent***.

Second, they ***cannot be healed***.

I've also said, all Personality-sized Disorders result from ***chronically*** painful experiences during the first year of life. As opposed to Event-sized Disorders which result from ***acutely*** painful experiences (startles) and can occur at any time in life.

This last pair of ideas is the critical piece of information here.

It points to the principal difference between Event-sized and Personality-sized Disorders.

The principal difference between these two categories of disorders is the degree to which they cause disorder in human relationships.

Event-sized Disorders create ***time-limited, event-based disorder***—and only in situations where people relive the small-slice of context from a startling event. Whereas with Personality-sized Disorders, ***there are no knowable limits to the disorder they create in relationships***. Neither time, nor place, nor relationship are, in any way, limiting factors.

In truth, the disorder caused by Personality-sized Disorders is so unpredictable that even with their best efforts, these folks cannot sustain even marginally healthy relationships. Not ever. Moreover, this unpredictability IS the reason you can never rely on symptoms or behavior alone to diagnose Personality-sized Disorders. Rather, as I've said a number of times already, you must begin with, and rely on, a comprehensive knowledge of early childhood development—specifically, the development which occurs in the first two years of life.

What I'm about to introduce will be but the barest of outlines of this development. Please note, none of what I'm about to say has ever been used to describe personality disorders, let alone used to guide their diagnosis. This all begins with a two-word phrase, which then bifurcates into a perfect pair.

The phrase?

Undifferentiated life experiences.

As opposed to what?

Differentiated life experiences.

Now consider how these two italicized words share the same root as the key word in all existing diagnostic manuals.

The word? The "differential"—the means by which we diagnosticians are supposed to make sense of that muddled mess.

How can we differentiate what we see if the core symptom is a lack of differentiation?

This is the point. We can't.

Ironically, nowhere does this muddled mess seem more impossible to pull apart than when trying to diagnose personality disorders. People with any one of those ten current personality disorders can present with each and every symptom referred to in that list of titles. For instance, as I've said, anyone with a personality disorder can present with significant narcissistic features. Not coincidently, every one of these people will also exhibit significant instability in their relationships.

How then are we supposed to diagnose this? Here is the five-cent tour.

Differentiation: the Key to Diagnosing Personality-sized Disorders

Based on things I've said many times already, what I'm going to say next may surprise and confuse some readers. This thing applies to all existing diagnostic manuals—and to the authors of these books. When it comes to the lack of clarity present in the sections on personality disorders, none of this is their fault. Rather, by omitting any mentions of personality in these manuals, these authors inadvertently omitted what turns out to be the diagnostic "Rosetta Stone" when it comes to differentiating personality disorders. Here, I'm referring to the developmental sequence which all babies face during their first two years of life.

The headline here is simple. At birth, babies have close-to completely, undifferentiated awareness of life. This means they have close to zero life skills when it comes to creating and maintaining human relationships. By year-one end though, according to the "great" me, the know-it-all author of the present book—all the rudiments of having a self will either exist or they will not. Similarly, by year -two end, all the rudiments of human relationships will either have developed or they will have not. And if those first-year skills have not developed by age two?

Then this baby ***already has*** a Personality-sized Disorder.

The thing is, because we do not expect babies to exhibit these kinds of interpersonal skills so early on, these deficits will continue to go by unnoticed—usually until around age twenty. Hence the diagnostic tradition not to diagnose personality disorders in children. Lacking what I'm telling you here about developmental stages, diagnosing Personality-sized Disorders becomes impossible.

Why age twenty? Because by this age, it becomes obvious, people either have or lack the skills to create or sustain well-organized human relationships.

What docs any of this havc to do with diagnosis?

Think back on how I've defined the word "disorder."

A "disorder" is a clinically significant lack of ability to create and sustain well-ordered interpersonal relationships.

Now as I just said, at the beginning of the first year of life, babies have none of the skills necessary to create or maintain well-organized relationships. Rather, all of the rudiments of these yet-to-develop skills lie in yet-to-be-differentiated life experiences. Talk about disordered lives.

Realize, the skills I'm referring to here are primarily those necessary to develop the first half of all relationships—the self. With a self, babies begin to know they, as persons, exist. Then, in the second year of life, babies must expand on their sense of themselves. Here they acquire the skills necessary to know the other side of the relationship coin—that other selves exist.

This is the critical tipping-point in learning to have interpersonal relationships. For these relationships to exist, they must exist between two selves. Only then can babies be said to be able to have interpersonal relationships. And without a sense of two selves, people become narcissistic—this is what this word means. It means the person only senses one self, and one self has no ***inter***personal life.

Obviously, we have a whole lot more to discuss before I can ask you to believe these claims. Before I do, I need to create a firmer foundation on which these claims can stand. This is what we'll do next, beginning with a brief review of the basics of early childhood development. As we go through this though, please try to keep the two words I've previously mentioned in mind.

One. ***Undifferentiated*** life experiences.

Two. ***Differentiated*** life experiences.

Information-Based Differentiation in The First Year of Life

As I've told you, there are two main things to consider when diagnosing Personality-sized Disorders—[1] the kinds of ***Information*** present and how it changes over time (the shape of the Information Line)—and [2], the kinds of ***Meaning*** present and how it changes over time (the shape of the Meaning Line).

Realize, babies become aware of these two things (Information and Meaning) slowly, over time. Thus both can be said to be "developmental." In this discussion, we'll limit what we look at to how the 4 kinds of Information develop—as this is part of knowing how to diagnose Personality-sized Disorders.

If you now look over at the drawing on the next page, you'll see the kinds of Information babies learn to sense during the first two developmental stages. In the first—***A Baby's Information at Birth***—babies perceive all Information as Feelings, nothing else. Then, in the second stage—***A Baby's Information at 6 Months***—babies begin to differentiate this Information into two kinds. Babies still perceive most things as Feelings. But they now occasionally sense some Information as Facts.

Recall, in this book, these two words have very specific definitions.

Feelings are defined as "Invisible Change."

Facts are defined as "Visible Unchange."

Attentive readers will immediately recognize these two things as a perfect pair. As defined here, they are perfectly defined. Facts cannot have any Feelings in them, and Feelings cannot have any Facts in them either. Also, Feelings and Facts are not literal "things." They're merely two of the mind's four viewpoints. This means, all Information can be viewed as all four kinds of Information. Depending on how you voice it, a Feeling can be viewed as a Fact, and a Fact as a Feeling.

Now notice the numbers One and Two in these drawings. These two numbers indicate the developmental order in which each kind of Information appears. Thus the number One means, all Information first exists as Feelings. And the number Two means, the baby's awareness then progresses to occasionally sensing Information as Facts. Please note, the word ***Feelings*** can apply to a lot of things. As used here, it refers to anything which can be said to be "Invisible Change." What does this mean? Before you answer, please consider what kinds of Information this phrase can refer to. A Feeling can refer to a physical thing, as well as to something mental.

For example, take anger. Anger— is invisible. Obviously, you can't see the anger itself. You only know it exists because you can feel it changing.

A Baby's Information at Birth

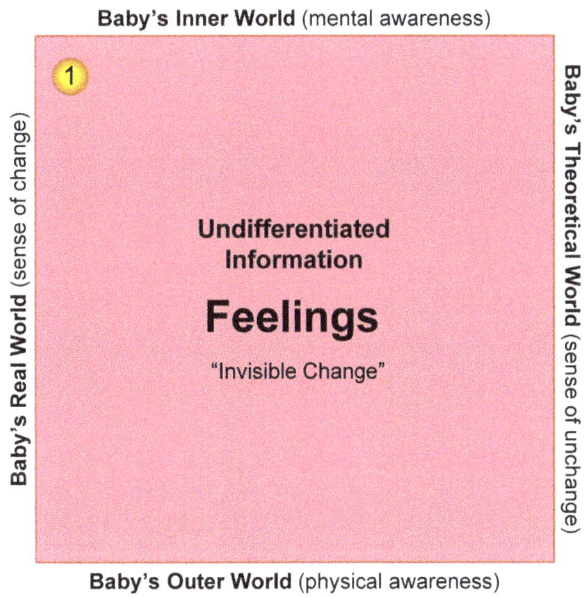

A Baby's Information at 6 Months

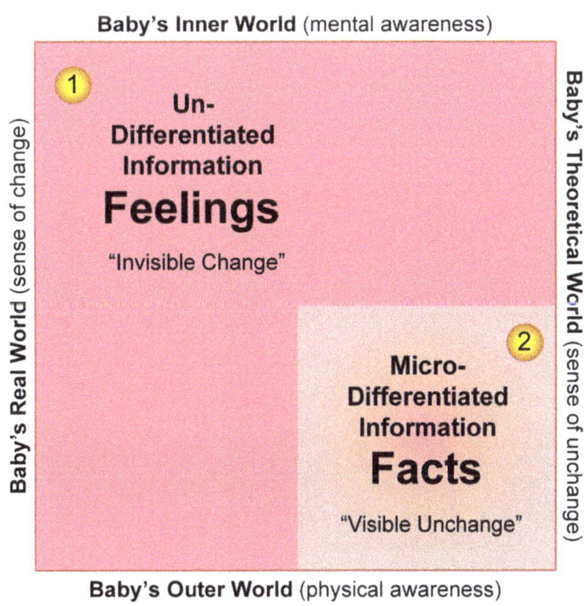

A Baby's Information at 9 Months

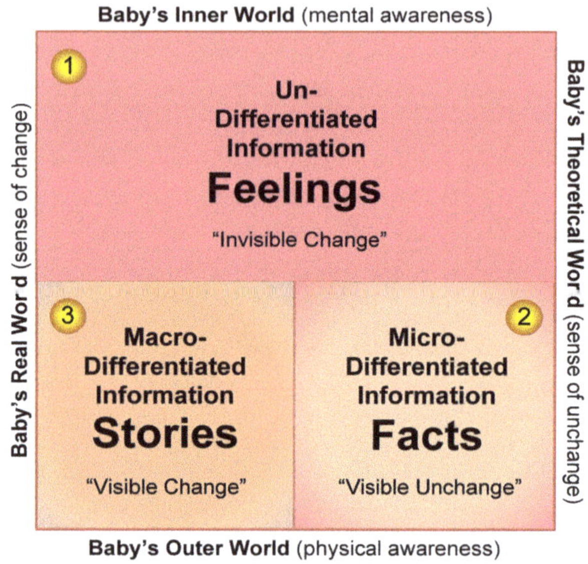

A Baby's Information at Age Two

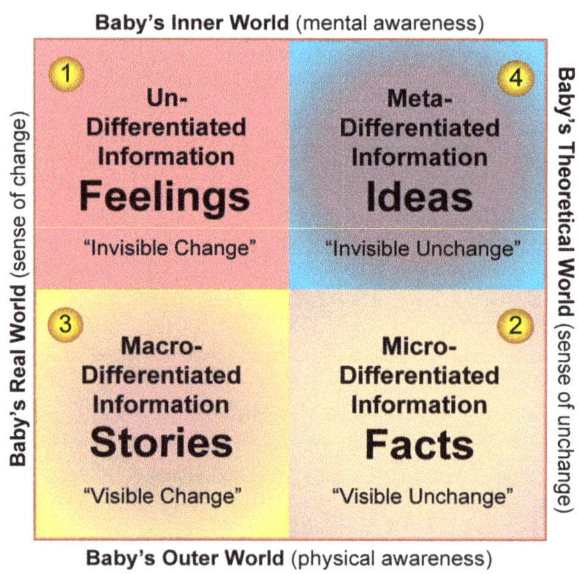

And if it stops changing? Then you stop feeling angry.

The same things apply to having an itchy nose. You can't see an itch. You only know it exists because it's changing. And if it stops changing? Then you stop feeling the itch.

This points to something important.

Information is simply "change sensed."

As for the word ***Facts***, it too can apply to many things. But while a ***Fact*** is not a ***Feeling***, it's also not a ***Story***. As I've said, a ***Feeling*** is "Invisible Change." Whereas a ***Fact*** is "Visible Unchange." So what is a ***Story***? A ***Story*** is "Visible Change."

When do Stories begin to appear? At about nine months old. And by age One, babies have a limited ability to sense all three of these kinds of Information. Then, in the second year of life, babies begin to sense the fourth kind of Information—***Ideas***.

What are ***Ideas***? ***Ideas*** are "Invisible Unchange."

Can you see it yet? As defined here, no other kinds of Information can exist. If not, try looking at this simple list. Can you see the two perfect pairs (visibility/invisibility and change/unchange) which bifurcate into the 4 Informations.

- [1] ***Feelings*** - Invisible Change
- [2] ***Facts*** - Visible Unchange
- [3] ***Stories*** - Visible Change
- [4] ***Ideas*** - Invisible Unchange

Realize, the idea that two-year-old babies can sense all four kinds of Information does not mean they can do this well. At this age, the actual distribution of these four kinds of Information still reflects a strong bias towards sensing Information as Feelings. Please keep this in mind as you study the four Information squares in these drawings. The sizes of these squares does not indicate how well babies can sense those kinds of Information. Rather children continue to differentiate these 4 kinds of Information throughout child development.

Now, before moving on, there are two more things I need to tell you.

One, all adults end up with unequal ***abilities*** to sense—and to publicly admit to having sensed—these four kinds of Information. Most often, people exhibit a bias towards offering Ideas—and a bias against revealing Feelings.

Two, anytime a person regresses to one of these early childhood times, there will be a bias towards sensing the Information present as the kind of Information which was developing at that time. And this effect is most visible in people with the two most extreme Personality-sized Disorders—Affective Bipolar and Schizophrenic Bipolar.

Indeed, based on the words in the titles of these two diagnoses alone, you should be able to know things about people with these two conditions.

People with an Affective Bipolar diagnosis experience chronic neglect or abuse during the first three months of life. So their bias is towards Feelings. Whereas people with a Schizophrenic Bipolar diagnosis experience chronic neglect or abuse during the second year of life. So their bias is towards Ideas.

Are you beginning to see how useful personality is when diagnosing?

This is not as hard as you might have expected it to be, is it?

Personality-Based Differentiation in The First Year of Life

Much of the theory behind what I'm going to discuss next has been described in detail in my prior books. Thus I will not be giving you much more than the barest of outlines here. This said, when it comes to diagnosis, even these bare outlines will be better than what's been described in existing diagnostic manuals. Know it's all rather simple, actually. In the first year, there are two developmental periods. And together, these two periods result in the baby having all the rudiments of a "self."

The first developmental period?

Most books will tell you that in the first six months, babies develop the ability to manage and use their five senses. And that by about six months old, they've acquired the beginnings of depth perception. What they do not say—because they haven't a clue that this happens—is that at first, those "five" senses are actually "four primary senses"—and that the fifth sense, vision, is an "emergent sense."

What the heck do I mean by an "emergent sense?"

Start with this.

I call the senses of smell, taste, touch, and hearing, the Four Primary Senses. For newborn babies, these four senses are almost completely undifferentiated. This means these babies are "synesthetes." And in case you've not heard this word before, it means, babies have yet to properly separate these 4 senses into four ***separate*** senses.

What must this be like?

Babies may at times feel sounds, hear tastes, or smell colors.

Based on this knowledge alone, it should be obvious, they cannot see things like we can see them. Can babies react to changes in their visual environment? Obviously, they can. But "see," as in, "define objects in their view?" Not so much.

Some readers may have come across an adult condition which uses a variation of the word "synesthetes." The formal name for this condition is "synesthesia." It's estimated that as many as 4% of adults have some form of it. Simultaneously hearing and physically feeling "nails on a blackboard" is a good example.

Know I spent some time looking for explicit mentions of this experience being interpreted as regression. Nothing I read mentions a time during early childhood where this condition is normal—let alone that synesthetic experiences are a return to this time. It seems, most medical people haven't made these kinds of developmental, personality-based connections yet either. Like mental health professionals who also have yet to make these connections, I don't blame these folks either.

Now consider what it must be like for babies to live in a state where their five senses are undifferentiated. It explains why most of their awareness is focused in on themselves, rather than out into the world.

These efforts also can't leave much headspace to begin to know that they, as individual selves exist. Indeed, the idea of having a self can't even have begun to exist at this point.

Said more simply, in the first six months of life, babies focus mainly on mastering their four primary senses. Where's my evidence that vision is not a primary sense? Babies gain the ability to see out into the world only after they acquire depth perception. This emergent sense then allows them to see a world which is separate from themselves. And this occurs only after the four Primary Senses have sufficiently differentiated.

Only then do babies turn their attention to what extends beyond themselves. Want to test for this in yourself? Then try this thought experiment. Try reading those last few paragraphs in your normal way of reading. While doing this, try to observe what doing this feels like. If you're normal, you'll be separating two of your senses. You'll almost imperceptibly be cycling between [1] taking in the physical words and letters with your eyes, then [2] following this visual process with hearing these words in your head, as mental sounds. And rinse, and repeat.

Now try doing this same exercise again. Only this time, as you read, try to visualize yourself doing the reading. Too hard? Then try becoming aware you exist as a person, while you read those words.

Not so easy, is it?

Most people rarely do this, let alone picture what they're reading. If this is you, don't worry. Nothing is wrong with you. You're perfectly normal.

So what do babies do? What is life like for them? To see for yourself, think back to a time you were watching a movie and lost track of where you were—a time you felt you'd been drawn into the scene.

This feeling—where you lose your sense of "out there" versus "in here"—is what babies feel like in their first year of life. Not coincidently, this is the state serious meditators aspire to learn how to do.

Finally, try to imagine being in that state once—a time you were sitting in a movie theater and you've been drawn into the scene. Realize this is far more likely to happen when the scene generated high levels of Feelings.

Did you just catch that?

A high level of Feelings.

And what developmental age is this Information most likely?

Between six months and age One.

Now if you've done this thought experiment well enough, you may have noticed something quite important. If you didn't—or don't know what I'm referring to, please don't blame yourself. The thing I'm referring to? That if you're drawn into a scene, you no longer sense anyone else sitting next to you. All that's left is a very blunted sense of self, one which gets more blunted, the more you're drawn into the scene.

My point?

If you were able to do this thought experiment?

Then you just experienced the loss of the self.

This is the state babies constantly cycle in and out of for that first year of life.

In their case, however, they've never had a sense of "self." So they can't feel they've lost it.

No sense of self?

Imagine?

Know this has many implications.

All of which apply to people with a Personality-sized Disorder.

What Happens to Babies in the Second Six Months?

What I've just told you is that the first year of life is roughly divided into two halves. And the tipping point for these two halves occurs at around six months. At this age, babies begin to develop depth perception—"seeing out into the world." This is the first great differentiation. Here, babies slowly begin their move towards knowing that "they" and "the world" are two different things.

This state of mind also has a name—solipsism: the state of mind wherein you are the world. Here again, despite my searching extensively for any mention of how this connects to early childhood development, I found none which refers to the kind of connections I just mentioned. What I did find, however, were many mentions of this state of mind in connection with diagnosing Schizophrenia—in particular, a central belief involving a clinically significant distortion in one's sense of self.

One theorist, Clara S. Humpston, says Schizophrenia is "fundamentally, a pathology of self-awareness"—which leads the person to adopt a solipsistic world view—"a basic and fundamental change in one's experiences of the self, and also, subsequently, the world." ***The paradoxical self: Awareness, solipsism and first-rank symptoms in schizophrenia, 08 Dec 2017, Philosophical Psychology, Volume 31, 2018 - Issue 2, Pages 210-231***)

Now add to this the idea that current primary diagnostic criteria for Schizophrenia focus on things like delusions and hallucinations. My point? Both of these things point to a baby's experiences during the second six months of life, as seen through the baby's "second year of life eyes." Both of these things are grounded in intense experiences of some or all of the five senses—including a notable lack of the Meanings that an older child, or an adult, would assign to this Information.

So what happens to babies in the second six months of life?

They build on what they've mastered in the first six months.

They use their newfound abilities "to sense out into the world." Here they begin to master their sense of physically manipulating the "things out there" as things. This differs significantly from the first six months, where the baby was the world. Now rather than experiencing these things as mere extensions of themselves, these things begin to feel separate and apart from themselves.

What Develops in Most Babies During The Second Year?

The tipping point into the second year? Learning to walk. This tips them into the next developmental stage. Only then can they begin to develop a real sense of separateness from the world. There are things they want to get to, and to get to them, they have to walk.

What are the main things babies want to get to?

Can you guess?

Mothers, fathers, and caregivers in general.

This desire is the driving force behind the developments which occur in the second year of life. The main realization? That others exist. Know that in the personality theory I'm drawing on as I write this book (Emergence Personality Theory), this change is referred to as a person's Character Type. Here there are four possibilities.

Adults can be a Character Type One, a Two, a Three, or a Four. Know each title refers to the patterns present in that year of life. A person with Character Type One has all the patterns we've just spoken about, including that they have yet to develop the sense that other selves exist. Rather, they, for their entire lives, experience others similarly to how babies in their first year of life experience any and all caregivers—as mere extensions of themselves.

This changes if, and when, babies develop second year of life skills.

Principle in this skill set is the awareness that other selves exist.

Here, by "other selves," I mean, other beings with needs similar to theirs. As opposed to the first year of life, where the baby is the only self with needs.

As I write this, I'm recalling the day I first recognized this change in a baby. I'd known and been around this baby, Jacob, since he'd been one month old. Two events mark the before and after tipping-points of this change in him. The first involved trying to prevent a ten-month-old Jacob from putting his hand into a cup of boiling hot tea. The second involved seeing Jacob exhibit a new pattern of attention, as he looked out at his mother and me.

Seeing a Baby Tip From First to Second Year of Life Development

The mother of this baby was a younger colleague who back then had an office in the same office suite as mine. Jacob was her first child, and I interacted with him numerous times during his first few years. Me being me, I became interested in—and so learned a heck of a lot about—child development during this time. In fact, I can even, in this moment, immerse myself in many visual scenes from that time.

The hot tea scene?

I was in this therapist's home, in her living room. She'd just made me tea and I'd set this mug on an end table. Baby Jacob had yet to learn to walk without aids. So he'd hoisted himself up on the couch and was walking himself towards that mug.

I was watching him to make sure he was OK.

However, when Jacob reached that end table, he suddenly tried to put his hand into that mug. I then managed to catch and prevent him from doing this several times in a row. But babies are nothing if not persistent. So he eventually burned his little hand. A clear mental movie of him doing this remains in my mind.

In this movie, Jacob kept trying to do this—and I kept catching his hand. But not once during this time did he look up at me. To him, I was merely an obstacle. And even when he burned his hand, he continued to look longingly at that mug.

Contrast this story with the second one I previously alluded to.

What happened then?

In this second story, I was again in that same colleague's living room, this time, sitting with her on her couch.

Notably, I cannot imagine a house being more baby-proof. Not one thing seemed to be something Jacob could get into and harm himself.

Know that at this point, Jacob had crawled into the next room. The only things in that room were a dining table and chairs and a large potted rubber tree plant.

What could he get into?

His mother and I wrongly thought, nothing. But a moment later, we both knew he'd gotten into something.

He was too quiet.

At this point, we both got up, slowly walked over to the doorway, and peeked in. And when we did, we saw that the little explorer had hoisted himself up on, and was holding onto, the rubber-tree-plant pot. In this moment, I saw, for the first time, what I've come to know as that developmental tipping-point.

Rather than pay no attention to us (as he did with me and the mug), this time, Jacob looked over at us both. Then he looked at the hand full of dirt he had in his hand, then back at us, and back at his hand.

Realize, Jacob already had a mouthful of dirt in his mouth. So that handful of dirt would have been the next mouthful.

Can you see the difference yet between the first story and this second one?

The difference lies entirely in "where Jacob looked."

In the first story, he only looked at the mug, never at me.

In the second, he first looked out at us, then at what he wanted for himself (the handful of dirt), then out at us again (where he wondered if we had needs). And for the first time, he hesitated because in that moment, he realized, "others who have needs" also exist. So in that moment, his becoming able to see "others with needs" moved him into Character Type Two.

What Then Is A "Personality Disorder"?

It never ceases to amaze me how a book listing ten "personality" disorders can make no mention of personality—not one word. How can they call these disorders, "personality" disorders, when they make no attempt to define what personality is—let alone offer the kinds of definitions I've offered in previous chapters.

There I told you, personality consists of what a person can remain aware of, after a sequence of five nested filters, existing in the mind, reduces his or her ability to experience life.

In effect, what the mind can no longer sense are the life experiences which remain undifferentiated. The mind cannot assign **Meanings** to undifferentiated life experiences. Life experiences only become **Information** when the mind has differentiated them. Only then, can the mind assign **Meanings** to them.

Is this making sense? What the mind filters out—the life experiences without **Meanings**—is what we normally can't be conscious of. The knowable patterns in what's left determine what we can be conscious of. Principle in all these patterns are those which enable us to have interpersonal relationships. And developmentally, our ability to recognize these particular patterns must occur during the first two years of life.

[1] In the first year of life, we must learn to recognize the patterns we need in order to know we have a self.

[2] In the second year of life, we must learn to recognize the patterns we need in order to know others have a self.

So what are we diagnosticians doing when we attempt to use symptoms and behavior to diagnose?

We're identifying assets and deficits in interpersonal relationships which do not appear to be well-ordered.

What does it mean to say we are "healthy?"

It means we can create and sustain reasonably well-organized relationships. Here "well-organized relationships" are those which are based on stable, consistent, visibly well-ordered patterns of interpersonal life experience.

People with a Personality-sized Disorder cannot create, let alone sustain, this kind of order in their relationships. And the notable features of the persistent patterns of disorder which are present then determine the specifics of their diagnosis.

For instance, take people who have a traditional "Borderline" diagnosis. As we'll explore in the next chapter, for these folks, the mere smell of being abandoned triggers a regression in them—a regression to a time wherein they cried themselves past their ability to breathe.

However, if you set aside the insanity which occurs during these times, something interesting surfaces. In between these times, much of what can be observed in their relationships appears to contain many of the rudiments of a well-organized life. Granted these rudiments have never led to fully developed, interpersonal life skills. But they do contain the skill levels of a baby in their first year of life.

This last idea explains a good portion of the almost magnetic attraction people with a Borderline diagnosis can exert on others. We humans are programmed to respond almost involuntarily to the needs, and wants, and faces, of first-year-of-life babies.

People whose Character Types begin in a You state (Twos and Fours) are especially susceptible to such interactions. No coincidence, this accounts for most of the people who attempt to have relationships with these folks.

What Must A Personality-sized Disorder Diagnosis Include?

To begin with, all Personality-sized Disorders should be defined and differentiated from each other using two things—both of which must be present and recognizable in order to diagnose a Personality-sized Disorder.

The first thing?

What all these diagnoses have in common.

The person's ability to access and organize both Information and Meaning must exhibit notable bipolar features (see the drawings on pages 1723 through 1727).

Moreover, in both cases, this bipolarity must be based on an easily recognized, primary pair of perfect opposites.

Information-wise, this means, all diagnoses must be based on this diagnostic category's primary pair—Affective vs Schizophrenic Bipolar. And Meaning-wise, this means, all diagnoses must include periods in which the Meanings assigned to this Information exhibit bipolar features. Here I'm referring to clinically notable changes which involve sizable movements between the two extreme States of Mind—Depression and Mania. Moreover, these movements must exhibit the recognizable features present in the shape of the Bipolar Meaning Line.

Information-wise, this is what we began to look at earlier in this chapter—in the drawing titled, "The Two Bipolar - Information Lines." There we looked at a drawing which visually describes the two most extreme examples of bipolarity. All other Personality-sized Disorders are a less-extreme subset of this pair. All other Personality-sized Disorders derive from either Affective or Schizophrenic Bipolar.

People with either of these diagnoses exhibit a gross inability to create and sustain interpersonal relationships. Why? Because significant portions of this Information are, and will remain, undifferentiated. In a future chapter, we'll look more closely at why these deficits are permanent. For now, let's continue with what these diagnoses must include.

Meaning-wise, the two drawings following that earlier page reveal correlations between bipolar Information lines and Meaning lines which together exhibit bipolarity.

Realize, these Meaning lines represent two important things.

One, the amount of Meaning assigned to this Information (the Information which has been ***differentiated***).

Two, the amount of this Information which is currently ***undifferentiated.***

Now consider the correlation between the experience of depression and the experience of undifferentiated Information. The thing is, experiencing depression does not in and of itself indicate that this person has never differentiated this Information.

Depression, in and of itself, merely indicates that this Information is currently undifferentiated—and not that the person's mind has never sorted it into recognizable categories.

As for the second thing, we've been discussing it for some time now.

These patterns of bipolarity must be present to such a degree that the person being diagnosed cannot tolerate, maintain, or experience well-ordered relationships of any kind. Moreover, the shapes of the lines representing these bipolar features, again, pages 1723 through 1727, must correlate well to the ways observable deficits (the missing Information in those drawings) occurs in this person's life.

This bipolarity must include periods—no matter how brief—wherein this person appears to have learned to create, and maintain, a well-ordered relationship.

Finally, A Few Thoughts On The Scientific Method I'm Using

Many readers, especially those who have spent their whole lives adhering to the conventional scientific method, will likely have bristled many times in this chapter—and even more so in this entire book. If this is you, I'd politely like to ask you to consider heeding Herbert Spencer's advice against "contempt prior to investigation"—by reading my third book, "The Science of Discovery" (2016). Admittedly, it's a tough read, even for me.

Considering I'm the author, that's a bold admission. This said, and in case it hasn't occurred to you yet, "diagnosis" is just a form of scientific discovery. Or at least it should be. And it could be, given you follow a few simple corollaries.

Here, I'll reference but one of these corollaries.

All trains of discovery must be developmental.

Ad hoc trains of discovery, such as what the present scientific method employs, guarantees your work will be built like a castle in the air.

Now consider how this book has been built so far.

I've tried to unravel, and map out, this somewhat circuitous path to diagnosis with as many carefully laid steps as I think would be minimally necessary.

One principle I've tried to adhere to throughout this process is that corollary—to always root my claims in developmental steps.

My doing this allows you to retrace my steps, if and whenever you get lost. It also gives you a good picture for how you would go about rediscovering these things for yourself.

This brings to mind a time, early in my career, when I'd scheduled a family meeting at the rehab. This was back in 1989. I was sitting in the hospital chart room when my supervisor came and asked me the purpose for this meeting.

I felt embarrassed.

I couldn't come up with anything other than I thought it would be a good idea.

That question, and my lack of a clear answer, changed my life.

That question is a large part of what I've just told you about my science.

Diagnosing human suffering should never be less than this.

It should always have a knowable purpose—and path. And to have a knowable purpose, it should always be developmental.

Always.

Human beings deserve nothing less.

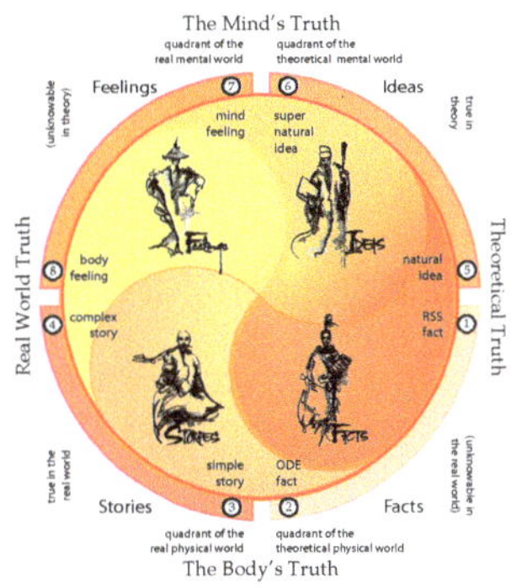

Chapter 5

Evidence Gathering (a guide)
(what can we learn about . . . ?)

How To Diagnose: Part One | Evidence Gathering

Based on this Chapter's title, you may think it will be a no-brainer. After all, who doesn't know what evidence is? In truth, this chapter may contain some of this book's most difficult concepts. There are fewer drawings, more words, and you'll need to rethink the math you use.

You'll also need to learn what kinds of evidence to include. Do this well and you'll help many more people. You'll also spare them the horrors of traversing through something many suffering people endure—multiple diagnoses. And when each diagnosis becomes ineffective, they're simply given a new one.

More often than not, the new diagnosis is just as useless as the old one. Over time then, these people feel less and less hope. You can help them to avoid this suffering if you can absorb, then use, what's in this chapter. Admittedly, there are several things which can make doing this hard.

Giving up and falling back on what you know is the worst thing you can do. Please try to not do that. Instead, when you get stuck—and you will get stuck, this chapter is a tough read—try rereading the takeaways I've left for you throughout the chapter. Each of them can make you feel more confident and enthused. More important, each one has the power to improve the chances you'll change a life. And isn't this the point of it all?

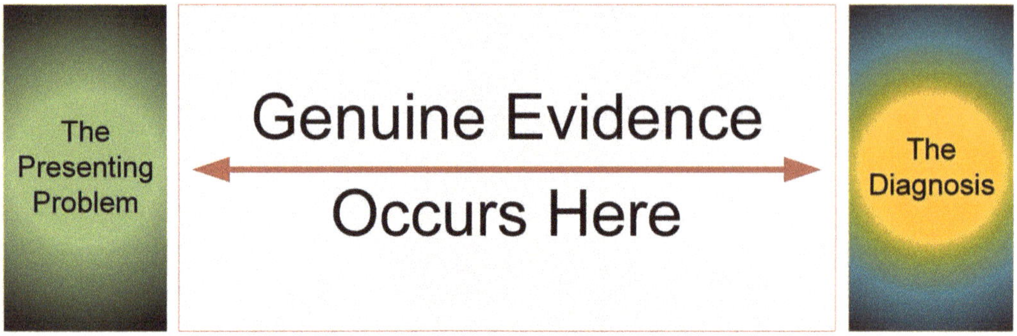

What Do I Mean By "Evidence?"

Some readers will read this subhead and wonder why this chapter even exists. After all, you've probably been collecting evidence for a long time now. But in this chapter, you'll hear some things about evidence you've likely never heard before—including that there are only two kinds.

One kind will quickly lead you to the heart of the matter. The other kind will cause you to make all manner of unintentional—and often overlooked—errors.

I call the first kind of evidence, "Genuine Evidence."

I call the second kind of evidence, "Inferred Evidence."

What makes evidence, "Genuine Evidence?"

Genuine Evidence is "the things you literally observe in your room."

In hindsight, you can picture these things, because you've actually witnessed them happen. These things can be true things, like seeing patients well up with tears—or the times patients wince or flinch. But they can also be things which patients insist are true, but which you suspect are false—such as them saying a spouse *always* or *never* says, or does, something.

Inferred Evidence, on the other hand, is evidence which diagnosticians and patients logically assume has occurred. The thing is, not having actually witnessed these things, you cannot know for sure they have happened. Either way though, once posited, from then on, these logical inferences will so distort the evidence gathering process that you may at times begin to question your skills.

The most insidious of these confusing times?

Feeling something about the diagnosis just doesn't feel quite right.

Realize, all diagnosticians feel this way at times, as all patients infer evidence. When patients feel pressured to answer questions, they can blurt out all manner of sketchy ideas. This often occurs, even when you reassure them it's okay to not have an answer. Human beings often have trouble not knowing things.

Know that diagnosticians, themselves, can also do this—especially in cases where great suffering pressures them to arrive at a diagnosis quickly. And diagnosticians being human, they then waste time trying to fit these inferences into the case.

This is often the case for diagnosticians who work in an acute care, psychiatric hospital setting.

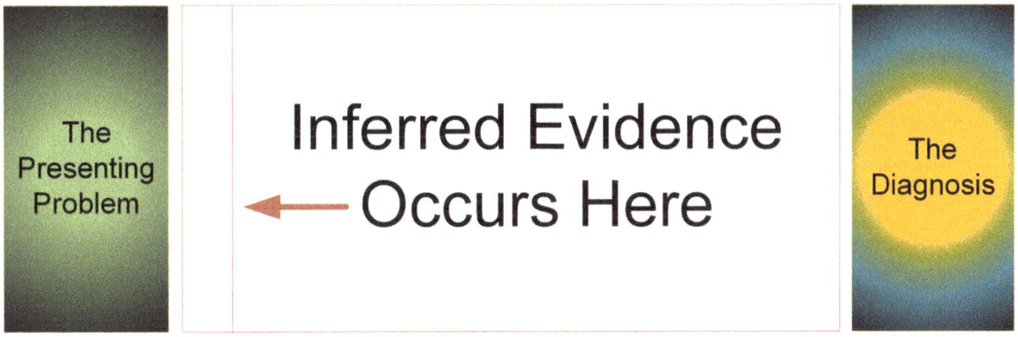

Ultimately, these inferred diagnoses just prolong the patient's suffering. This said, some readers may be misinterpreting what I'm saying as that you should never include inferred evidence.

Actually, I am not saying this. While diagnosticians themselves should strive to never infer evidence, the inferences they hear patients make can be helpful.

Why?

Because everything diagnosticians *witness* is literally Genuine Evidence. Again, Genuine Evidence includes everything diagnosticians directly observe in their therapy rooms. This not only includes literally true things like observations of the patient's affect and mood. It also includes things patients believe are true, even when you know they are incomplete, misinterpreted, or just plain false.

Here then is the first of many things to take away from this chapter.

Every single thing you literally witness should be seen as diagnostically relevant.

Big things. Small things. Seemingly irrelevant things. Discard nothing. Every single thing you see should get put into the diagnostic funnel.

The thing is, under pressure, diagnosticians often try to infer what is and isn't relevant. Ironically, in my years as a diagnostician, I've often been surprised by how something I'd assumed was irrelevant was the key to a case. This means you should try to never assume you know what's relevant or how this evidence fits a diagnosis. Each and every piece of evidence must eventually be accounted for, and these pieces must fit into a single cohesive visual picture. And if you can't do this, then you must assume, the diagnostic process is as yet, incomplete.

What About Using Scientific Inferences (Hypotheses) As Evidence?

Already, some readers may see where I've been going with all this. The idea? That to be a proper diagnostician, you must become skilled at setting aside professional assumptions. In doing so, you leave space for the diagnosis to emerge from the evidence *naturally*—all on its own. As opposed to creating a hypothesis based on logic, inferences, guesses, and first impressions—and in doing so, skipping passed most of the legitimate evidence gathering process.

What's wrong with using a hypothesis to diagnose? Oh, where do I begin?

As I think about it, a story which has been told many times comes to mind.

What will help here is if you can picture this story as I tell it.

The main quality all Genuine Evidence has in common is that you can literally picture it. So to be a skilled diagnostician, you must get good at picturing things.

As for the story, it's about a drunk diagnostician who has lost his car keys. Forgive me if you've already heard it. But even if you have, you may not have realized what it means. It's a story about what happens when you infer evidence. It's also a story which points to one of the main flaws in the present scientific method.

What's Wrong With Hypotheses? (The Drunk Who Lost His Keys)

Picture a well-dressed, seriously-drunk man—about forty—standing under a streetlight. His car is parked across the street from where he's standing and it's night. Know that if you're actually picturing this scene, this man's car will have a color. Please picture this car and silently, in your head, say the name of the color you see.

Except for the streetlight, it's very dark, and this man appears to be looking for something on the ground. Beyond this streetlight though, the street and surrounding trees and houses are hidden in close to pitch black night. Only the ground directly under the streetlight is clearly visible—the rest is hidden in darkness. And at some point, this man's friend, also drunk, arrives at the car.

This second drunk sees his friend searching for something on the ground, and not knowing what he's doing, asks him, "What happened?" Drunk Number One then tells Drunk Number Two, "I'm looking for my car keys. I lost them." The friend then asks the logical next question. "Where did you last see them?" Drunk Number One then says, "Over, by the car."

The story then continues to logically unfold as the friend asks, "Then why are you looking for them over there, under the streetlight?" To which, Drunk Number One answers, "Because I can see better under the streetlight."

This is what beginning with a hypothesis does for anyone seeking to arrive at a diagnosis. It limits the diagnostic evidence to what you already see as relevant. Ironically, this all but guarantees you will not arrive at a proper diagnosis. A proper diagnosis has a distinct sequence. We'll talk about what it is in a moment.

Admittedly, a diagnostician may, if talented enough, guess the correct name of this diagnosis. But guesses make you forever question the validity of your work, especially if someone asks you for your evidence.

As for why people use hypotheses if they lead to so many problems, for one thing, because the present scientific method claims they're the best place to begin.

Also, without a hypothesis, it can seem, there's no limit to where you'll need to look for evidence. Know this is untrue. Admittedly, I need to offer proof for this claim. Know we'll look at this and the many flaws in using hypotheses throughout this chapter—as well as exploring a better path to take during the diagnostic process.

With this in mind, I want to begin with one of my favorite metaphors for a proper diagnostic process—the train station metaphor.

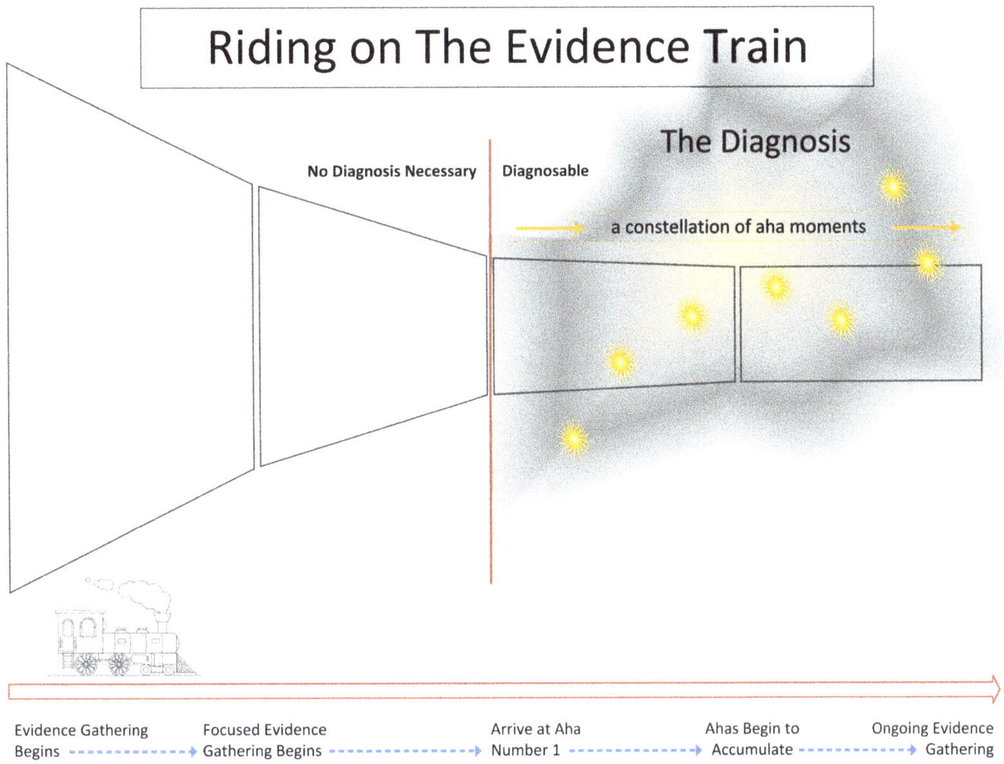

How Is The Diagnostic Process Like A Journey?

One way to think about how you arrive at a diagnosis is to picture riding on a train. Why? Because you *arrive* at a diagnosis the same way you arrive at a train station. Obviously, you can't make the train go faster. Once you're on it, you have to just let it take you there. So in one sense, a train ride is "developmental." It has a knowable natural progression, especially if you've ridden on this train before.

Another thing to know about arriving at a diagnosis is that it's a kind of "light bulb moment." Arriving at train stations feels the same way. Think about it. When a plane lands or a train arrives, we often say, "We made it."

We logically knew this would happen. Yet somehow, it still surprises us.

My point?

Arriving at a proper diagnosis feels the same way. To properly diagnose, you must learn to trust the Diagnostic Process—in the same way you learn to trust a train to take you to your destination.

In both cases, you cannot make the process go any faster. Rather, you do what you must, then just let it take you there.

What do I mean when I say "you do what you must"?

This is what we'll address next.

Before we do, please note, this section's takeaway.

This is this chapter's first takeaway—*you must learn to trust the process.*

A Few Things You'll Need To Do During The Diagnostic Process

[1] To begin with, ***you'll have to revisit the "scientific method" you've been using.*** To do this, you'll need to become familiar with—and learn to use—an alternate method. By now, you've no doubt heard me say the name of this new method.

"Constellated Science."

You've already been exposed to this new method, in this book, many times.

Obviously, deliberately choosing to diagnose this way will require a leap of faith. Know that using the old science has been making you overwork—every time. The thing is, you have it in you to learn this new method. I promise. And once you do, as they say, "You can never go back."

The biggest part of learning to use this new method? Accessing your "baby mind." Why? Because being in this state of mind is how babies learn so much, so quickly. In effect, learning to do this will allow you to access your sleeping genius.

Think I'm bullshitting you here?

Maybe I am.

Then again, perhaps you just may be far smarter than you think.

[2] ***You'll also need to learn to use a new math*** called, "tipping-point based" math. Everything in this book has been based on this math. What's wrong with the old maths, e.g., statistics, scale-based maths, and counting math? I suspect when we look at that question, you'll be surprised by how much you never realized. And if you're math-phobic? Then you're in luck. This math is as easy as flipping a coin.

[3] This next thing I tell you may be the most critical consideration of all.

Y***ou must divide the Diagnostic Process into two clearly-defined parts.***

Know these two parts cannot be prematurely intermingled. Mix them up and the Diagnostic Process falls apart. Also, these two parts cannot be done out of order. Part One must be well under way before Part Two begins.

[4] What is Part One? It goes by several names. Learning to do it is the focus of this chapter. Its main name? **Evidence Gathering**. But you can also call it **Diagnostic Pre-learning.** Or you can call it, "accessing your baby mind." Whatever you call it, **Evidence Gathering** is the most important part of diagnosing. From the sound of it, you may think you've been doing it already. I'm claiming this is different. My proof? When you're **Evidence Gathering** (part one) you're not looking to know the diagnosis. You're simply doing what babies do every minute of their lives—in an unrestricted way, you're just taking in what you see.

[5] **Arriving at a Diagnosis** (part two), on the other hand, is a by-product of Evidence Gathering—so it's NOT something you do. Rather, it's something that just happens to you. In a sudden flash of insight, you suddenly realize you've discovered a constellation of patterns in the data. So you can't arrive at a diagnosis logically any more than you can logically make a train arrive sooner.

Rather, at some point, the diagnosis just dawns on you.

Said in other words, no amount of intelligence or will power can force a diagnosis to appear. Moreover, unlike what many diagnosticians get taught to expect of themselves, you certainly can't figure it out. Rather, a diagnosis is something which just occurs to you during the latter part of the evidence gathering process. This means you must learn to trust the process and just "let it happen." And to do this, you must have faith in yourself.

Why Divide The Diagnostic Process Into Two Parts?

To some readers, it may seem obvious why I'm dividing the Diagnostic Process into two parts. It's like dividing a journey on a train into the same two parts. In one part, you look out the windows (you gather evidence). In the other, you arrive at your destination (you arrive at the diagnosis). Unfortunately, most diagnosticians never get taught to separate these two parts.

Sometimes this intermingling begins the minute they hear the patient say a few words. Sometimes they do it just based on the way a patient's voice sounds in the first phone call. Doing this is like trying to begin a train ride at the destination. Obviously, this can't be done. No more than you can gaze out at the scenery on a train ride after you've arrived at your destination.

The point here is simple. Beginning the Diagnostic Process at a diagnosis is just as illogical. Evidence Gathering must come first. This is similar to the way you can't look out of train windows and observe the scenery after the fact. You have to do it along the way.

A good way to see why this matters is to imagine you've arrived at your destination. You see a friend on the train station platform, waiting for you. She then does what most people would do—she asks you how your trip was. The thing is, you were asleep most of the way. So you don't actually know.

Because you've been asked though, you say what you assume it was like. Later you feel squirrelly about having done this. Diagnosticians who begin with assumptions feel similarly squirrelly about the diagnoses they give. To avoid this, you must remain awake the whole time—so you can see the evidence for yourself.

Some people will, at this point, still be questioning why I'm claiming you shouldn't create a ***hypothesis***—especially one based on years of training and experience. I'm saying this because as I said a few pages back, a hypothesis is just another form of logically prejudging an outcome *before gathering the evidence*. If you do this, you've not only already closed your mind to all but a few possible diagnoses. You've also already decided what kinds of evidence you should be looking for.

Can You Recall The Five Things You Need to Keep In Mind?

Before we turn to other things—including the problems with ordinary maths, I'm going to briefly review the five things you must do during the Diagnostic Process. As you review this list, please notice—the ***first*** two reminders refer to math.

After we finish this short summary, I'll do my best to explain this math to you.

If you then look at the ***last*** two reminders you'll see, together, they refer to the structure of a natural diagnosis. No hypotheses. No logical inferences. Just baby-minded exploration.

Finally, please notice how the ***middle*** reminder refers to how these four things are to be used. As I said, the last two reminders refer to the Diagnostic Process, while the first two refer to the science and math behind this process. So the last two reminders refer to ***what*** you do during diagnosis, while the first two refer to ***how*** you do what you do.

The list?

- To begin with, ***you'll have to revisit the "scientific method" you've been using.***
- You'll also need ***to learn to use a new math*** called, "tipping-point based" math.
- You must then ***divide the diagnostic process into two clearly-defined parts.***
- **Part One— Evidence Gathering (also called Diagnostic Pre-learning).**
- **Part Two— Letting the Evidence Speak For Itself.**

Next we're going to take a look at how the maths diagnostician's use confound and complicate the diagnostic process. Like each gender often says about the other gender, with these maths, you "Can't live with 'em. Can't live without 'em."

Can Math Ever Accurately Measure People?

If I toss a coin and after it lands, I ask you for the result—as long as you can see the coin, you'll be one hundred percent certain of the outcome. Amazingly, if you extend this simple truth to all real world measurements, you end up with the same certainty about your mathematical results.

There is a caveat though. Your measurements must measure naturally occurring, tipping-point based outcomes. With coin tosses, doing this is easy. Coins are two-sided and physical. But sometimes creating these tests is hard, like when you're trying to measure a patient's anger. Like all feelings, anger is invisible and by itself, doesn't have two sides.

Given you know how to do this though, why would any science-based endeavor—including diagnosis—use any other math? This is what we're about to discuss. Realize some of this may seem so hard that you fear you may never be able to get it. And some of it may seem so easy that you may experience what I call, the "Jesse Effect." This occurs when you think things are so obvious that all you need do is skim them. But in doing so, you fail to grasp, let alone retain, most of it.

What can help here is to try to picture the examples I offer you. Do this well enough and you'll retain most of it, and doing this will help you to change lives.

What's Wrong With Using Existing Maths To Measure People?

Most of the errors in existing diagnostic manuals can be traced back to just two things—shitty definitions and using maths in the wrong way. If we ignore these errors, we doom our attempts to gather proper evidence right from the start.

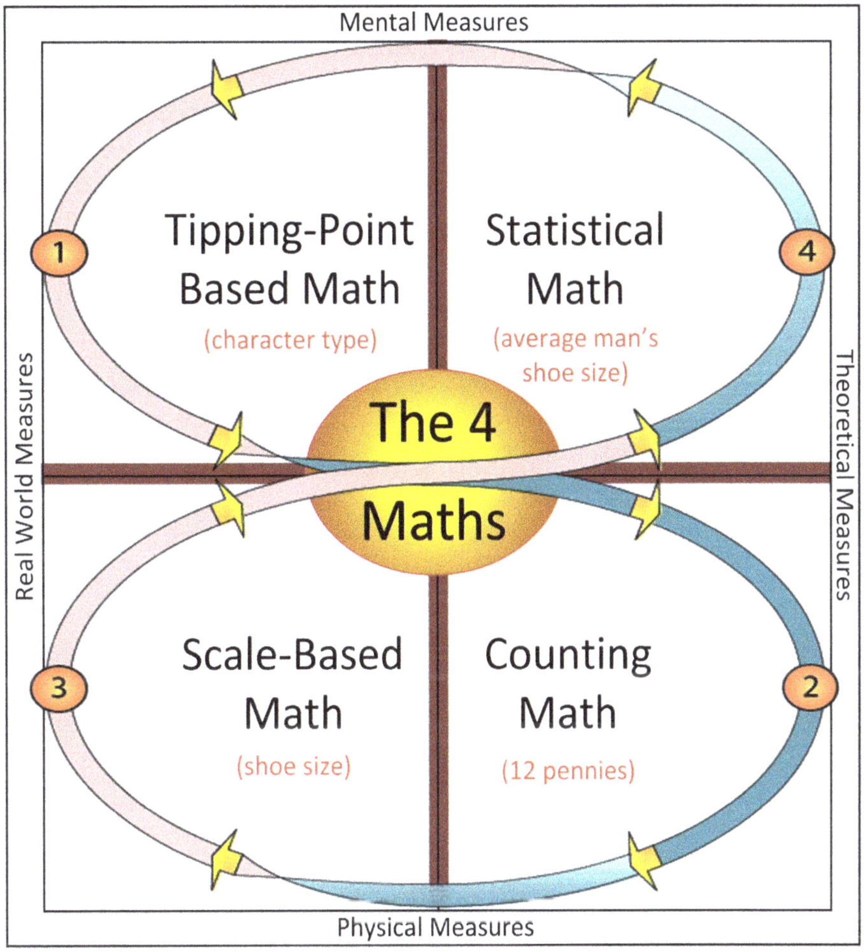

There is a solution though. This solution has two parts.

One. Use pairs of perfect opposites to define all words and terms—perfect opposites are complete sets. Then two. Use these definitions to create tipping-point based tests which result in accurate real world measures of individual people.

In this book, we've used logically geometric drawings—like the drawing you see above—along with sets of colored, shaped lines—to address the first of these problems. These drawings result in clear, scientifically measurable definitions.

The thing is, even with properly defined terms, we still need to be able to properly measure these things. The problem? The idea that the maths we use to measure people are so inaccurate, that even when we measure well defined ***theoretical*** things, our measurements often do not translate well in ***real world*** situations.

For example, take the math the authors of existing manuals base most of their claims of scientific validity on. In theory, statistics, used correctly, should have some validity in the real world. At the same time, anyone who has taken a college statistics class should immediately see the flaw in using statistics to diagnose people.

College Statistics 101 classes clearly state, you need a large enough sample size for outcomes to be considered valid. Said in statistical language, you need a big enough "N" in order to smooth out the bumps in real world variations.

Have you ever thought about what this statement actually means?

It means "N" cannot be one person. Not ever.

How can diagnostic manuals have been based on statistics then?

Because if you have a large enough sample size, you have a built in "fudge factor." And given a high enough "F" factor, those authors can claim their books are scientifically accurate.

Obviously, these claims of scientific accuracy are bullshit of the highest order.

Diagnosticians don't diagnose large groups. We diagnose individuals.

Oddly, this idea—that statistics isn't supposed to be applied to individual cases—is the idea most college statistics professors begin semesters with. Based on the titles of those books, I guess the authors of existing diagnostic manuals never got the notice. Then again, even people who have taken college statistics classes rarely question the work of people who choose to ignore this warning. Why not? Because as we all know, statistics is one of the most difficult classes to pass.

This leads many people to assume professional statisticians simply know more than they do. This is untrue. Indeed, have you ever asked yourself why statistics classes are so difficult? Because of all the maths, statistics is the one which is based on, and contains, the absolute highest level of unintelligible bullshit.

Think I'm wrong?

Consider what Jacob Bernoulli, the man who wrote the first book on statistics (Ars Conjectandi | The Art of Conjecture, 1713), had to say.

In his book, Bernoulli warned against treating statistics as equal to real world evidence. Rather, he said, statistics (stochastically derived evidence) equates to a rough guess about what the real world evidence would be—if we could actually see it.

Not a very reassuring thought.

What about maths like counting math and scale-based maths though? Are they any better? After all, they're much more understandable.

Unfortunately, when used to measure real world things, surprisingly, they're not. Know we'll be looking at a few examples of these maths—shoe size and the number of apples needed for a pie—in a bit. And yes, seeing these two maths as flawed as well may be hard.

We use them to make personal decisions almost every day of our adult lives.

Even so, I'm going to claim, all three of these maths are so seriously flawed that they should never be used to measure individual people. No coincidence, legitimate scientists so often mock and ridicule our efforts to measure things like people's feelings. Admittedly, in cases like counting apples and trying on shoes, these flaws don't really matter. We can pick different apples and try on different shoes and in doing so adjust for any errors on the fly. But when it's people's suffering we're measuring, we can't just pick another person—let alone diagnose them based on some statistical averaging. Ironically, scientists (and yes, we diagnosticians are scientists) are some of the most careful people on the planet. How then can I claim, the way we measure people is riddled with errors?

This is what we're about to look at.

How Accurate Is Math In General?

[Warning: What you're about to read is really hard shit. So do go slow. Or skip it if you need to.]

One way scientists claim their measurements are accurate is to say the results always come out the same. They see this "scientific sameness" as proof, these claims are accurate and true. Oddly, most practitioners of the old science never once question this belief—let alone realize, this claim is based on statistics.

What's wrong here? These people are claiming this reliability makes something true. ***Yet nothing in the natural world ever repeats the same way twice—and they're claiming they're measuring real world things.***

So when they get reliable outcomes, what does this prove? Nothing more than that their experiments are contrived, which is why they spend so much time carefully designing their experiments. In truth then, scientists rarely test things in real world contexts—whereas this is all we diagnosticians do. Clearly, we cannot use their method to diagnose. It doesn't work. To them, the "best designs" are those which yield the most "reliable" results. To us, the only ones that matter are the ones that help our patients.

Then there's the claim most scientists make that their measurements neither miss nor overlook anything important. According to Gödel's Incompleteness Theorem, however, this idea is also bullshit. Don't worry if you haven't met Gödel yet. The core idea here is also simple. His theorem states—"any theory capable of expressing elementary arithmetic cannot be both consistent and complete."

WTF does this mean?

It means counting math (or anything based largely on a system of mathematics, such as diagnosis) must be able ***to account for*** all possible cases—***or be considered incomplete***. To be honest, it took me a long time—and a lot of hard work—to understand what Gödel's saying here. Like most people, I'd, for so long, assumed these maths were true, that it took me years to accept they could be flawed.

So how can a thing as simple and believable as counting math be incomplete?

By including things it cannot define. And you cannot measure undefined things.

For instance, in simple arithmetic, the answer to dividing anything by zero is considered to be undefined. Translation. Simple arithmetic cannot solve this problem. So this statement has no meaning to mathematicians.

Mathematicians fudge their way around this incompleteness by claiming that dividing any number by zero will always give us a zero.

This claim is clearly bullshit as well. Can you see why?

Dividing anything by zero literally means "you are not doing anything."

And "not doing anything" includes that you are not doing math.

Are you having trouble seeing how this applies to diagnosis? Wait for it. I promise, it's coming. But I first need to digress for a moment.

This time, I need to say something similar about the way we use words. Here, I'm referring to the work of the philosopher, Ludwig Wittgenstein. Wittgenstein proved the same incompleteness exists for anything expressed in words.

His most famous quote?

"Whereof one cannot speak, thereof one must be silent."

WTF does this mean?

He's telling us, if we can't perfectly define our words, that we should shut the fuck up. In other words, he's saying that for most part, words are so vague and nebulous, that it's rare for two people to have the same exact meanings for the words they use.

He then adds that if you can't say a thing using perfectly clear, logical words, then don't bullshit and just keep your mouth shut. No surprise, Wittgenstein is considered to be one of the most acerbically harsh philosophers in history. And yes, he is mean. He certainly is. At the same time, can you see that he is right?

Shouldn't we either be correct in our words or be silent?

No coincidence, Gödel's and Wittgenstein's ideas both had a strong influence on me. I frequently imagined them calling "bullshit" on my claims—and for much of my life, they'd have been right. This led me to spend years developing Logical Geometry, the first math to define all things—including both numbers and words—without incompleteness. In a way then, these two challenges were a big part of everything I've done.

Fortunately for me, Logically Geometric maps answer both challenges. These maps create perfectly measurable sets of perfectly defined numbers, words and terms. This allows us to design tests which measure real world things accurately. Clearly, this applies to what we diagnosticians are mandated to do. We need to be able to measure people and their inner lives, with perfect accuracy, in the real world.

Before I explain how this is done, I first need to do as I've promised. I first need to explain, in a bit more detail, why I'm claiming existing maths are flawed.

We'll begin with the simplest math—counting math.

What's Wrong With Using Counting Math to Diagnose People?

The first of this trio of three flawed maths is what's commonly called "counting math." Counting math is what you use when you go to the supermarket to buy things like apples. For example, imagine you're making an apple pie and the recipe calls for 8 to 10 apples. My question to you is this.

Why can't the recipe call for a scientifically accurate number of apples?

Meaning what? ***That this statement literally assumes, all apples are identical.*** Yet in the real world, no two apples will ever be alike.

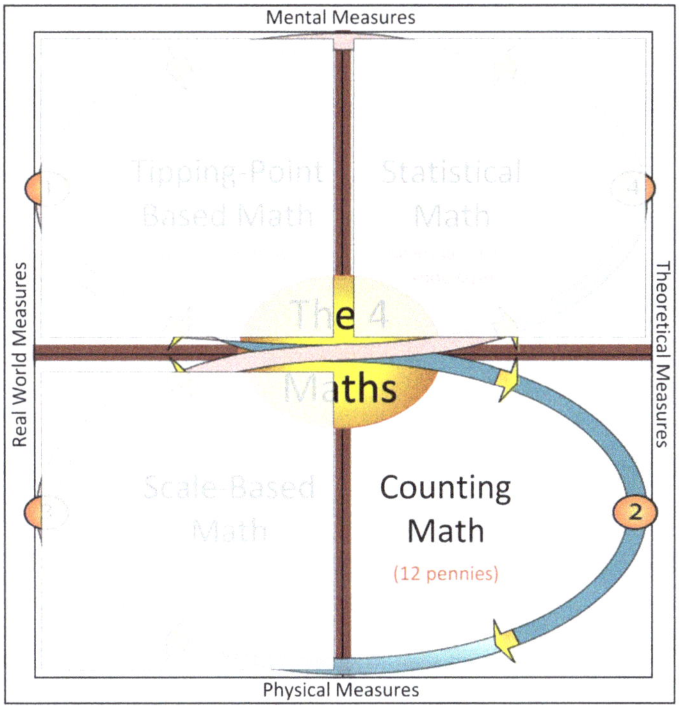

Does this make sense? Think about it. Have you ever gone to get eight apples and had the first eight you picked be the ones you bought? If all apples were identical, you could do this. But this isn't true. So you can't.

But if this isn't true, then how can we claim we've bought "eight" apples? The same way we diagnosticians can claim we can use counting math to diagnose.

We fudge it.

Do you see it yet? We diagnostician's often ask things like, "How many times did you do such and such?" Given this number is significant—or if the patient answers "always" or "never," we often assume this answer is accurate. But these kinds of answers are no more accurate than saying we've bought eight apples. For instance, consider what it would be like to ask a patient how often (how many times) they feel depressed.

Which kinds of questions would be more accurate—counting the number of "yes" answers to a bunch of ill-defined, vaguely-phrased questions—or having a patient point to the depression line and saying, "A lot." Know that recently, someone I supervise who does diagnostic intakes in an acute-care mental hospital showed a new patient a drawing of the Four States of Mind lines. She then asked this patient, a teenaged boy who was presenting as severely mentally ill, to draw a line to explain how he felt.

This boy had never previously seen any of the lines we use to describe states of mind. Yet all on his own, he, without hesitation, drew a line he'd not seen before.

Which line? He drew an accurate Bipolar One meaning line. His diagnosis? Bipolar One. Are you realizing what this means?

A severely mentally ill teen with no training whatsoever accurately described his diagnosis. Moreover, this occurred before he'd even been given this diagnosis.

What's Wrong With Using Scale-Based Math to Diagnose?

Ever used one of those scale-based questionnaires to assess for depression—for example, the founder of CBT, Aaron Beck's, ***Beck Depression Inventory***? How about the World Health Organization's ***Major Depression Inventory***? Or ***The Edinburgh Postnatal Depression Scale*** (EPDS)?

Did you know these questionnaires were developed by psychiatrists?

Do you find it strange that none of them were practicing personality theorists? Yet despite their lack of expertise, they still claim to know how to measure people. Even grandmas know, fake scale-based assessments suck on people. Have you ever wondered how they know? This is what we're about to explore.

To begin with, the ***Beck Depression Inventory*** asks things like, "Are you sad?" Possible answers?

(0) I do not feel sad.
(1) I feel sad.
(2) I am sad all the time and I can't snap out of it.
(3) I am so sad or unhappy that I can't stand it.

Never mind that they never define the word "sad," even though no two people would ever see it exactly the same way. Do you see the numbers? They do not begin with one. Rather, they begin with zero.

This means these folks aren't using counting math. They're using scale-based math. What's wrong with using scale-based math?

To begin with, consider the patently stupid ways these questions are phrased.

Mentally ill patients routinely fail to recognize symptoms in themselves. So how can you expect a mentally ill patient to know something like, "I do not feel sad"? What does this sentence even mean to a healthy person? Does it mean "never," "rarely," or "intermittently?"

This also does not account for the relief patients often feel when they finally sit across from a caregiver. So if they answer, "I do not feel sad," are they saying this because they're finally feeling someone cares?

What about that last question—asking whether the person "can't stand it." Do all people tolerate sadness the same way? Obviously not. So how in the hell can a linear scale represent things which are all over the place?

All of it is simply more bad science. Just pretend all people, like all apples, are the same. Then there's the scale Beck uses to rate the results. Where do these numbers come from? Is there any science behind them? Beck never says.

The numbers?

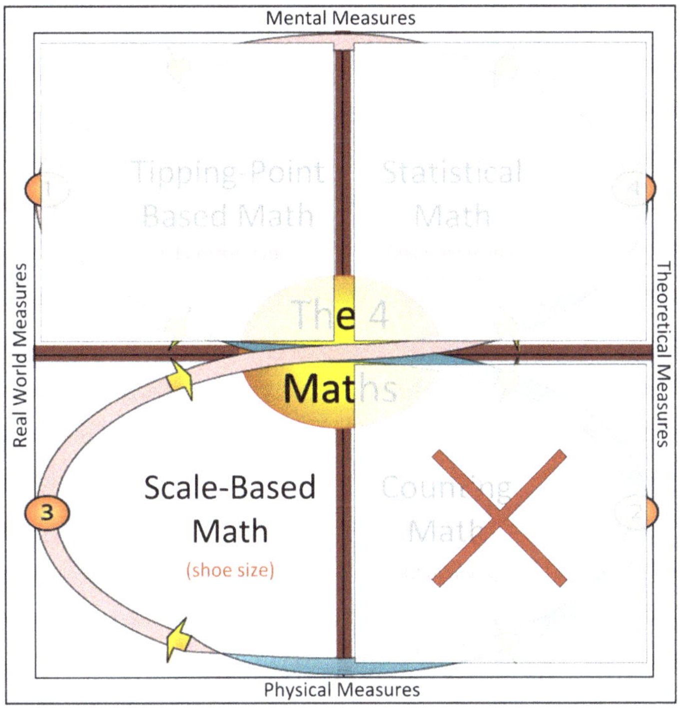

- 0–9: indicates minimal depression
- 10–18: indicates mild depression
- 19–29: indicates moderate depression
- 30–63: indicates severe depression.

Picture these four ranges as increments on a funky ruler. 0-9 is nine small ticks. 10-18 is another nine. But 19-29 is ten. And 30-63? Well you get the idea.

Where do these ranges come from?

From psychiatrists making guesses about something they know nothing about. No science here. None at all. Then again, all fake scales are bad science.

Think I'm wrong or being unduly harsh on Mr. Beck? Then consider this.

After CBT being touted for decades as the most thoroughly vetted talk therapy, multiple studies now show how improvements from this treatment do not last. For instance, a paper in the journal Psychological Bulletin claims CBT is becoming less effective over time. And after analyzing 70 studies conducted between 1977 and 2014, researchers Tom Johnsen and Oddgeir Friborg concluded, CBT is now roughly half as effective in treating depression as it used to be.

The real reasons I'm claiming CBT is bullshit?

Right away, I can think of three problems.

The science used to claim it's effective is riddled with ill-defined terms, ridiculous scales, and statistical nonsense.

My evidence for this?

It's a simple, straight-forward, easy-to-see idea.

There is no such thing as a "standard person."

There's not even a "standard" lab rat.

So while treating rats like this may be acceptable in the name of advancing science, treating suffering human beings like this is—to be blunt—fucking stupid. The point? Using scale-based math to measure people assumes there is a standard person. There isn't. So let's just move on.

What's Wrong With Using Statistics to Diagnose People?

No need to say much more than I've already said.

Using statistics to diagnose is like using a fire hose as a waterpik.

A more relevant question is, why are people not more troubled by these flaws?

The answer. Because human beings tolerate wrong answers better than they tolerate having no answers.

In effect, people rationalize statistics as being better than nothing. Admittedly, when you're designing an agency wide policy, sometimes, it is. But when you're diagnosing a single human being? Not so much. Want to see this for yourself? Here's a simple test. This test involves answering a few short questions.

Do take your time answering.

[1] Would it be OK with you if the only TV programs you had access to, or the only books you were allowed to read, were limited to what statistics said most people your age normally liked?

[2] Would it be OK with you if the doctor you went to was statistically decided for you as well?

[3] Would it be OK with you if a computer statistically determined what kind of hair cut you got or what kind of clothes you could wear?

[4] How about a spouse or where you should live or what you should be doing for a living? Would you be OK with this being statistically decided for you as well?

Is this how you want the treatment for you or a loved one to be decided—by a statistical computer model? Obviously, no sane person would agree to do any of these things. Yet the "science" behind most diagnoses is entirely the same. Worse yet, most of the statistics behind these manuals don't consider personality at all—let alone, whether the things you do or don't report are based on personality or wounds.

Ok. Let's try a more serious test. If you can pass this test, I'll agree to publicly embrace statistics (hand me that puke bag, please).

The test?

Literally, in your mind, picture five of your patients—*all five at once.*

Know you'll need to offer me proof that you are actually picturing these five people—*all five at once.*

The proof?

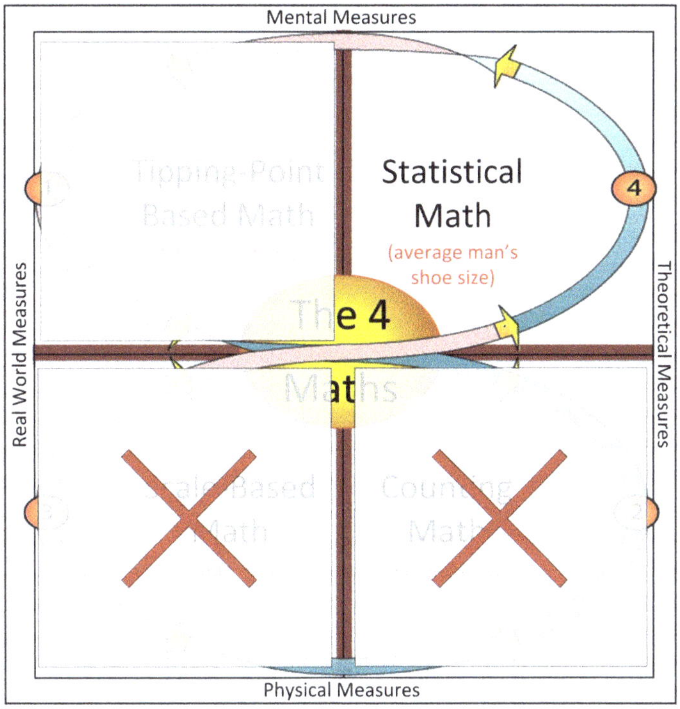

If you are able to do this, then you can simultaneously see all of their eye colors. Literally—you'll be able to see these colors, not just think of the words.

Keep in mind the specifics of what I've just asked you to do. I've asked you to picture all of their eyes—*all at once*.

If you're simultaneously picturing all five sets of eyes, then you can't be switching between them, not even quickly. Rather, you need to be picturing all five of them simultaneously, all at the same time.

Did you actually try to do this?

If not, please do try to do it now.

Knowing what the outcome would in theory be changes nothing.

The outcome?

Clearly, doing this is humanly impossible. Even seeing a photo of all five together would require you to switch between their faces to see their eye colors.

My point here?

Could you diagnose multiple people, all at the same time?

Obviously not.

Can you now see why I think, all existing diagnostic manuals with the word "statistical" in their titles should be relegated to the shit heap, post-haste?

Suffering people deserve personal attention. And to give them this personal attention, a diagnostic manual would need to scientifically address individual cases.

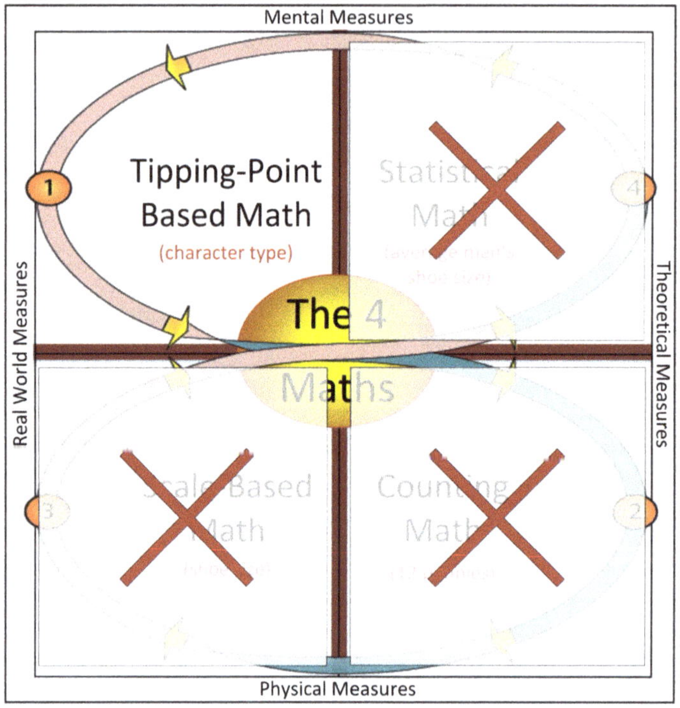

What About Tipping-point Based Math? Any Flaws There?

We've already spoken about tipping-point based measures a number of times in this book. Here, my favorite way to refer to them is to say—you decide which one of a pair of perfect opposites a person, place, or thing best resembles.

Obviously, any tipping-point based test is far simpler to execute than tests based on the previously discussed maths. Like coin tosses, the outcomes of tests based on pairs of perfect opposites are easily determined. And even when measuring real world things, you can be 100% certain of the results.

Admittedly, setting up coin-toss tests is easy. But coming up with perfect opposites in personality can be hard. Not nearly as hard as trying to make the Beck Depression Inventory match what's happening in people's minds though. As for the specifics of ***what*** you'll need to measure, we'll discuss that in Chapter 6. Before we do, we'll first need to discuss ***how*** to gather the evidence we'll be measuring—including how you'll do this in a sequence of four separate steps.

Evidence Gathering: Introducing The Four Steps

Finally, all that agonizingly difficult math stuff is behind us. We can now turn to the topic at hand. Here, we'll be looking at the four steps diagnosticians must take to arrive at accurate results. Please know, like the kinds of things people learn in a painting and art school, parts of diagnosis will always be an art. At the same time, a proper diagnosis should always be well-grounded in real science.

I call what I'm going to introduce you to ***The Four Steps for Evidence Gathering***. Know these steps are only meant to be a rough guide. Used well, they function like draw organizers, where empty compartments help you to decide what and where to put things in this drawer. The compartments closest to the front of this drawer naturally function best for the stuff you use most. And those which are at the very back of the drawer? Well you get the idea.

Know I've arranged these four steps similarly to the way those drawer organizers work. I've arranged them in the easiest to use, most natural order. By this, I mean, this order optimizes the chances a diagnosis will emerge from the evidence naturally—all on its own. Thus doing the first step first matters the most—and so on.

Keep in mind, the more you use these steps, the more using them will feel natural to you. In Chapter 6, we'll look at some cases from actual Grand Rounds groups my colleagues and I have held. We meet once a month, for two hours, in part, to reinforce this method in each other. Why? Because like Evidence Gathering, there's always more to learn. And the more we use these steps, the more we learn.

Evidence Gathering's Four Steps: The Importance of This Sequence

At this point, we're ready to begin to explore how Evidence Gathering works. And since we'll be looking at some real life examples in the next chapter, this will be but a brief look. I suggest you try to read these words *without trying to understand or memorize them*. We'll talk more about why I'm saying this before we end this chapter.

The Four Steps?

- **Step One** - **Use Initial Data to Begin to Set The Diagnostic Baseline**
- **Step Two** - **Have the Patient Slowly Elaborate the Presenting Problem**
- **Step Three** - **Construct a Detailed Mental Image of the Disorder Present**
- **Step Four** - **Note The Direction of The Patient's "Internal Tide"**

Step One - Use Initial Data to Begin to Set The Diagnostic Baseline

In step one, you acquire the new patient's [1] name, [2] age, and [3] presenting problem ***in the client's own words***. Obviously, getting the first two things is easy. It's the last one which gives most diagnosticians trouble.

Why say this?

Because rather than literally writing down the client's own words, most diagnosticians—almost immediately—reduce what clients say to professional language. These restatements then reduce the patient's words to the "over-cooked string bean" version of what's been said.

They also almost entirely derive from inferences. Up to this point, the patient has barely spoken. Yet by restating things, the diagnostician has already posited a hypothesis about the nature of this patient's problems.

Can you see how doing this equates to looking for your car keys under the streetlight, across from your car? Here, rather than waiting until you've gathered sufficient evidence, you're assuming you already know where to look.

This will then cause you to look for symptoms which fit a diagnosis, rather than fitting a diagnosis to the patient's symptoms.

Suffering human beings never present exactly the same way twice.

Interviewing this patient two days later could result in a very different picture.

Bonus Points - Have the Patient Write Down Their Problems

Give yourself extra credit if you have the patient write out their reasons for coming ***in their own words***. Know that in the next chapter, I'll demonstrate this in action, by offering you a number of examples of gathering evidence both ways.

Finally, give yourself extra bonus points if, instead of having them do this in a text or an email, you get them to handwrite these words and bring them in. Know it's not that emails or texts are bad. It's just that the client's handwriting can be valuable evidence as well. In fact, in the next chapter, I'll describe a case where the client's handwriting held the key to the case.

∞

Step Two - Have the Patient *Slowly* Elaborate the Presenting Problem

At this point, you have the three most important pieces of evidence you'll need for any case. A name. An age. And the presenting problem, stated—and better yet, handwritten—in the patient's own words. When a new patient calls for the first time, these three things should be your main goals. Empathy? Yes. Listening with an open mind? Yes. But other than contact information, these three things are all you should record. Nothing more.

I'll explain why in Chapter 6.

What do you then do in the first face-to-face?

Here is where Step Two begins.

The best method?

Given the patient doesn't arrive so overwhelmed that they have trouble being clear, hand them a deck of 3x5 cards.

Then say, "I'd like you to write down why you're here, one idea to a card."

Then add, "Know that what you're about to write just may change your life."

Bonus Points - Physically Document and Separate the Gathered Evidence

Why use 3x5 cards? So the patient can list the parts of the presenting problem—one part per card. No need to have them write out small details or complete sentences either. Best is one to two short phrases. The goals? To get the person to reveal patterns in the way they communicate, while focusing on learning to better understand themselves. Also, hopefully, these cards will include the names of the significant people in their life.

Why do this? It's simple. To arrive at a proper diagnosis, you need to see how this person does in relationships with others. Using people's names also personalizes the process and gives you a better picture of the patient's life. Also, pictures, not words, should always be the diagnostician's ultimate goal. If you can't picture what a patient says, then you cannot, and do not, know this patient.

∞

Step Three - Construct a Detailed Mental Image of the Disorder Present

If you've done the first two steps well enough, you've begun to picture the basics of this patient's life. In doing so, you've managed to create the beginnings of a diagnostic baseline. Now it's time to begin to collect pictures of the disorder which is bringing this patient to therapy.

Ask this patient to picture times when this disorder did and didn't trouble them.

Keep in mind, if you can get the patient to voice this data as pairs of opposites, you will gain a lot. This includes gathering a broad spectrum of responses to this part of the patient's life. For example, say you ask your patient about his marriage and he tells you, "We fight all the time." Get him to picture a time they were fighting. But then ask him to picture times when they were getting along.

Another example would be if your patient reports she came to therapy to get over being depressed. Avoid asking her something mind-numbingly stupid—like why she thinks she's depressed. Evidence Gathering should not include requests for hypotheses. Instead, ask the patient to try to picture times she felt depressed. Then ask her to picture times when she was not depressed.

Bonus Points - Bookending & Complex Event-sized Disorders

If you limit the evidence you gather to "words which create pictures in your mind," you will eliminate most extraneous or misleading data. For instance, asking the patient whose marriage is troubling him, "where he met his wife," will bookend this set of questions. Here, by "bookend," I mean, it will create a working continuum on which to further explore the disorder. Why do this? Because quite often, what initially brings a couple together points to the Complex Event-sized Disorder which will eventually threaten to break them apart. This too can be the key to the case.

∞

Step Four - Note The Direction of The Patient's "Internal Tide"

Imagine your patient is riding in a boat on a river, and that you are looking down at them from above. This vantage point should allow you to see tides in this person's life. Here, by "tides," I'm referring to patterns which can point you towards the patient's "personality constellation." In particular, you should be looking to discover as much as you can about this person's personality.

Is this patient Mind first or Body first? You should be looking for this evidence throughout these four steps. You should also be looking for evidence as to whether this patient is Me first or You first. And if, as you're reading this, you have no clue what these terms mean? Then at this point, don't worry. Just know, these ideas refer to some of the things you'll use to create a proper diagnostic baseline.

Bonus Points - Spend Time Learning Measurable Personality Measures

Many of these measures have been at least briefly mentioned in previous chapters in this book. This said, you may want to explore ways to measure personality more deeply. My 2011 book, *Unraveling Human Nature*, is a good place to begin.

Know I'll also have a lot more to say on this topic in the next chapter.

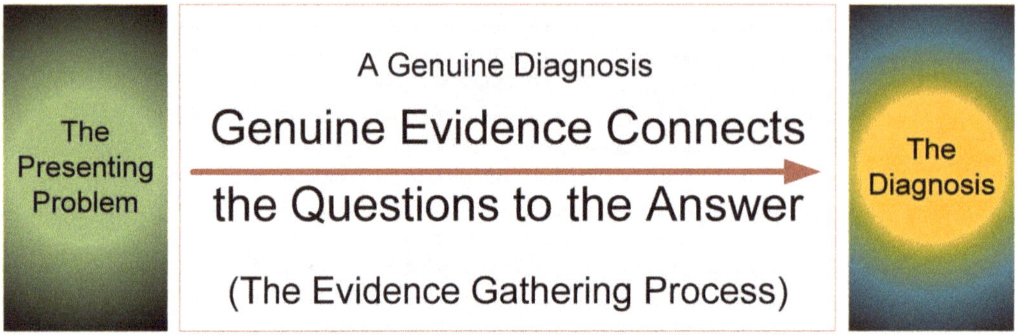

Four Things *to Keep in Mind* As You Begin to Gather Evidence

Having given you a basic outline for the Evidence Gathering Process, I want to briefly review a few other things to keep in mind. It's likely none of this stuff got taught to you back in school. Rather, these things all derive from the train metaphor I mentioned a few pages back. The first thing to keep in mind? It's simple.

[1] All train journeys begin at a starting point. ***The starting point for all diagnostic journeys should always be where the patient is at.*** By this, I mean, gathering evidence should always begin with paying attention to the small details present in patients ***as they arrive.*** Seemingly insignificant details can hold the entire key to a case.

The second thing to keep in mind?

[2] All train journeys occur on a continuous, pre-defined path. All diagnostic journeys occur on a well-defined path as well. The well-defined path in diagnosis? The timeline of the patient's life. ***Here, as each new piece of evidence appears, it should always be placed onto this timeline, before asking any more questions.*** This is why you've asked for the client's current age. Asking for their birth date then creates this timeline. Then each piece of evidence gets placed onto this timeline. Doing this ensures the path from presenting problem to diagnosis will emerge over time.

The third thing to keep in mind?

[3] All train journeys include twists and turns. All diagnostic journeys do too. There are no naturally-occurring, straight lines out in nature—there are none in the mind either. This means, during diagnosis, you must resist any urges to reshape the path of the patient's thoughts. Rather, ***you should always honor the naturally-occurring twists and turns in the patient's mind, as these deviations can reveal a lot.***

Finally, the fourth thing to keep in mind?

[4] All train journeys end at a destination—but only *temporarily.* All diagnoses are similar. Thus ***all diagnoses should be seen as provisional diagnoses—remaining in effect only until the patient returns for the next evaluation.*** What do you gain by doing this? Something quite important. The idea that no diagnosis needs to be perfect. Why? Because like trains, all diagnoses return to their starting point at the scheduled next appointment, when they begin their journeys once again.

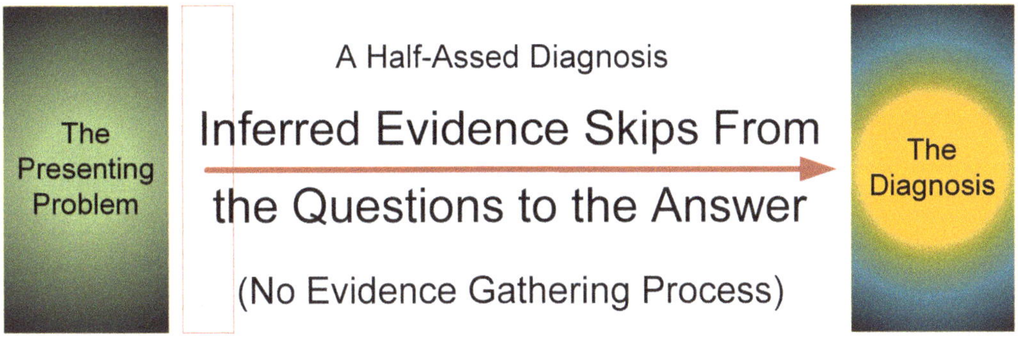

Four Things *to Not Do* As You Begin to Gather Evidence

Something which I rarely see diagnosticians do is to deliberately create pairs of diagnostic opposites. With Evidence Gathering, I've already introduced you to the main pair of diagnostic opposites—***Genuine Evidence*** versus ***Inferred Evidence***. Here gathering Genuine Evidence is what you *should* do—and gathering Inferred Evidence is what you *should not* do. And while logically, this oppositeness should be easy to understand, you'll need to picture both sides or it won't sink in.

With this in mind, here is a list of Inferred Evidence's four "to-not-do's."

[1] You can't begin a train journey at the final destination. You can't begin diagnosis this way either. Thus you should ***never begin the Diagnostic Process by assuming you know what the diagnosis will be.*** This will introduce a confirmation bias into the process which will impair your questions. Never a good thing to do.

[2] A train journey can succeed only if the train stays on the track. A diagnosis must do this as well. ***Even Genuine Evidence will fail to lead to a proper diagnosis if you don't first create a proper path on which to arrange and organize this data.*** Here, a proper diagnostic path extends from the patient's present age back to his or her birth. Also, all train journeys have historical precedents leading back in time to why this path was chosen—all diagnostic timelines have similar historical precedents. And if made visual, these precedents will reveal the story of how the patient's presenting problems came to be.

[3] No train journey exists on a straight line. No diagnostic assessment does either. People do not do things for reasons. They do them because they have personalities, inhibitions, and at times uncommon sense. The point? ***Honor the patient's story by allowing it to sit on the timeline in the order in which the patient tells it to you. This story, and not some contrived logic, is what reveals the true origin of this patient's problems.***

[4] Train schedules can, and often do, change. Diagnoses can and do too. A diagnosis is only as good as the direction it supplies for the therapeutic process. With this in mind, never begin an evaluation by assuming the past dictates the present. Rather, ***please begin each evaluation with a clean slate and an open mind.***

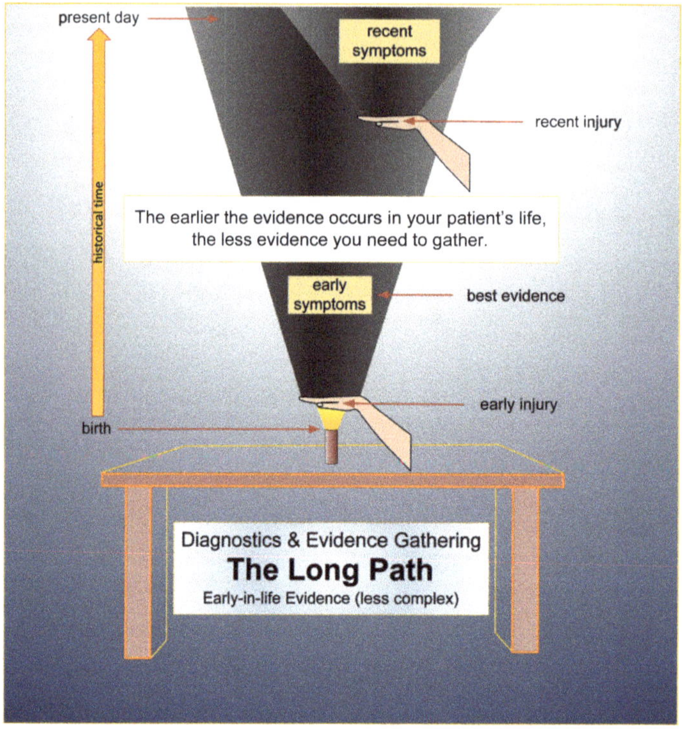

The Flashlight Metaphor (Is All Evidence Developmental?)

What you see in the drawings on this page and the next is one of my favorite metaphors. For obvious reasons, I call it the "Flashlight Metaphor." Here, the two flashlights represent a patient's birth moment—the beginning of all life experience. And the ever-expanding light cones then represent how their life experience expands and grows after that.

Look closely. Can you see the differences between these two drawings? In both drawings, there's a hand inserted into the light cone which blocks some of the light. On this page, the first hand is almost touching the flashlight. So it's blocking almost all of the light. Whereas the only hand in the drawing on the next page is near the top of the light cone. So it's blocking very little of the light.

What does any of this mean? To see it, imagine being in a large, completely dark room, with a table in the middle of this room. On this table is a flashlight, standing upright, on end. Can you picture what this light cone would look like if you were standing back from it, maybe twenty feet away? Likely, this light would reach all the way to the ceiling. This represents a completely uninjured, fully conscious, life.

Now imagine putting your hand into this light cone only inches away from the flashlight itself. How much light would doing this block? This is what's happening in this page's drawing. Now imagine standing on a step stool, and inserting your hand into this light cone, near the top of the light cone. How much more light would your hand block? This is what's happening in the drawing on the next page.

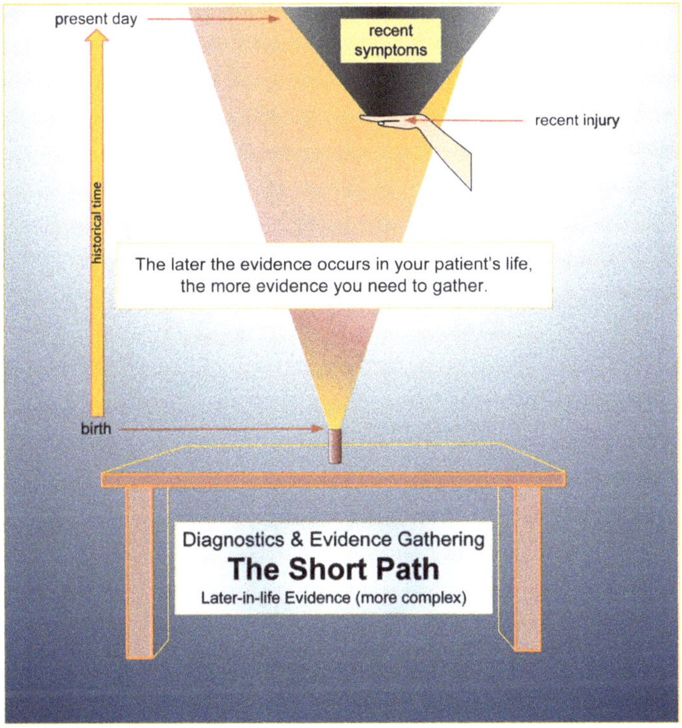

Please keep this metaphor in mind as you gather evidence. Why? Because given the evidence you gather is accurate, in most cases, the earlier it occurs, the more weight you should give it, as compared to evidence gathered from the present day. Why? Because the closer the evidence is to the patient's birth moment, the more this evidence will affect all the rest of the patient's life events, including recent ones.

The point is, ***Genuine Evidence is always developmental.*** So earlier occurring evidence will, most times, have a greater effect with regards to causing disorder. In truth, all things in personality, including injuries and symptoms, are developmental in nature. This is what the hands blocking the light represent. So if the patient's life experience begins at the flashlight's tip, then flows up—the older the patient gets, the more complicated the trail of evidence gets. And vice versa.

The earlier in life an event occurs, the less complex it will be.

This idea—that all things in personality are developmental in nature—is one of the more important considerations in diagnosis. Strangely, few diagnosticians get taught this. So it's often overlooked. If you keep what you see in these two drawings in mind though, you'll avoid many mistakes. For instance, on this page is what I call "the short path to the disorder." Here, the evidence you gather is coming from relatively recent times in the patient's life. As opposed to what you see in the drawing on the previous page, where the evidence is being gathered on "the long path." In general, evidence on the long path is a better guide to what's happening in the present. Why? Because it offers a clearer evidential trajectory. This means it creates a clearer, less complicated picture of the patient's life patterns.

The Idea That Evidence Exists on Two Experiential Time Lines

This idea—that genuine evidence is always developmental and that diagnosticians should give earlier evidence more weight—brings us to the next thing to keep in mind. As you gather evidence, you'll need to pay attention to how your questions affect your patient's two *experiential* ages. Meaning what?

Each time you ask patients to access a particular *chronological* age, this will cause them to access a particular, often different, *developmental* age. In some cases, these two ages will intersect. In some, not so much. And sometimes your patients will regress.

Why does this matter? Because each experiential age affects the words patients use. We use different words at different ages, and these differences create different impressions of the evidence. These changes in what the evidence seems to mean can then give different diagnostic impressions. And in some cases, this will cause patients to focus away from, or overlook, certain things, while focusing on others.

Three-year-olds and eight-year-olds may both know what a dog is. But an eight year old, if asked, will report additional things. What a pet is. That they require care. And perhaps, that they themselves may be responsible for some of this care.

My point is, paying attention to your patient's current experiential age will add a lot to your ability to diagnose. For one thing, you'll be far less likely to misinterpret your patient's responses. For example, say your patient seems to be having "difficulty answering questions." Some diagnosticians might see this as that this patient is "reluctant or refusing to answer questions." But they could be regressed. How would this interpretation affect the diagnosis you give? Can you imagine? The point here is obvious. Noting your patient's current experiential age is a critical part of correctly assessing evidence. So do try to keep this in mind.

Composite Triggers | A Kind of Falsely Reported Evidence

Now let's talk about a few other things which can also derail your evidence gathering efforts. Admittedly, these things can at times be quite hard to sort out. Fortunately, learning to see them in real time can help to minimize these problems.

The first kinds of problems? Something I call, "Composite Triggers."

What are "Composite Triggers?"

Composite triggers exist whenever two or more Event-sized Disorders interact.

Realize this situation can exist within a single person—or between two people in a close relationship. Either way, these problems always involve someone who has been startled. As I've previously told you, anytime a person gets startled, he or she ends up getting an Event-sized Disorder. What causes the disorder? The once-normal patterns which occurred in the three-to-five seconds just before this startle.

Getting startled changes these once-normal patterns into triggers. From then on, similarly to how gene splicing permanently alters the nature of a thing, these triggers alter our reactions to these events. With gene splicing, scientists extract a small chuck of DNA out of the context of a larger, complete set. They then splice these genes into the DNA of a completely different thing. The hope here is that doing this permanently improves the physical nature of that second thing. And sometimes it does. But sometimes, it doesn't. Scientists never know until they try it.

Getting startled literally causes a similar thing to happen in the mind. The person's mind extracts a small set of patterns out of the context of a much larger, mental event. From then on, as I've said, these patterns function as triggers. But the thing is, they also do something far worse. From then on, this person's mind can splice this small chunk of mental DNA into any number of other, often dissimilar, mental experiences.

Each time this happens, like gene splicing, the nature of these other experiences permanently changes. Unlike gene splicing though—where the changes can sometimes be positive—with startles, the changes are always negative. In every case, these changes lead to an increase in mental disorder. So in a way then, these chunks of mental DNA function like mental viruses. Once injured, people not only get triggered in similar events. They also get triggered during all manner of dissimilar, otherwise innocuous, present-day events.

The thing is, if someone else sees this person relive this startle, and if this other person gets startled by what they see—from then on, each time the first person relives this wound, they'll feel certain the other person got triggered. Are you getting this? I know. It's complicated. Know the drawing you'll find on the following page may help. Before looking at it though, let me take one more shot.

To begin with, picture someone reliving a wound. Do try to actually picture this person. Now imagine a second person seeing this first person reliving this wound. Now imagine this second person was once wounded by seeing someone else have this same reaction. Now add to this that the first person was once startled by seeing someone get startled, by seeing them getting startled.

Are you getting this? Yes. I know. As I've said, it's seriously complicated. Know I've described an actual case, along with the drawing I mentioned, on the next page. In it, you'll see a diagram of what's happening, including that ***both people are being triggered by their own triggers.*** But they're also ***both being triggered by seeing the other person react to them getting triggered.***

This means, each time one of them gets triggered *in the presence of the other,* a feedback loop will form between the two of them. This interpersonal feedback loop will then cause all kinds of hell to break loose. Why? Because like the feedback loops we looked at in Chapter 2 (the Nature Of Wounds), all feedback loops amplify and distort whatever is in them. And these changes then create chaos and disorder in these people's lives.

Realize too, it won't matter which person gets triggered first. Each time one gets triggered, the other will also get triggered. This interpersonal triggering will then bounce back and forth between them until whatever they're saying to each other begins to sound like squealing-feedback in an auditorium. Only here, the squealing will be the two people yelling at, screaming at, and arguing with, each other.

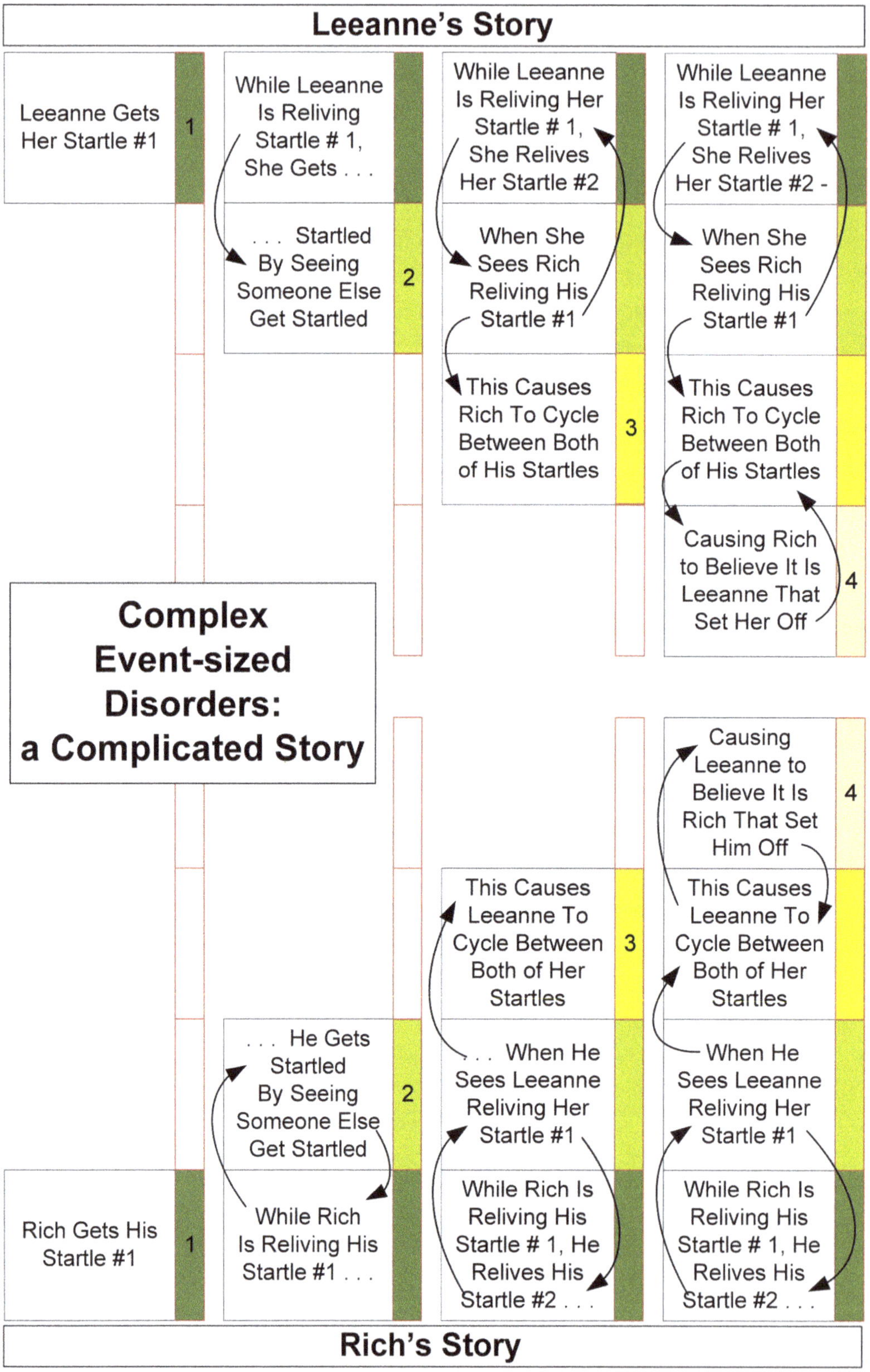
Leeanne's Story
Leeanne Gets Her Startle #1
1
While Leeanne Is Reliving Startle # 1, She Gets . . .
. . . Startled By Seeing Someone Else Get Startled
2
While Leeanne Is Reliving Her Startle # 1, She Relives Her Startle #2
When She Sees Rich Reliving His Startle #1
This Causes Rich To Cycle Between Both of His Startles
3
While Leeanne Is Reliving Her Startle # 1, She Relives Her Startle #2 -
When She Sees Rich Reliving His Startle #1
This Causes Rich To Cycle Between Both of His Startles
Causing Rich to Believe It Is Leeanne That Set Her Off
4
Complex Event-sized Disorders: a Complicated Story
Causing Leeanne to Believe It Is Rich That Set Him Off
4
This Causes Leeanne To Cycle Between Both of Her Startles
3
This Causes Leeanne To Cycle Between Both of Her Startles
. . . He Gets Startled By Seeing Someone Else Get Startled
2
. . . When He Sees Leeanne Reliving Her Startle #1
When He Sees Leeanne Reliving Her Startle #1
Rich Gets His Startle #1
1
While Rich Is Reliving His Startle #1 . . .
While Rich Is Reliving His Startle # 1, He Relives His Startle #2 . . .
While Rich Is Reliving His Startle # 1, He Relives His Startle #2 . . .
Rich's Story

Composite Triggers | An Example: Rich and Leeanne

Do realize, I know, what I've just described will likely have been incredibly hard to follow. This is why I'm going to give you an actual example to picture. This case has been taken from my private practice. Hopefully, the drawing on the previous page will help you to follow it. As you can see, this case involves two people—Rich and Leeanne. (Obviously, those names are not their real names.)

In Leeanne's version of this incident, she told me she was mad at Rich. Why? Because when they argue, she said, he only ever uses logic.

She also said, he never tells her that he feels hurt during these arguments. She further claimed that if Rich would tell her he was hurt, that she would not get set off.

Was she right about this—that she would not get set off if Rich told her he was hurt? Probably not.

How can I know this? Because of what Rich told me. Rich claimed he does say this to her—all the time. And based on the evidence I'd gathered, I believed him. But if Rich had been telling Leeanne he'd been hurt, then why was she saying he never says this to her? Because if Leeanne was getting set off by seeing Rich get set off, then it's likely she wouldn't remember much, if any, of what Rich had said. Reliving a startle always causes the person's mind to go blank. And anything involving Composite Triggers makes things even worse.

Rich, in his version of the story, then added, if Leeanne told him she was sorry, that he wouldn't be mad. He then claimed, "She's never told me she's sorry for anything—not even once."

Did I believe Rich when he said he wouldn't get set off if Leeanne said she was sorry? Like what I felt about Leeanne's claim, not really. Why? Because like Leeanne, Rich, too, had been getting set off by Composite Triggers as well. So he likely would have heard little if any of what Leeanne had been saying to him either.

Do These Few Details Tell Us Anything Useful?

Given the level of confusion this evidence has likely caused in you, what can you possibly know about this relationship? Any takeaways? Yes.

Things which point to a "measurable aspect of human nature" require very little evidence to be diagnostically relevant.

Complex Event-sized Disorder is one of these things. It always masks much of what people say. For instance, in Leeanne's version of this story, Rich only uses logic and never tells her he feels hurt. Whereas in Rich's version of the story, Leeanne never tells him she's sorry, not even once.

Both claims are versions of the "always" and "never" problem—which is a measurable aspect of human nature. Whenever you see this pattern, it makes people's claims questionable. Why? Because "always" and "never" are words people use when they're in a Baby State of Mind. And since a baby's sense of time is limited to a single, "present moment," if they didn't hear, "sorry," then it *never* got said.

What's happening here?

When people are in a Baby State of Mind, they experience the present moment as the only moment to have ever occurred. This prevents them from being able to contrast and compare this event to any other times. This lack of perspective then distorts and exaggerates the meanings of anything they experience during this event. Some things take on much greater meanings; some, much smaller meanings. Either way, all decision-making becomes a mess.

How does decision-making differ for people in an Adult State of Mind?

In an Adult State of Mind, the meanings of most things remain right-sized. Why? Because for these folks, things exist on a historical timeline. This timeline allows them to mediate any perceptual distortions—by creating sensible contrasts and compares across time. This vastly improves their decision-making abilities, as it allows them to see greys and shadows, even in the best of times.

Know we'll discuss these two states of mind, in depth, in the next chapter. In many ways, this topic is one of the more useful measures a diagnostician can ever learn. Conversely, if you fail to account for these two states of mind, your sense of the evidence you collect will be seriously flawed. So much so, in fact, that it will be difficult to determine what is, and is not, diagnostically relevant.

Can you see yet why I am calling these situations, "Complex Event-sized Disorder?"

To begin with, go back to the drawing you looked at two pages back. Can you identify the two main feedback loops which formed between Rich and Leeanne?

Like all feedback loops, the myriad possible interactions within these loops can seem infinitely complex.

This is why it's so important to get people's ages when beginning diagnosis—and even more so in times where a diagnosis involves Complex Event-sized Disorder.

An Exception To The Warning Against Inferring Evidence

It occurs to me, I may have confused you as to why we've been talking about Rich and Leeanne's case.

In part, I've mentioned it to point out the myriad feedback loops which form in these cases. But I've also had a second reason. I've raised this case to point out an exception to my advice to not interpret things patients say. My normal advice? Avoid restating and reducing what patients tell you to some dry, professional summary risks. Doing this risks distorting your diagnostic impressions. So to avoid this, I've advised you to write down your patients' exact words. However, there is an exception to this advice. This exception involves cases of Complex Event-sized Disorder.

In these cases, there are at least four, and often more, feedback loops in play. Two feedback loops exist within each person—and at least two exist between them; interpersonally. And like all things in feedback loops, this will distort any and all things patients report. Think about it.

Can you imagine how many ways these multiple feedback loops could distort and exaggerate the things a patient reports?

Realize too, this is especially true in cases where couples repeatedly fight the same fight. This pattern is yet another measurable aspect of human nature. Even the best patients—people who are normally willing to look at themselves and who can articulate fairly well—will have trouble reporting what's happened in these times accurately. And in some cases, the more intelligent the patients, the more they'll tend to infer logically sounding, but false, evidence.

In these cases then, for obvious reasons, you should limit the evidence you see as relevant to the things you can—with reasonable certainty—derive from tipping-point based tests. Even here, there is yet another, even more insidious problem to watch out for here.

This problem does not involve distortions in the evidence you actually collect. It involves times your patients completely and utterly—but unintentionally—fabricate evidence.

Always and ***never*** are common examples of this kind of problem.

Couple's repeatedly fighting the same fight is another.

In cases involving Complex Event-sized Disorder, however, there is another, even worse problem. This involves times where you realize what your patient is saying is quite clearly fabricated, because it seems completely unrelated. Despite your seeing this clearly, all efforts to get the patient to see this error result in useless and unpleasant arguments.

What's going on here?

This is the topic we're about to explore next.

False and ***unrelated*** evidence which, to the patient, feels absolutely real—but which in truth, never actually occurred.

A Second Example of Composite Triggers: Derrick and Nicolette

Before we discuss this second case, please note, I've placed a drawing of this story on the next page. Like Rich and Leeanne's drawing a few pages back, this second drawing is there only to guide you in case you get lost.

Know the takeaways from both drawings are the same.

The main takeaway?

The complex web of interpersonal feedback loops. This is why neither drawing includes any details of these fights. These details do not matter.

What does matter?

That you begin to see how these feedback loops effect the evidence gathering process.

The names of the two people in this case? Derrick and Nicolette.

Again, this case is taken from my private practice and involves Complex Event-sized Disorder. Again, these names are not their real names.

What happened?

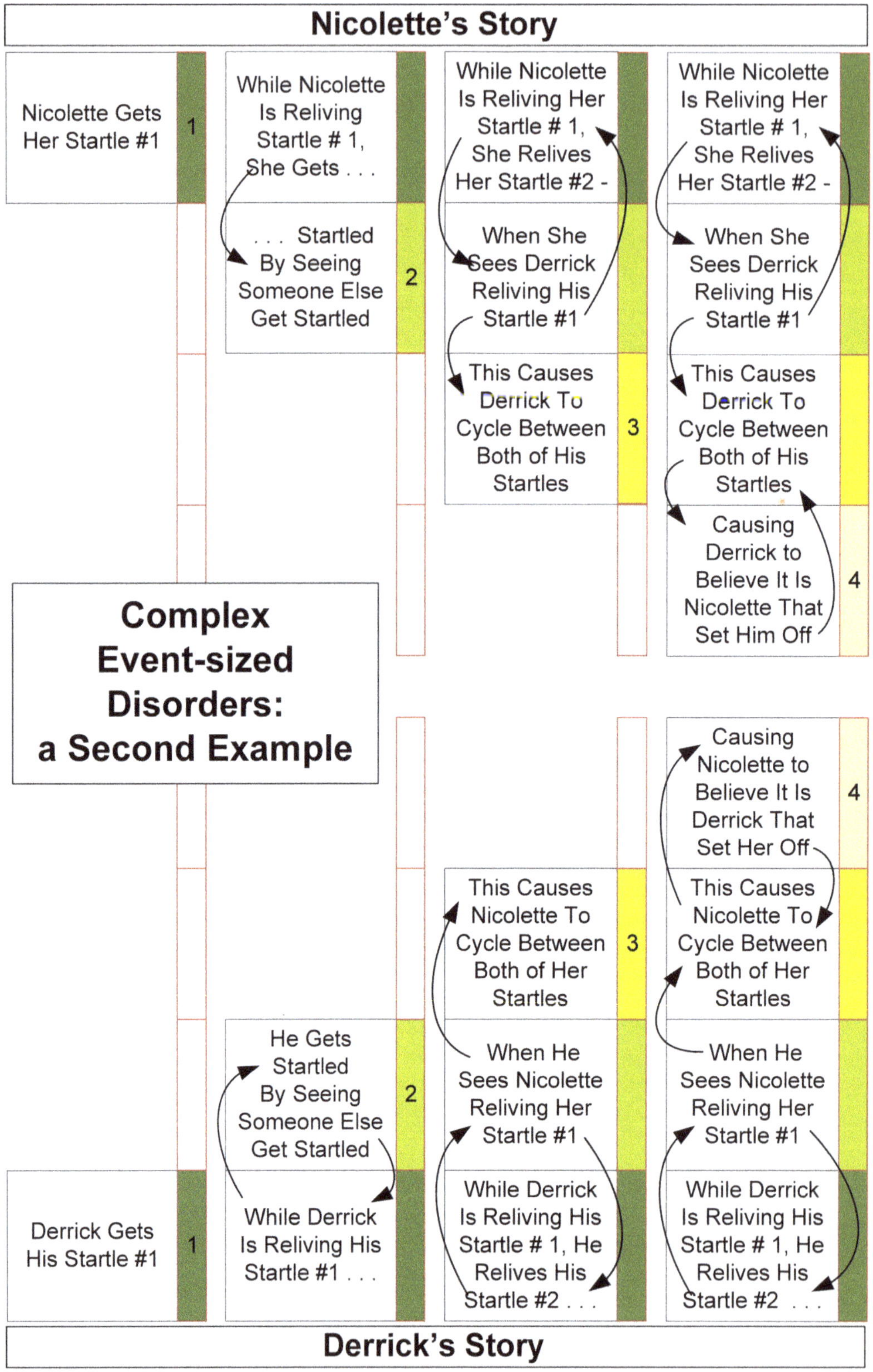

Nicolette's Story
Nicolette Gets Her Startle #1
1
While Nicolette Is Reliving Startle # 1, She Gets . . .
. . . Startled By Seeing Someone Else Get Startled
2
While Nicolette Is Reliving Her Startle # 1, She Relives Her Startle #2 -
When She Sees Derrick Reliving His Startle #1
This Causes Derrick To Cycle Between Both of His Startles
3
While Nicolette Is Reliving Her Startle # 1, She Relives Her Startle #2 -
When She Sees Derrick Reliving His Startle #1
This Causes Derrick To Cycle Between Both of His Startles
Causing Derrick to Believe It Is Nicolette That Set Him Off
4
Complex Event-sized Disorders: a Second Example
Causing Nicolette to Believe It Is Derrick That Set Her Off
4
This Causes Nicolette To Cycle Between Both of Her Startles
3
This Causes Nicolette To Cycle Between Both of Her Startles
He Gets Startled By Seeing Someone Else Get Startled
2
When He Sees Nicolette Reliving Her Startle #1
When He Sees Nicolette Reliving Her Startle #1
Derrick Gets His Startle #1
1
While Derrick Is Reliving His Startle #1 . . .
While Derrick Is Reliving His Startle # 1, He Relives His Startle #2 . . .
While Derrick Is Reliving His Startle # 1, He Relives His Startle #2 . . .
Derrick's Story

To begin with, the week prior to the explosion, Nicolette and Derrick had been, for some time according to her, trying to eat healthier. This was further complicated by the fact they had, at one point, gone away for the weekend. While away, Derrick asked Nicolette if he could deviate from these efforts—by buying a few donuts from an exotic donut shop. In that moment, Nicolette ***instantly*** reacted by telling Derrick, he wasn't being supportive.

I later learned, he'd told her he only wanted the donuts for himself. But evidently, this had done nothing to ease Nicolette's unease. Please realize too, it's likely some readers will identify with Nicolette and with her struggle to eat healthier. If this is you, do try to set these feelings aside. Do take note however of the onset speed of Nicolette's reaction. The word, "instantly" tells you this.

Why focus on this word? Because anytime a person experiences an "instant" reaction to something, this indicates they've entered a Baby State of Mind. As such, their reporting about this event is, at best, seriously flawed.

What about Derrick? Did he also enter a Baby State of Mind? When I asked him how Nicolette's outburst affected him, he reported being fine. And I believed him. Why? Because he was easily able to picture the whole thing—and while recounting it, he did not speed up. Nor did he wince or flinch.

Why mention wincing and flinching? This is yet another takeaway.

The only time people wince or flinch is when they are reliving an Event-sized Disorder. Diagnostically, this makes locating injuries relatively easy. Anytime you see a patient doing either of these two things, they're, in that moment, reliving an injury.

Fast forward a week. Derrick and Nicolette were again talking about food. And by Nicolette's reporting, Derrick first blamed her for something—then he abruptly ended the conversation and left.

By Derricks reporting, he did leave ***abruptly***. So it's likely he did, ***at that point***, relive something. But when I tested him, prior to that point, Derrick was easily able to picture everything before he left, with no wincing or flinching.

What made Nicolette feel so sure Derrick had blamed her before he left?

This question is the point for me telling you this story.

To begin with, by now, I've likely seriously annoyed you by repeatedly describing how wounds happen. The triggers in Event-sized Disorders derive from a "three-to-five second" chunk of mental context. This chunk of mental context originally existed in an event—and occurred right before—the person got startled. Also, this chunk of mental context always contains more than one trigger—and the closer to the startle it occurs, the stronger a trigger gets.

Now note, in the case of Simple Event-sized Disorders, ordinarily, people need to relive multiple triggers in order to get triggered into reliving this event. The more triggers they relive, the more triggered they get. However, because Complex event-sized Disorders create multiple feedback loops, sometimes even a single trigger can be enough to cause the person to ***completely*** relive this wound.

Further complicating this problem is that in these cases, a single trigger can make a person feel certain they've experienced all the triggers. This is likely what happened to Nicolette in that event. She'd felt certain Derrick had blamed her, even when he hadn't.

Can you imagine trying to make sense of these events without knowing how Complex Event-sized Disorders work? Ordinarily, people need to experience multiple triggers in order to relive a wound. In these complex cases though, a single trigger—if sufficiently powerful—can recreate the entire wounding-event context. And when this happens, the person feels sure they've experienced all of the triggers.

Worse yet, they HAVE ***experienced*** all the triggers. So no amount of discussion can convince the person the other triggers didn't occur. No coincidence, this is often what's behind those frequently-recurring fights all couples have at times.

This is also one of the more difficult situations diagnosticians face when gathering evidence. How can you know what was present and what was not? How do you decide what's even missing?

We will explore these situations in depth in the next chapter. For now though, just know this. If you suspect this is what's happened, then know there are likely things which this patient can't report accurately. What can you do? Just do your best to let this go. Why? Because even just knowing this is possible can help you to overcome your urges to fill in the blanks with false evidence.

Correcting "Assumed to Be False" Evidence | A Diagnostician's Error

In the category of false evidence we just spoke about, diagnosticians gather false evidence from patients who are experiencing a Complex Event-sized Disorder.

In the category of false evidence we're about to discuss, we'll look at false evidence diagnosticians themselves create.

The gist of this problem? The pressure diagnosticians feel to arrive at a diagnosis quickly. Diagnosticians who feel this pressure often make inferences in order to fill in what appear to be missing links in the evidence.

In a moment, I'm going to talk about a particularly difficult case in which I somehow managed to avoid this problem. Before I do, I first need to briefly review the differences between Inferred Evidence and Genuine Evidence. If you wish to become skilled at gathering evidence, you must become an expert in telling these two things apart.

The differences?

Inferred Evidence is "the things you assume or guess at about your patient, ***but never actually see***." Often these things are based on some amount of Genuine Evidence. But then the diagnostician, under pressure, uses this evidence to ***leap*** to a conclusion.

Genuine Evidence, on the other hand, is "the things you literally do see and observe in your patient. You can actually picture this evidence, as it's things which you have actually seen occur."

The Case of The Piece of Shit Boyfriend

The case I just mentioned?

I once had a new patient—a 28-year-old nurse—come in.

Her name? Lydia.

Her presenting problem?

I'd been told by her referent that her younger brother had recently died of a drug overdose—and that she was drowning in grief.

Being this was her first session with me—and being I knew she'd be overwhelmed—I decided to do "paper therapy." So after a few minutes of introductory talk, I handed her a deck of 3x5 cards and a Sharpie pen.

I then asked her to write down the things that were bothering her, one to a card.

When she'd finished, I asked her to lay these cards face up, in front of us.

I then asked her to pick the card she wanted to work on first—she'd written four cards.

For obvious reasons, I'd assumed she'd written one regarding her brother. This assumption turned out to be right. No surprise here.

The thing is, I'd also assumed she'd pick that card to work on.

Would you have done the same?

I'd guess, most diagnosticians would have assumed this as well.

In part, I'd assumed this because, on the initial call, when she'd told me about her brother, she had broken down.

In truth, I'd been so sure this was what she'd choose that I was floored when she didn't pick that card.

Can you guess what kind of a thing she did ask to work on? Know I've purposely told you nothing about the other cards. Why? To see if, despite having no evidence, you feel pressured to infer what it was.

Some readers will feel this way. Some will simply hurry to get to the answer. Either way, if this is you, know this kind of pressure is what causes diagnosticians to infer evidence.

Realize too, any time you give in to these urges, this will bias your sense of everything your patient then tells you.

Worse yet, many patients will assume you know more about them than they do. So they'll just follow your lead—then base what they say on whatever you've asked for.

Thank goodness, in this case, I'd done the right thing, by asking this woman to use the cards—this despite the fact that I rarely, if ever, use 3x5 cards in a first session.

It can seem too cold.

Why had I chosen to use them that day? I had chosen to use them for several reasons.

For one thing, I had chosen to use them because, as I said, I knew very little about this patient.

Mainly though, I'd chose to use them for two other reasons.

The first? The one I've already mentioned. Paper therapies slow down the patient's racing thoughts. But I'd also chosen to do this because I wanted to give my patient the ability to make this choice for herself.

In situations like this one, where people feel out of control, paper therapies can help patients to feel they are regaining some control. Admittedly I'm glad I did, as the card she chose was far more important than the brother-dying card.

What kind of card did she choose?

The one she'd written about her current boyfriend.

How could what her boyfriend was doing possibly trump her brother dying? It turned out to be a rare case of Human Garbage, DSM 318.765, Level 3.

Her boyfriend had been mocking her for feeling sad about her brother dying.

Can you imagine? This piece of shit had been mocking her for grieving the death of her younger brother. Specifically, she told me—each night, when she got home from work, as she walked in—he would say, ***"What's the matter? Your dog die?"***

To my credit—and unlike many diagnosticians who, having made an assumption, might have had trouble changing direction—I immediately went with what the patient had chosen to work on. As I should have. Patients should always be given this respect, even in extreme cases.

I readily admit, though, that I was, in some sense, lucky here. Had I not used those 3x5 cards, I might have been more invested in continuing with what I'd assumed. In the end, this woman and I did great work together in that session. This work then set the stage for her to do the grief work she clearly also needed to do, but at a later time.

In a moment, I'll describe what we did in that session. Before I do, let me ask you this.

What do you think would have happened if I'd pushed her to do that grief work in that initial session? Also, would this have been wrong? After all, she'd have likely left feeling better. My answer? Yes. She'd likely have left feeling better. But then she'd have gone home, only to have that piece of shit mock her yet again when the grief resurfaced in her.

And then what?

Then she'd likely have cancelled her next session and never come back.

Know I've seen this happen many times.

When a patient's hopes get raised in therapy—only to be followed by these hopes getting dashed—this often leads this person to go from hopeful to feeling resigned. The person then tries to accept that this problem will never change—so why try. Hence like diagnosis, interventions also have a best path, and this path should not skip steps.

Doing this only risks the train running off the rails.

Finally, here's this section's takeaway. Know there are two parts.

For one thing, ***diagnosticians can infer evidence just as easily as patients can. So don't assume you know what a patient sees as the problem, without first gathering genuine evidence.***

Also, ***please never forget the patient's right to self-determine the work. You may know more. But this doesn't give you the right to encourage or pressure the patient to skip steps. Diagnosis and therapy both have a natural path. Best to keep this in mind.***

Does Determining The Truth of What Patients Tell You Matter?

This leads us to yet another thing I've yet to address.

This thing also often biases and confuses many diagnosticians.

This thing?

The pressure diagnosticians feel to determine the *literal truth* of the things patients tell you. For instance, in the story I just told you, could the woman have misheard her boyfriend's intentions?

Could he have been trying to relieve her suffering, by making her laugh?

Know I ask this as I, myself, frequently use these kinds of interventions in cases of serious violence. Absurdity, if well-timed—and tempered with kindness, can jump-start the healing process for some pretty significant wounds.

Case in point, in Lydia's story, this is exactly what I did. Keep in mind though that in this case, I was doing both diagnosis AND therapy. With diagnosis alone, you would never do what I did here, certainly not in a single session.

So what did I do for Lydia? Here's her story.

∞

After Lydia chose the boyfriend card—and after she briefly told me what he'd been doing, I asked her to stand up. Why? Because she'd been standing in the scene in her story. And because the body has memory.

Having her be in the same position she'd been in during her story added to her ability to picture what had been happening to her. So after she stood, I used Visual Dialogue—the principle style of Emergence Psychotherapy—to explore further.

I began by asking her to picture arriving at the door to her apartment. I had her picture as many small details as she could. The color of the door. The color of the doorknob. The temperature in the hallway. Any sounds she could hear. I then told her to picture a remote control in her hand—then told her, she had the power to freeze what she saw at any time.

I then added that I would be standing right behind her the whole time. Then, when she'd been sufficiently drawn into the scene, I had her imagine opening the door. I then had her picture her boyfriend coming to meet her, then asked her to imagine hearing him say the dreaded sentence.

"What's the matter? Your dog die?"

I then had her imagine pressing the pause button and freezing the scene. At this point, she looked nervous. I then began to introduce the counter-violent intervention into this scene. What did I do?

I asked Lydia to look down at her hand and to picture a Number Two pencil. Emergence Psychotherapists call what I'd asked her to do, "the windup." In the windup, you get the patient to imagine something which expands their sense of the dynamic range of what's happening in the scene. Often, you do this by asking them to ***consider*** doing something violent to their abuser.

This is what I was about do to with Lydia.

Continuing with the windup, I asked her to look more closely at this pencil. What color was the shaft? (Orangey yellow.) How worn was the eraser? (It was new.) What color was the number two? (Silver).

I then asked her to touch the point and asked her how sharp it was. (Very sharp.) Then I—very slowly, introduced her to the counter-violent moment of this intervention. I told her to take this pencil and then, after a long pause, told her to drive it all the way into her boyfriend's eye.

∞

I fear I may have just triggered some readers by saying what I've just said. If this is you, then you might want to read more about doing Visual Dialogue in my 2020 book, ***Therapy for Therapists (a guide to changing lives)***. Here, the only valid question to ask in these cases is, "Did doing this help the patient or not?" And in case this doesn't make sense, you need to do your best to hear my answer.

The question? Did this intervention help Lydia? To be honest, at first, I couldn't tell. Lydia stood there, silent, for almost two minutes. Finally, though, she calmly spoke a single sentence. To be honest, having never worked with her before, at this point, I got a bit nervous. But then, slowly, deliberately, calmly, Lydia spoke a sentence I will never forget. Slowly, calmly, and with an inner strength, she asked me, "***Can I have another pencil?***"

She left this asshole not long after that.

How The Novelty of An Event Affects A Patient's Sense of Truth

Now comes the point of this story. There's a lot to discuss. So go slow.

Obviously, the violent thing I had Lydia picture herself doing never actually happened.

But if it never happened, if it wasn't true, then how did it change her life?

To see, we need to briefly talk about two things—[1] how memory works, specifically, how it's ***the amount of deviation from a patient's perceived normal*** which dictates whether people experience something as memorable or not—and [2] how memory connects to, and determines, a patient's perception of what's true.

We'll begin with memory. Start with this. You learned in a prior Chapter that there are four kinds of Information. ***Feelings*** (invisible change). ***Facts*** (visible unchange). ***Stories*** (visible change). And ***Ideas*** (invisible unchange). All memories are "the ability to recall some variation of a story." So you don't remember a fact, idea, or feeling. You remember recalling a fact, an idea, or a feeling. And recalling stories is the act of recalling "changing combinations of the other three Informations."

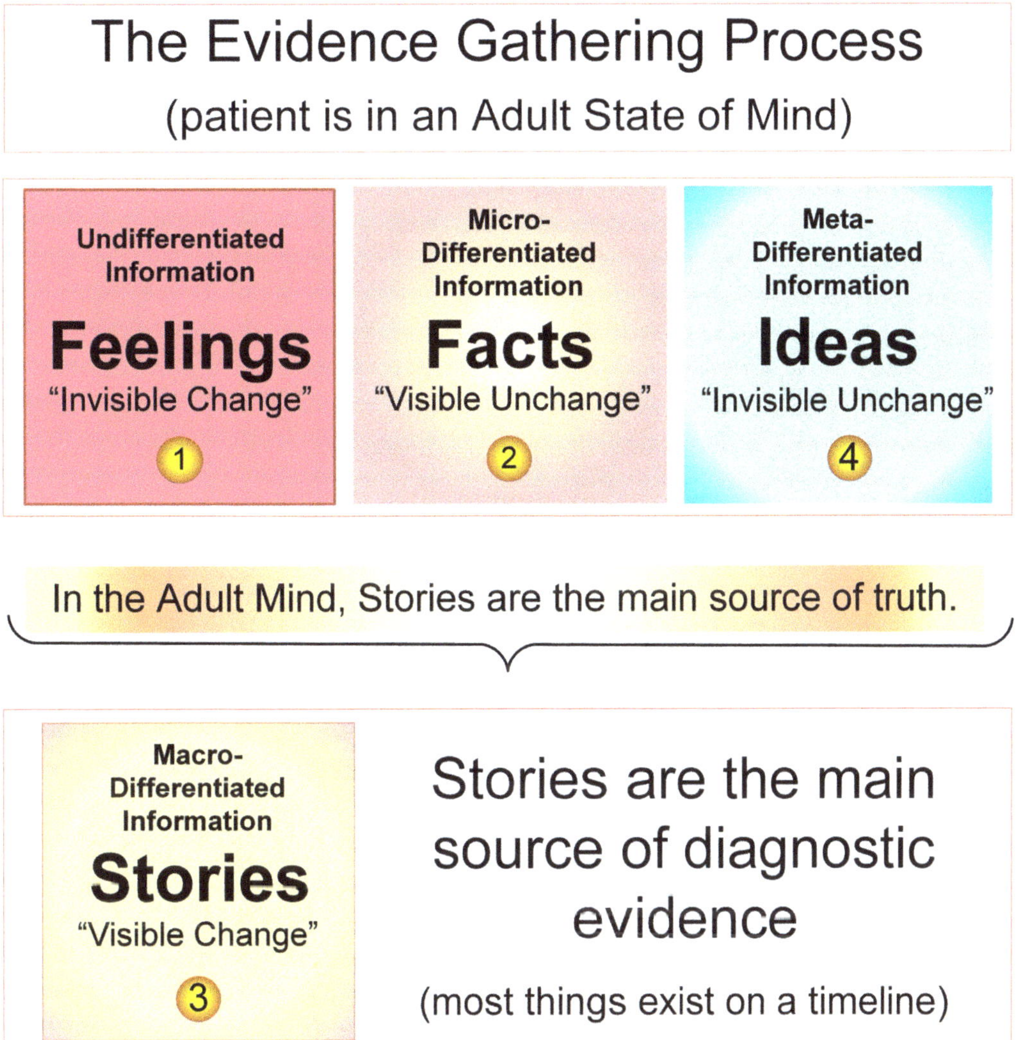

This simple concept is one of the most significant in this book.

Diagnostically, it's the key to understanding many things.

For one, it explains why, in most cases, it's a waste of time to try to determine literal truths. After all, we're mostly diagnosing our patient's *experiences* (perceived stories), not merely documenting medical measurements (facts).

Making this distinction is incredibly important when diagnosing. We cannot *directly* read minds. If we could, we'd be directly observing facts. This makes the ability to read minds *indirectly* a major portion of the skill of diagnosis. So we must know where to look. And patients have three sources for the Information they draw on to create their stories—the three places we must look at. [1] Their ***physical bodies*** (changing patterns of physical sensations). [2] Their ***nonphysical minds*** (changing patterns of mental representations). And [3] the combined experience of the ***observing self*** (changing patterns of physical and mental patterns intermingled).

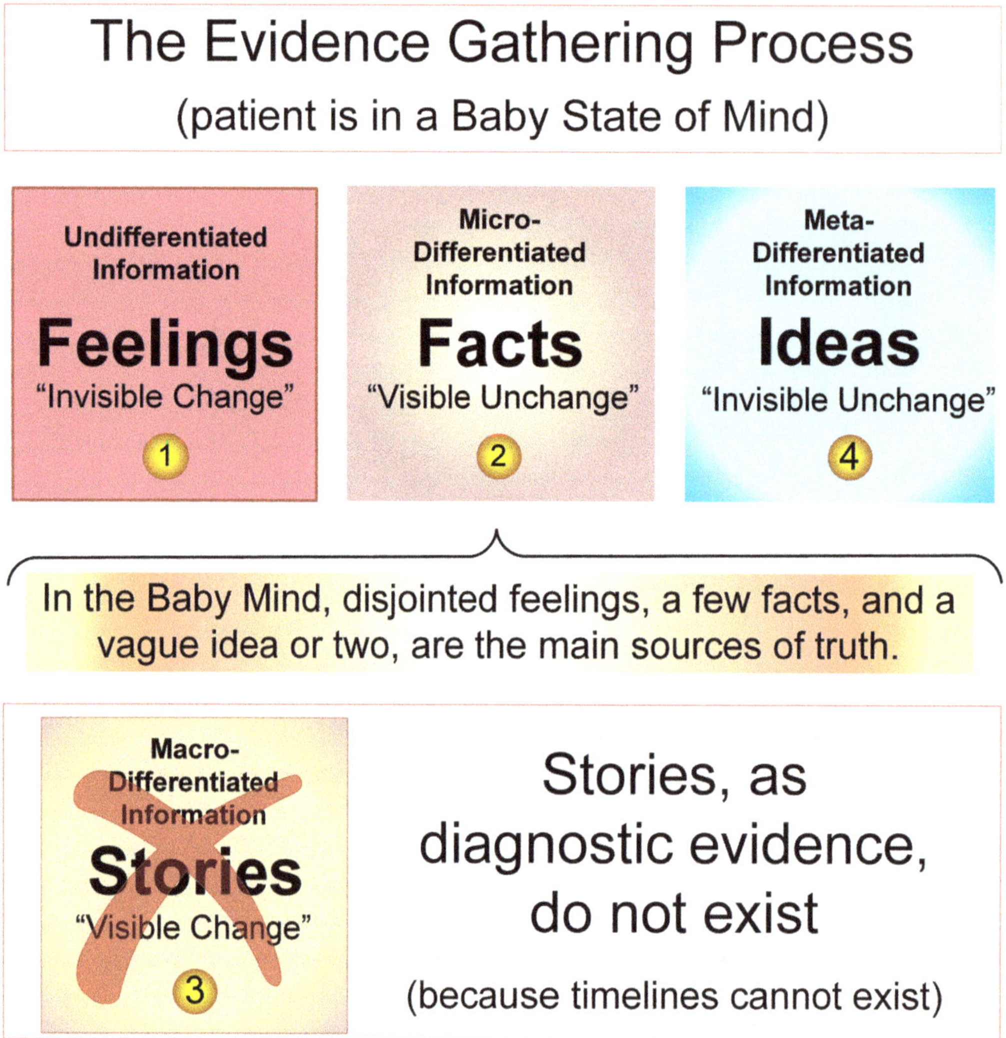

This means all patient memories derive from these same *three sources.* Patients can recall things changing in their bodies, as *physical* memory. They can recall things changing in their minds, as *mental* memory. And they can recall combinations of these changes as if they've been observed "from above," as the "*observing self.*"

Now add to this that there are two Mental States of Time—the Adult Mind (a timeline exists) and the Baby Mind (no timeline exists). These two states of time determine the kinds of Information we can gather.

From patients in an Adult Mind (see the drawing on the previous page), we mainly gather Stories (blends of the other three Informations). And from patients in a Baby Mind, we can only gather disjointed or undifferentiated feelings, a few primitive facts, and an occasionally parroted idea or two.

Here, from what I've said, we can see, there are two kinds of Patient Truth. The Adult Mind versions of Patient Truth—things mostly based on patient's stories.

And the Baby Mind versions of Patient Truth—where truth is whatever disjointed feeling, fact, or idea is currently front and center in their minds.

Now take a moment to consider this idea—that to patients, the truth of things depends on two things. First, the source of their memories—the kinds of memories they're currently accessing—body, mind, or observing self (mind and body intermingled). Second, the dynamic range of these memories as in how much they deviate from the patient's perceived normal. Here, the Information which deviates the most from the patient's perceived normal will feel the strongest. Thus these things will feel most true.

For most human beings, Adult-minded Information forms the basis for most experience. So when people experience Baby-minded Information, since this Information so obviously deviates from the norm, to most patients, Baby-minded Information feels stronger and so, more true to them. This in part explains why reliving early-childhood injuries so easily co-ops people's complete and utter mental focus. It also explains why diagnosis requires us to thoroughly explore the earliest accessible, memorable events in a patient's life.

The intervention I used in Lydia's case is a good example of this power. This includes that my intervention focused on doing something two-year olds would laugh at if they saw this in an animation. What I had Lydia do caused her mind to create such a powerful memory of what she imagined, that it became indistinguishable from any actual, literal memory.

This idea reveals the force and mechanism behind using imaginary scenes to heal wounds. It's what makes these interventions possible. But it also points to why the patient's truth, rather than some literal truth, is the most important diagnostic truth of all.

The patient's truth is what we diagnosticians must identify. Why? Because the patient's truth is what therapists must look to heal.

The Patient's Truth: The Takeaway

To some, it may seem I am implying that you'll need to allow, and adjust for, the truth of all of these things and more. I am not saying this. What am I saying then?

I'm simply refining my description of the nature of Genuine Evidence.

To patients, all three of these truths ARE literally true. So each and every one of them is diagnostically relevant.

What does this mean? That in most cases, the "literal truth" doesn't matter. This is especially true in cases involving Composite Triggers, where trying to dissemble and logically process symptoms *literally* is often a complete waste of time. For instance, take Lydia's case. Her story involved a couple experiencing Complex Event-sized Disorder. Moreover, she'd been unable to speak up for herself. So I fabricated an intervention which side-stepped this inability. My use of a completely fabricated intervention then led to her being able to leave her abusive boyfriend.

The takeaway here? It's simple.

Gathering the details of patients' stories—without needing to judge the **literal** *truth of what's being said—has great diagnostic value.*

It's also a necessary part of a legitimate, evidence gathering process.

For one thing, it gives you accurate indicators of the patient's state of mind.

For another, patients frequently shut down—and stop offering evidence—when they think you don't believe them. Questioning their truth is the main way this happens.

What comes to mind here is something I was taught early on when dealing with patients who exhibit delusions, psychosis, and hallucinations.

Never try to correct these distortions by arguing about what is true.

Instead, use patient's beliefs to learn the true nature of their problems. How? By stepping into them and asking patients to describe their inner-world view.

Indeed, because all diagnostic cases involve distortion and dissociations, this idea should be the rule rather than the exception. Rather than treating diagnosis as some attempt to determine what's literally true then, it's far better to see the evidence gathering part of diagnosis as a separate step which sets the stage for whatever therapeutic interventions may follow—all the while knowing that therapeutic interventions must all begin with, and address, the patient's current truth.

The Idea That "Evidence Gathering" Is "Pre-Learning"

As I write this, I've now spent close to forty years trying to make the discovery process more science than art. Here, I define "discovery" (natural learning) *as* "learning by witnessing surprises, rather than by memorizing." Think about it. Young babies don't give a shit about tests or memorizing things. Rather, they spend every waking hour exploring everything that they can see, all the while seeking surprises.

If you wish to be a good diagnostician, then you should be doing the same. Why? Because diagnosis—if you're doing it properly—follows the same path as the learning process babies use. In the case of diagnosis, obviously, the learning focuses on discovering the two things I've previously mentioned. First, this learning focuses on learning *who* this patient is, by patiently gathering visual evidence. Second, it focuses on *letting the evidence you gather speak for itself.*

"Speak for itself?" What does this mean? Here, a few words about how we humans learn may clarify what I'm saying.

In essence, there are two ways we human beings try to learn new things.

I call the way most adults try to learn, the *traditional* learning process.

I call the way young children learn, the *discovery-oriented* learning process.

What is the "traditional" learning process? It consists of memorizing and regurgitating words about other people's ahas. You can tell the learning is this kind if recalling things later takes effort. There's also no observable pleasant surprise when it's recalled. So it's not as joyful. In truth, it's a lot of hard work.

What then is the *discovery-oriented* learning process like?

It consists mainly of *visually-oriented* pre-learning (evidence gathering).

Babies may not know they're doing this—but that doesn't prevent it from happening. They spend every hour engaged in pre-learning.

Why do they do this?

Because they so love the feeling of discovering things.

This means they don't mind doing the work. More important, they also don't want to stop. My proof for this? Have you ever seen a baby who has to be pressured to engage in pre-learning? Obviously not.

Now contrast and compare this pattern with how you normally look to gather evidence. Does it feel like work, or does it feel like something you love?

This simple test is a good one to take now and then.

How about now? How do you measure up?

Why Do Babies Love Pre-learning?

So why do babies love pre-learning? The main reason?

On its own, pre-learning always leads to having pleasant surprises. And who doesn't like to be pleasantly surprised? In addition, there's the added benefit that this kind of learning lasts for the rest of your life. It's the "learning to ride a bike" kind of learning.

Another benefit involves what it's like to later recall this kind of learning. Recalling and using natural learning is close-to effortless. Contrast and compare this with what it's like to recall and use traditionally learned, memorized data and ideas. Recalling that kind of "learning" almost always requires significant effort.

Is this making sense? Are you seeing the differences yet? Surely you've been pressured and forced to memorize an awful lot of empty things in your life. Wouldn't you like to return to the kind of learning you did as a young child, where everything felt new and exciting? Imagine how feeling like that would affect your ability to diagnose?

Now think back to what "learning to diagnose" felt like back in college. How does the horrible shit you had to endure back then compare to what babies spend their lives doing?

Now realize, this is the point.

When you use pre-learning to diagnose, ***you don't try to mentally determine the patient's diagnosis.*** Like what happens to babies when they pre-learn, ***a diagnosis simply dawns on you at some point, during the pre-diagnosing process.***

Of course, for this to happen, you must be familiar with the possible diagnoses. Given you are, then at some point during the evidence gathering process, a diagnosis just emerges in you. To me, I imagine this is what Freud must have been referring to when he asked Jung to swear to fight the "tide of occultism." Have you ever been taught what Freud meant by this phrase?

His use of the word "occultism" didn't refer to black magic. Rather, it referred to doing bad science.

This includes having to guess at diagnoses.

What was Freud urging Jung to do instead?

He was urging Jung to base his diagnoses on *observable*, scientifically-gathered evidence. In this book, this kind of evidence is rooted in the Four Kinds of Change lines you learned to picture in Chapter 2. Can you picture any of them? Hopefully, you can at least picture the "getting wounded" line. Every diagnosis in this book begins with ruling this line in or out.

Then there's the idea that of those four lines, only two of them change the mind permanently. The shape of the "getting wounded" line is one kind of permanent change. The shape of the "having an emergence" (healing) line is the other.

Why mention this here? Because when you arrive at a properly constructed diagnosis, your experience will have followed the shape of that second line.

You'll know this because you'll have felt pleasantly surprised by this realization.

If you haven't, then what you've arrived at is a contrived, logical, and largely inferred "diagnosis."

The Two Ways to Learn Who The Patient Is: Questions and Guesses

Speaking of contrived diagnoses, another way to see diagnosis is as "learning who the patient is and is not." Here, there are two ways you can go about doing this. You can learn who the patient is by literally ***asking this patient questions*** and ***by limiting the evidence to what you see and hear*** (the long way). Or you can skip many of these questions (and think you're saving time), by using "professional" assumptions and pre-conceived notions (the even longer way).

This seems simple, yes?

Actually, there's a lot to unpack here.

We'll begin with something I just said which may have confused you.

Why say that using "professional" assumptions and pre-conceived notions is the "even longer way" to a diagnosis?

One way to see this is to imagine yourself functioning as your patient's end-of-year tax accountant.

Now consider the case where your patient gives you only 70% of their annual expense receipts. How would you go about getting an accurate Standard Form 1080 from this 70%?

Let's say you have years of experience and ten prior years of this patient's tax returns. Obviously, you could choose to simply review these earlier returns, then estimate the missing numbers by averaging those returns.

Real accountants end up having to do this all the time. Most people do not keep perfect records and most times, doing this will be fine. Can you see why? In part, because not all—or even most—tax returns get audited. But in the case of diagnosing patients, every single "return" gets audited. By who? By life, that's who. And when life says "pay up," there's no appeal process.

Either you arrive at a proper diagnosis—or your patient suffers unnecessarily.

Avoiding the Logic Trap: Why Logical Diagnoses Fail

Before moving on to Chapter 6: ***Part Two: Arriving at a Diagnosis***, I first need to annoy you yet again, by talking about why you shouldn't use logic to guide ***Part One: Evidence Gathering.***

Logic, in general, reduces a question to an "already, assumed to be true" outcome. So if you make logical assumptions as to jump to an assumed diagnosis, then you'll also assume the kinds of evidence you should be looking for.

This makes ***beginning*** the diagnostic process with a logical assumption like skipping ahead to the last page of a book. Most times, doing this with books will ruin your enjoyment of the book. Doing this during the diagnostic process is much worse though. Here you risk wasting your patient's time and worse. You risk misdirecting the entire course of their treatment.

A second problem with diagnosticians making logical assumptions during the diagnostic process is that logic leads to evidence largely created by inference alone.

Emergences cannot include inferences. Inferences are the thing Freud warned Jung against—a way to skip ahead without evidence.

To diagnose properly then, you must limit your evidence to genuine evidence. Know the need for this becomes obvious when you consider why actual discoveries (emergences) always surprise you.

Why do they surprise you?

Because they can never be logically predicted. Not ever. To see what I'm saying here, consider the nature of ordinary water—good old H_2O.

Taken apart, water consists entirely of two gases—hydrogen and oxygen. But when these two gasses are connected in just the right relationship, something not previously present emerges. This thing is a property no gas ever has.

Do you know what this property is?

Wetness.

In the case of water, "wetness" is an emergent property. It appears only when you marry these two gases in just the right way. Moreover, since no gas has the quality of wetness, the best logic in the world could never predict this would happen. We know it happens only because it's an observable pattern which emerges after the fact.

Something I was recently surprised to learn is that our skin contains no receptors which sense wetness. Did you know that? This means our sense that something is wet is yet another emergent property. Thus wetness, like proper diagnoses, is something that exists primarily in our minds. And if you've been following all this, then something else may have just emerged in your mind. The idea that all proper diagnoses must emerge naturally—that they can never be contrived. They only happen because the human mind is programmed to have these kinds of ahas.

This makes diagnoses arrived at using logic, by comparison, mere shadows of those arrived at using genuine evidence alone. This is why those half-baked diagnoses require great effort to arrive at. They also never feel as solid or real as diagnoses which naturally emerge. Just something to keep in mind.

A Few Final Hints About What to Watch For

[Lordy. Will he ever stop repeating himself? Ed.]

Please forgive the following repetitions regarding ***Inferred Evidence***.

Clearly, I've already told you most of these things, many times, by now.

For one thing, I've repeatedly warned you against restating or reducing a patient's words to professional language. A patient's own words often reveal a great deal about who this person is and how his or her mind works.

Case in point, in the next chapter, I'll offer a number of cases where the patient's words were the key to the case. As opposed to obfuscating this nature by putting a logical spin on how patients describe their problems.

Why must you avoid doing this? Because as I've also repeatedly said, patients do not do things for logical reasons. Rather, they do them because it has become natural for them to do these things.

This, in fact, is what diagnosis looks to address. Diagnosis looks to discover these patterns in our patient's natures. Only by doing this can we hope to properly direct the path of any future treatment.

Here, the word "proper" refers to a diagnosis which "exposes the true nature of the patient's suffering—and does this to such a degree that the treatment does more than merely mask symptoms."

Another common situation where diagnosticians infer things occurs when patients can't think of anything to say when you ask them a question. In an "effort to help the patient," the diagnostician then begins to ask leading questions.

For instance, say you've asked your patient to describe how they've been doing—and they respond with anything resembling, "I don't know." Many diagnosticians then begin to ask leading questions like, "Have you been feeling depressed?"

All questions which include the word "feelings" will potentially result in compromised evidence. We'll explore why, in depth, in the next chapter. But in this case, if the diagnostician suspects this person has been depressed, a better approach would be to inquire about common symptoms of depression—things which can be pictured. Here the diagnostician might ask open-ended questions about specific activities of daily living.

For example, instead of asking, "Have you had trouble sleeping?" you might ask, "How have you been sleeping?" Similarly, inquiring about a patient's motivation would likely elicit vague results as well—"motivation" is just another way to refer to feelings.

Better would be to ask, "What kinds of things do you usually do?"

Then follow this by asking, "Have you been unable to do those things lately?"

Does Diagnostic, Evidence Gathering Ever Get Done?

Yet another of the many problems ***Inferred Evidence*** creates is that it prematurely assumes you know the diagnosis. In effect, you act like you've found the 4 corner pieces of a 1,000 piece puzzle. So you believe you already know what the puzzle is.

Worst case, you make these assumptions at the very beginning of the diagnostic process. From then on, either the evidence gathering process is biased—or the diagnostic evidence gathering window closes entirely.

Genuine Evidence on the other hand, consists of "an *open-ended* collection of scientific observations." Here, "scientific" means these observations are either based on responses to tipping-point questions—or on actual things you've seen or heard your patient say in your therapy room.

Know that to properly gather this kind of evidence, you must be able to assess at least the basics of a patient's ***personality***.

You must also be able to construct a proper ***diagnostic timeline*** using early childhood milestones.

Recall that I've told you, your questions must be tipping-point based.

Why?

Because they give you evidence for both what is—and what is not—present. This greatly decreases the chances you'll infer missing evidence, as these questions create a continuous spectrum of ***Genuine Evidence***. This spectrum then accounts for all possibilities, while at the same time ruling out things which do not apply.

Did you get that?

This process rules things IN and rules things OUT.

And the *open-ended* part?

Obviously, you cannot be expected to continuously gather evidence. So at some point, you must say, "At this point, this is as much as we can know." At the same time, "open-ended" means the evidence gathering window never permanently closes.

What it does do is, "it finishes the evidence gathering process *for now*."

This raises yet another of this chapter's takeaways, one we'll revisit many times—***the idea that all diagnoses should be considered "provisional diagnoses."***

> *"At this time, this is what we can say, based solely on the Genuine Evidence gathered so far. But should something come up later on—especially something which does not fit the diagnosis already given—then at that time, we must reconsider the diagnosis until we come up with one which accounts for all of the evidence observed."*

Here then is one of the more significant differences between these two kinds of evidence.

Inferred Evidence gathering focuses on quickly reaching some sort of conclusion—whereas ***Genuine Evidence*** gathering honors the process, is never hurried, and never results in a closed topic.

For example, if a patient, at a later date, says something which cannot be accounted for within the constellation of things already observed, then the evidence gathering process restarts and the entire diagnosis must be reopened and reconsidered.

And if someone pressures you to overlook this new evidence?

Then picture your patient's well-being and tell this other person to "fuck off."

When Do We Get To The Diagnosis?

In the sixth and final chapter, we'll expand on what you've learned about Evidence Gathering. There we'll look at how to use Emergence Personality Theory's five fractal patterns to set the baseline for a diagnosis. These measures exist in all human beings. So we'll use them to discern the difference between *clinical insignificance* and *health*. We'll then look at how the distributions of these five qualities allow us to discern between "Majority Personalities" and the four "Minority" variations.

Is autism really a pathology? How about ADHD? OCD? The answer lies in knowing that under it all, personality IS NOT patterns of behavior. Rather, personality functions like a set of five successively nested filters which hide things from our awareness. These filters function sort of like colored cellophanes, each subtracting part of the visible light. So we see less, not because we don't try or are broken. Rather, this is just part of being human.

At this point, we'll be ready for Part Two of the evidence gathering process—**Letting the Evidence Speak For Itself.** This will be our focus in Chapter 6. There I'll teach you how to let the natural patterns in evidence emerge in your mind *without help*. Admittedly—at first—you may struggle to let go and let this happen. You'll also need more than my reassurances to trust that doing this will work. You'll need to see this in action for yourself. This is why I'm spending so much time on Part One. Part One is the action step in diagnosis.

Finally, a few more words about letting the diagnosis emerge in you naturally (Oh, my God, is he never going to stop?). As I previously told you, in the language of an education expert, Part One of the diagnostic process—Evidence Gathering—equates to my concept, pre-learning. Here, ***pre-learning*** is defined as, ***"giving your mind unrestricted access to follow (be led around by) your curiosity."***

Part Two is then defined as, ***"letting the evidence speak for itself."*** In other words, in this part, you discover the meanings hidden in the pre-learning.

What are these hidden meanings? What exactly gets spoken?

An emergence, an aha moment, a sudden realization—where you suddenly know how all the evidence points to a patient's diagnosis. The thing to keep in mind here is that ***you should not try to make this happen***. Rather, you must let this be a side effect of doing Part One—Evidence Gathering.

What may help you to see why I've been annoying the shit out of you about this has to do with how I'm defining the word "emergence."

An emergence is ***"a pleasant surprise arising from a sufficient amount of pre-learning."*** Moreover, it's always a ***side-effect of this pre-learning—and never a deliberately induced outcome.***

Keep these two ideas in mind and you'll be diagnosing like a champ in no time.

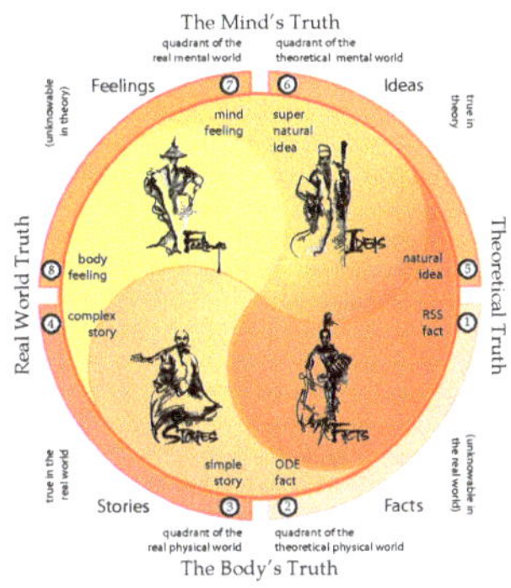

Chapter 6

Letting The Diagnosis Emerge
(what can we learn about . . . ?)

Diagnosis | Part Two - Allowing the Evidence to Speak For Itself

If you've made it this far, you've likely begun to see a few patterns emerge. If you have, do give yourself a proper at-a-boy or at-a-girl. Reaching this point without making assumptions as to what a patient's diagnosis should be means you're well on your way to becoming a world class diagnostician. No easy task given the amount of pressure you likely felt, back in school, to diagnose quickly.

In this, the final chapter, I'm going to do my best to pull it all together. To be honest, as I think about having to do this, I'm feeling a bit nervous. How can I possibly explain what I've learned about diagnosis during my past thirty years? Then again, as I check in with myself, I realize, I know this feeling.

I felt this way back in school, when I got told, "Get to the point. What's your diagnosis?" No pressure at all. Just make sure it's what we approve of.

Argh . . ., does this, "I don't know enough" feeling ever go away? My answer may surprise you. No, it does not. The real question is, "Does this mean you should start looking for an easier career?" My answer this time? Absolutely not. Indeed—hopefully—right about now, you're beginning to feel more like you've chosen the right career. And yes, revisiting so much of what you thought you already knew can be challenging. Then again, if you've made it this far, I know you have it in you to finish the job. Then too, you can always call "bullshit" on me for what you don't agree with. This said, we're almost done. So please, hang in there just a bit longer.

What will we focus on in this chapter? For one thing, we'll look at excerpts from a Grand Rounds group I and my colleagues recently held. Hopefully, this real life example will help you to see this stuff in action. Want to up your chances to gain from doing this? Then watch for [1] ***First Name***, [2] ***Chronological Age***, and [3] ***Presenting Problem stated in the client's own words—with nothing added.***

Why just the patient's "first" name? Because you should always be on a "first-name basis" with your patients. After all, you're diagnosing suffering human beings who clearly need your help. Also, if you want to be treated with respect, then you'll need to give respect as well. And being you're the diagnostician, this responsibility begins with you. Please do keep this in mind.

Why the patient's age? As I've previously said, this creates the patient's diagnostic timeline. Using Chapter 5's train metaphor, this timeline amounts to the railroad tracks stretching between the departure (birth) and destination (chronological age) stations. Once defined, the "Developmental Bingo Cards" can then help you to determine the developmental ages of the things your patients tell you. You then note when this evidence occurred on a second "developmental" timeline.

How will you determine these ages? As I said, you'll use the Developmental Bingo Cards. These cards use 4 groups of 5 developmental qualities, each of which identify 4 developmental periods. Now if you look over on the next page, you'll find the Title Card for this deck. This card includes a brief explanation of what you'll be doing. Realize, there's a lot to understand here—so please go slow. Start with the first words—"***Diagnostically Possible, Developmental Qualities***." These words tell you, you'll be using personality—and specifically, some developmental qualities of personality—to identify the developmental ages of the things your patients say.

And the next phrase; ***"Birth to Age 4?"***

This defines the overall range of ages you'll be choosing from.

Know this range of ages is broken down into 4 periods of early child development. Here, each list focuses on different developmental periods. The periods?

- Age Birth to Six Months (list 1)
- Age Six Months to Age One (list 2)
- Age One to Age Two (list 3)
- Age Two to Age Four (list 4)

The rest of what's written on this Title Card explains the point for doing this. Why do this? Because when patients struggle, they often regress. When they do, they lose access to the life skills they acquired *after* that age. If they regress to age two? Then they'll only have access to the life skills they had up to, but not beyond, age two. And if they regress to five months old? Well, you get the point. How does this help you to diagnose? In two ways. It allows you to tailor your words and questions to what a person that age would understand. And it creates a ***visual diagnostic history,*** allowing you to better organize and process the patient's answers.

The 5 Senses	The 4 Informations	Sense of Objects & Beings	Character Type	Sense of Self and Others

Diagnostically Possible Developmental Qualities

Birth to Age 4

All diagnostically-gathered evidence should reference both the patient's current, and developmental, ages. Diagnosticians can then use their patients' current "diagnostic age" to better voice questions.

The 5 Senses	The 4 Informations	Sense of Objects & Beings	Character Type	Sense of Self and Others
birth				
Comfort		Bluntness	Physical Gender	
The four **Primary Senses** begin to differentiate	**Feelings** (invisible change) begin to exist	No ability to see **Objects** or **Beings**	Unfocused & Strong **Me State**	No sense of **Self**
6 mo				

Child Development

Diagnostically Possible Developmental Qualities

Birth to Six Months

Life is "learning to get comfort"

Identifying "Birth to Six Months," Using Developmental Qualities

On the previous page, you'll find the first of the four **Developmental Bingo Cards**. Each card has its own unique **horizontal list** of the same 5 developmental qualities. These lists will help you to determine which of the four developmental ages best fits the things your patients say. The five developmental qualities?

- The patient's access to **The 5 Senses (Primary 4 Senses vs All 5 Senses)**
- The patient's access to **The 4 Informations (feelings, facts, stories, ideas)**
- The patient's **Sense of Objects & Beings (objects aren't persons, beings are)**
- The patient's **Character Type (who has these needs, Me or You?)**
- The patient's **Sense of Self and Others (neither, self, others, self and others)**

This particular card lists the **Birth and Six Months** versions of these 5 developmental qualities. Identifying even a single quality from this list can improve your questions and enable you to better understand your patient's answers. For instance, say a patient exhibits a strong need for physical **Comfort** *when he or she is under stress*. Then it's likely this patient will also exhibit other things on this list as well—including that *Feelings* will likely be their **Information** of choice.

What if you find your patient does tend to make *Feelings* their **Information** of choice (the 2nd column)? Then realize, your patient will likely struggle to find words to describe these feelings. At this age, babies have yet to *differentiate*, let alone assign word labels, to their feelings. So if your patient does struggle here, do remember to tell them to "take their time." Also keep in mind, at this age, babies have yet to *differentiate* their **4 Primary Senses** (hearing, taste, touch, smell). Nor have they developed their sense of **depth perception**. This means they will sense no separation between their inner world (themselves) and the outer world. These two worlds remain merged. This means they cannot perceive "other people or things" as "objects or beings" (the 3rd column). Patients who present like this often report feeling distanced and apart from objects—and from people, including themselves. As a personal experience, this refers to what you see in the 4th column—**Character Type**—which on the Birth to Six Months card, is an *Unfocused & Strong Me State*.

Finally it's likely this person will also have *little to no sense of self* (the 5th column) when he or she is under stress. Babies this age define themselves only through the eyes of others.

Why Am I Calling These Cards, "Bingo Cards?"

Why call these cards, "bingo cards?" Because of how they're used. You place mental bingo chips (or physical chips, if you print these cards) on each quality you identify in your patient. Here even one chip can be helpful, as this can point to which card you're going to use. And if your patient has trouble picturing things? Then this person may struggle with one or more of the 4 Primary Senses. Vision—as a sense—exists only when people can sense all 4 Primary Senses. Clearly, there's a lot to unpack here as well. So for now, just set aside any questions you may have.

The 5 Senses	The 4 Informations	Sense of Objects & Beings	Character Type	Sense of Self and Others
6 mo				
Neatness		Correction	Sexual Gender	
Vision (the fifth sense) emerges	**Facts** (visible unchange) begin to exist	The ability to see **Objects** begins	Focused and Weak **Me State**	A vague sense of **Self** begins
1 yr				

Child Development

Diagnostically Possible Developmental Qualities

6 Months to Age One

Life is "learning to interact with objects"

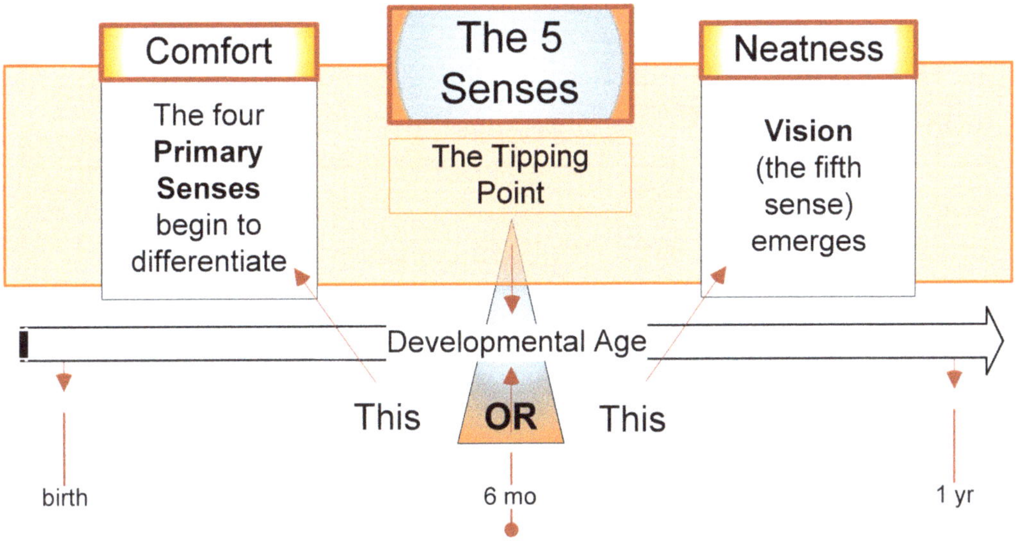

Identifying "Six Months to Age One," Using Developmental Qualities

On this Bingo Card is the list of developmental qualities unique to **Age Six Months to Age One.** To make use of this list, you'll need to contrast and compare it to the list on the previous card. The measures in each of the 5 vertical columns are tipping-point based. This means, *ruling in* a result in one age's list rules out the results in the other lists.

For example, contrast and compare the **5 Senses column** in these two developmental age lists. A few pages back, I told you that *Vision* (in the **5 Senses column**)—and specifically *depth perception*—can exist only after the *4 Primary Senses* develop. So the tipping-point based measure here is, "Can your patient picture the thing they're saying?" (Six Months to Age One). Or not? (Birth to Six Months)? If they can't? Then what they are saying likely lies in the **Birth to Six Months** era. But if they can? Then what they are saying lies in the **Six Months to Age One** era—*or older.*

Keep in mind, when assessing for vision, there is a second tipping point which must be ruled in or out. Can the person ***gradually*** picture things, or not? Becoming able to see something ***gradually*** means your patient is in a normal state of mind. But ***suddenly*** picturing something means your patient is reliving an injury.

The point here? These tipping-point based Bingo card measures only apply to things patients experience in an unwounded state. For vision, the unwounded state means ***gradually*** picturing things. ***Suddenly*** picturing something means this information can't be used on the Bingo cards. Just something to keep in mind.

Now contrast and compare the tipping-point based measures in the other four vertical columns. *Facts* vs *Feelings*. *The ability to see Objects* (or not). *Character Type* (a strong Me State vs a Weak one). And *Sense of Self or Others* (no clearly defined senses vs having the 5 senses but no sense of beings - self or others). Again, each measure is tipping-point based. So only one answer can be ruled in, at a time.

The 5 Senses	The 4 Informations	Sense of Objects & Beings	Character Type	Sense of Self and Others

Child Development

Diagnostically Possible Developmental Qualities

Age One to Age Two

Life is "learning to interact with Objects with Needs"

1 yr

Understanding		Precision	Psychological Gender	
Experiencing "vision over brief time" emerges	**Stories** (visible change) begin to exist	The ability to see people as "**Objects with Needs**" begins	Unfocused & Strong **You State**	The sense of **Self** and **Others** begins

2 yr

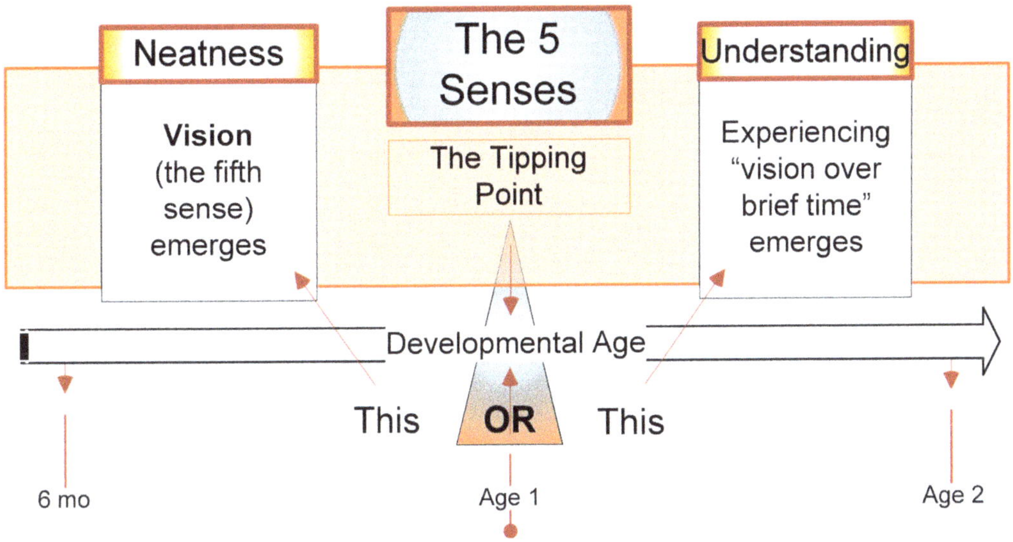

Identifying "Age One to Age Two," Using Developmental Qualities

Now we'll look at the third Developmental Bingo card. This time, the list refers to the developmental qualities unique to **Age One to Age Two**. Again, notice the five column headings. Now contrast and compare the tipping-point based measures in each of the vertical columns to those on the previous cards. Can you see how they tip, meaning, how only one answer can apply in each column, at a time?

For instance, take the ***Sense of Self and Others*** column. There are now three cards. Thus there are now three possible results. [1] "No ability to see ***Objects*** or ***Beings***." [2] "The ability to see ***Objects*** begins." Or [3] "The ability to see people as ***Objects with Needs*** begins." Only one of these results can be true in any given moment. No in between measures exist—hence the idea that these three measures are tipping-point based.

Granted, to understand what these phrases mean, you'll need to learn to recognize the kinds of visual clues specific to each of these developmental ages. For example, babies, at about Age One, begin to see that other "objects" have needs. What I'm saying is, at this point, babies begin to see themselves and all other beings as separate objects. Observing how a sixteen-month-old girl responds to having needs offers evidence for this. When most (not all) sixteen-month-old baby girls want something, they first look out at their mothers, then back at what they want, then back at their mothers. This kind of looking back and forth does not normally exist in babies before Age One. This means, if you observe it, then this baby is at least one year old. This means, if you witness this kind of behavior in patients, then it can indicate, they are currently experiencing life through the lens of the developmental stage at Age One to Two. Keep in mind, learning to process these kinds of cues will be a career-length, ongoing process. There are always more ways to see the signs that your patients are regressing to specific developmental ages. So please go slow with learning this, be patient with yourself, and take your time.

The 5 Senses	The 4 Informations	Sense of Objects & Beings	Character Type	Sense of Self and Others

Child Development

Diagnostically Possible Developmental Qualities

Age Two to Age Four

Life is "learning to interact with pairs/groups of people"

2 yr

Freedom		Digression	Social Gender	
Experiencing "lack of vision over brief time" emerges	Ideas (invisible unchange) begin to exist	The ability to sense people as "other beings with needs" begins	Focused and Weak Me-You & You-Me States	Sense of self **as** different from others begins

4 yr

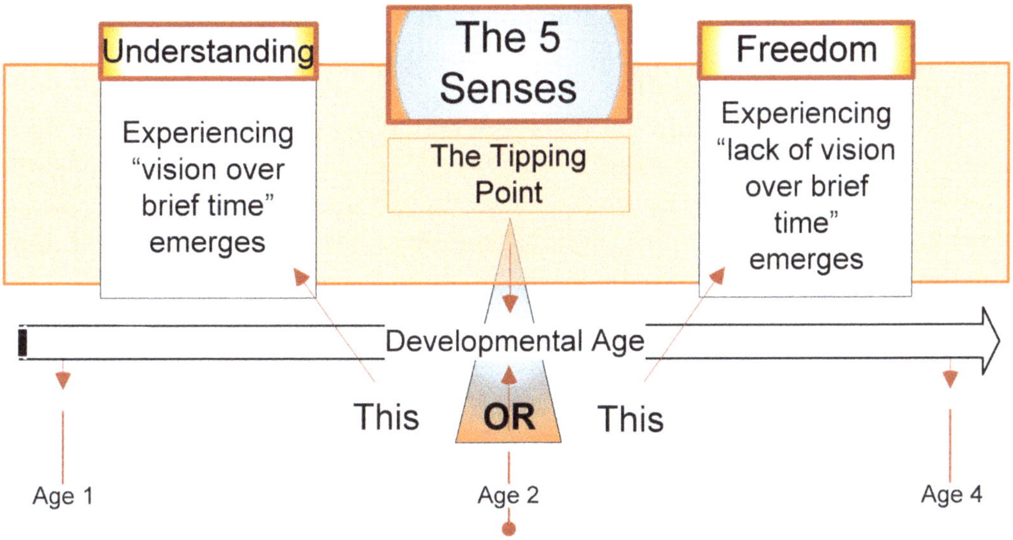

Identifying "Age Two to Age Four" Using Developmental Qualities

Finally, we come to the fourth and final Bingo card. This one lists the developmental qualities unique to **Age Two to Age Four**. By now, hopefully, the point for using these cards has become obvious to you.

You decide which qualities best fit the things your patient is telling you.

Will this be easy to do?

Not at first. Determining the developmental ages of the things patients say and do can, at first, seem beyond complex. What can help here is to keep in mind, you are only looking to choose based on tendencies—not on every nuance. Moreover, sometimes, the way in which a patient tells you something can switch between two developmental ages in a single sentence. When this happens, the thing to keep in mind this time is simply this.

You do not need to account for everything patients say.

You need only do this for the things which seem diagnostically significant to you.

And if none of what I've told you has made sense?

Then for now, just let all this go, knowing we'll talk more about it before we finish this chapter.

Grand Rounds Case #1 - Introduction

What we're going to look at next is an actual case from one of our once-a-month Grand Rounds groups. Our main goals in these groups? We have three.

[1] To improve our abilities to gather ***genuine evidence***.

[2] To learn to avoid gathering ***inferred evidence***.

[3] To improve our abilities to allow the critical diagnostic patterns to emerge from this evidence naturally, ***on their own***.

Before we begin though, I want to offer a kindly phrased, soft spoken caution. Please do your best to heed this advice.

There are a shitload of things going on in this transcript. So you'll likely need to read through it several times. Even then, you'll likely come away with only a modest sense of what's going on.

Despite my saying this, every bit of evidence will have come from only three pieces of information. First name. Current age. Presenting problem, in the client's own words. So you wish to improve your diagnostic skills, then as you read, please try to keep this in mind. Can you maintain your focus on the three principal things I've just mentioned? I believe you can. Also, do try to notice when you feel urges to infer evidence. Doing this can really help you learn to let the genuine evidence speak for itself.

And when you forget or feel lost—or when your mind wanders?

When this happens, just know this.

We'll discuss and explore what was said in this group, in depth, when this transcript finishes. Rereading the transcript—followed by rereading the analysis—several times through, can help a lot. Even here though, remember, this has taken me years to learn. So do know, you'll likely need to have your own real life experiences in order to connect these things to how you practice.

Finally, do keep in mind, you have one goal here—to pre-learn. Thus please do not try to understand, let alone memorize, any of this. My goal here? To expose you to a more efficient, more personal way to diagnose your patients. To properly use this way of diagnosing, you'll need to do something diagnosticians find really hard.

You'll need to let go of any desire to *learn* what's happening here.

What I'm saying here is, please do your best to simply let these words wash over you. This means, do your best to make no effort whatsoever to learn what I'm presenting. And yes. This can sound crazy. In effect, I'm asking you to try to let go of any need to learn. Instead, try to connect to—and get a personal experience of—these clinicians, all this without needing to retain a thing.

What should become apparent during this Grand Rounds dialogue is that we're each in our own way struggling to do the same thing. We're struggling to keep seeing this patient as a suffering human being. If you can join us in doing this, then you'll likely gain some new skills. Again, do your best. That's all I'm asking.

And now, the transcript.

Linda's Case – A 13-Year-Old Girl Named Alyssa (pre-case intro)

Steve (to the group): So you already know the three things you need to focus on when you're presenting a case—the patient's [1] First Name, [2] Current Age, and [3] Presenting Problem—as stated by the patient at the intake.

Why these particular pieces of information—and why in this order?

Why first name, not last?

Why current age?

And why must the presenting problem be stated in the patient's own words?

Maria: Because this begins to give you some sense of the patient's story?

Steve: Yes, Maria. That is part of it. But why these particular three pieces of information? And why in this order?

Sam: Because it makes the patient, a "person?" Using the patient's first name makes him or her a human being?

Steve: That's right, Sam. And to see this in action, try to recall a time when you were talking about somebody, but didn't mention this person's name. Shelby, you're smiling. Can you tell me the time you're thinking of?

Shelby: I can picture stumbling over the pronouns in a sentence and not being able to keep what I'm trying to say organized.

Steve: Okay.

Tom?

Tom: I was going to say, at my job, I don't use first names. I call everyone, "patient." This means I feel detached from them. Is this wrong?

Steve: Not at all. You work in a mental hospital, where crossing that line can invite patients to expect inappropriate things from you. Using a patient's first name in a case presentation is different though. There's a big difference between referring to a person as a "patient" (while also knowing their name) and actually saying this person's first name. And to properly diagnose, we need to paint a picture of the patient as an actual, living person.

For instance, I could say "the guy in the green shirt" (a reference to Sam). Or I could say "Sam." Or I could say "the guy in the gray sweatshirt with the beard and the "semi waking-up hair" (a reference to Jesse). Or I could say, "Otis's father" (another reference to Jesse—Otis is Jesse's one year old son). Or I could say "Jesse."

Can you hear the difference; how a person's first name creates something important? It connects you to this person and them to you. Conversely, last names tend to create impersonal distance and interpersonal biases. Strangely, these effects often get overlooked, both by diagnosticians and patients alike.

Most diagnosticians feel pressured to get right to the problem. This often leads to them overlooking the suffering human being, as they focus on finding this problem. Also, when people tell stories, they often talk about "a person," "my friend," or "my boss." Here they're referring to people based mainly on their roles (my boss)—or to a time in life when they knew this person ("somebody from my childhood").

Saying the patient's first name can accomplish something none of these things can do. It creates a picture of this person in your mind. Again, we are diagnosing people—not objects, times, or roles. So no picture, no personally accurate sense of who the diagnosis applies to.

What about stating their current chronological age?

Why must we do that? Sam?

Sam: It gives us a way to create a timeline for the person's life? So say my patient is currently 29 years old. I could use this age to create the end point of their chronological timeline. I could then ask myself, "What year were they born?" Knowing this year would then tell me a lot about their early childhood influences.

I could then contrast and compare this chronological age to the developmental ages of the things this patient tells me. Do they line up? Are they significantly different? This would reveal a lot.

Steve: This is excellent, Sam. Obviously, this information is deeply meaningful, and it tells you a lot about the patient's current developmental influences. Also, like Maria, you've told me how you'd use this information. This said, you've still not told me *why* the patient's current age matters.

Jesse, you had your hand up. Thoughts?

Jesse: I, too, was thinking about the patient's chronological timeline. But I feel more interested in putting things they say on their developmental timeline.

Steve: . Okay. Again though, while doing that gives us a lot of good information, it still doesn't point to *why* we look to do this. Linda, how old are you?

Linda: 56.

Steve: 56. So birth to 56 defines the limits of both of Linda's timelines—her ***chronological*** timeline and her ***developmental*** timeline. This age also sets the maximum age for the evidence we'd need to gather. We would not need to look beyond her age 56. Also, since the patient's most recent experiences of presenting problems exist at the patient's current age, we'd not begin looking for evidence at Linda's age 31. We'll begin our questions at age 56.

Why do this? Because *a patient's current age* [at the onset of treatment] *anchors the end-date of the presenting problem.* Here, with the patient's ***chronological*** timeline, we'll be looking to place whatever gets said, but especially the presenting problem—chronologically—based on their current age. With the patient's ***developmental*** timeline, however, we'll be looking to see how this problem resembles earlier events developmentally. This is why we need to make two timelines for every patient.

We need a birth to the present age—***chronological*** timeline.

And we need a birth to the present age—***developmental*** timeline.

So say your patient is currently age 42. You'd need to look for signs of a mid-life crisis in the air, and how this may be affecting the presenting problem. This crisis normally occurs between ***chronological*** ages 41 to 43. So the presenting problem may have been triggered by this. But if your patient is ***chronologically*** between ages 29 and 31? Then you'd look for signs of Erikson's "death of immortality."

Can you see how these two ages are each in their own way diagnostically significant? In both cases, the patient's age will developmentally color everything the patient says. So if your patient has just turned 30 and she mentions her father died at her age six? Then you'd make a note on her chronological timeline, at age 30, and look for signs of Erikson's "death of immortality"—and another note, at age six, on her developmental timeline—the date of her father's death.

Why write notes on both timelines? Because it's likely she'd be experientially alternating between these two ages as she speaks to you. Here you'd need to watch for the developmental signs of both ages, age 30 and age 6. And if you do see these signs? Then you'd need to voice your questions with this in mind.

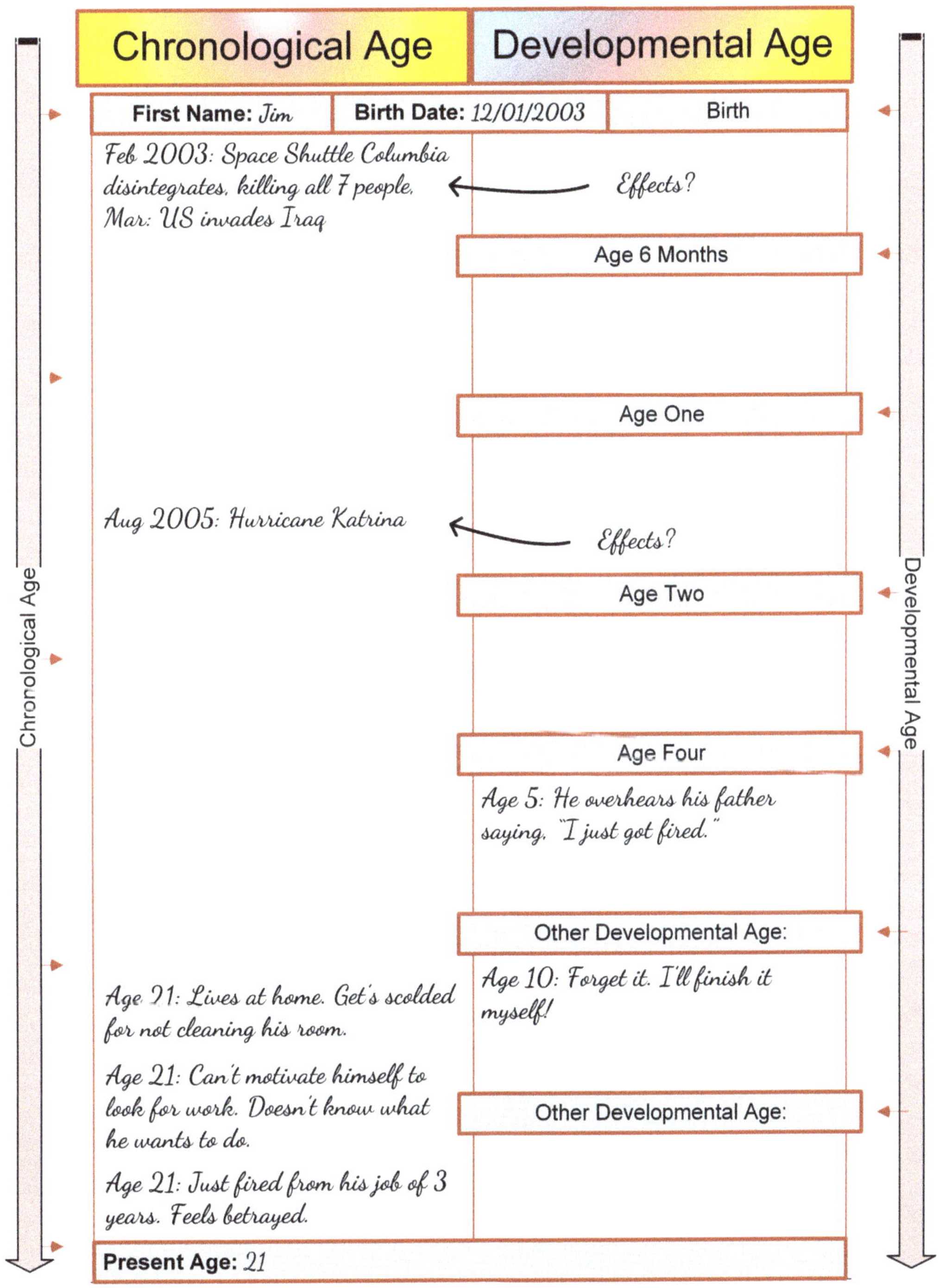
Chronological Age
Developmental Age
First Name: Jim
Birth Date: 12/01/2003
Birth
Feb 2003: Space Shuttle Columbia disintegrates, killing all 7 people.
Mar: US invades Iraq
Effects?
Age 6 Months
Age One
Aug 2005: Hurricane Katrina
Effects?
Age Two
Age Four
Age 5: He overhears his father saying, "I just got fired."
Other Developmental Age:
Age 10: Forget it. I'll finish it myself!
Age 21: Lives at home. Get's scolded for not cleaning his room.
Age 21: Can't motivate himself to look for work. Doesn't know what he wants to do.
Other Developmental Age:
Age 21: Just fired from his job of 3 years. Feels betrayed.
Present Age: 21
Chronological Age
Developmental Age

For instance, say you saw signs this patient was looking through the lens of her current age. Then you'd voice your questions in words typical to people this age. But if you then saw signs she was seeing life through the lens of her six-year-old self, you'd adjust your language and demeanor to best speak to her six-year-old self.

Another benefit of doing these two timelines has to do with the ability to backdate the patient's *chronological* age to the year they were born. What major things were happening in the world in that year? You'd also need to consider what occurred in the decade that followed this birth year. And together, these things would tell you a lot about the ***outside influences*** which invisibly affect much of what your patient will say—including how they will voice why they're there and what they expect to get from treatment.

Now consider the patient's ***developmental*** age, and how it creates the ***inside influences*** through which he or she will process their ***outside influences***. Say your patient—we'll call him, **Jim**—age 21, tells you he just got fired. Say he then adds, he felt like he'd been betrayed when they let him go. He'd worked for this company for three years and had worked really hard. Asking Jim if this event reminded him of any other time he'd felt betrayed might offer important diagnostic clues.

Could he be reliving something from when he was age 10, say a time when he was working on something with his father? Say he'd tried really hard that day to please his father. But in the midst of these efforts, his father abruptly said, "Forget it! I'll do it myself." Even though this would diagnostically have had more to do with what was going on in Jim's father that day, age 10 is the "age of heroes." And when your hero dismisses you, this experience sticks.

Notably, this—and all abrupt changes in early childhood—point to possible Event-sized Disorders. You'd need to look for this. So you'd record the current "being fired" event on the ***chronological*** timeline at age 21—because that's when it occurred. But you'd also need to note the earlier age 10 event on this patient's ***developmental*** timeline. Then you'd watch for signs that told you Jim was regressing to age 10 while he spoke to you about his getting fired.

Can you see why both of these ages would be important to watch for?

If, while reporting a recent event, the patient relives something significant from age 10, then you'd need to consider and watch for these two diagnostic influences. One, this patient's expectations from his ***outside*** world, at age 21. And two, this patient's ***inner*** experience of regressing to what he knew about life, at age 10.

What might this look like in Jim's case—responding to the outside world at age 21, and through his mind and its inner lens at age 10?

Say Jim still lives at home and he report's frequently being scolded for not cleaning his room. Could this in some way be related to the time his dad sent him away from "a job" at 10 years old? How about to his experience of getting fired?

Are you beginning to see how connecting a *presenting problem* to a *developmental event* gives you additional evidence? The possible diagnostic influences here are endless.

Can you also see how noting these connections would add to the genuine evidence you collect? Keep in mind, though, to get the full benefits from your doing this, you'd need to create these kinds of visual reminders on both timelines. You'd also need to look for more signs, including how these two influences interact.

Why?

Because these kinds of interactions often lead to "big picture" kinds of diagnostic patterns emerging during diagnostician/patient conversations. And a diagnosis is simply a kind of mega, "big picture."

∞

So—[1] name—[2] chronological age, which then creates the chronological timeline, birth to the present age—and then, [3] the presenting problem. You then add to this any observations wherein the patient regresses to an earlier, developmentally significant, event. Realize most regressions will be to times which occurred at or before the patient's age 7—before the patient learned to tell time. This will cause your patient to be unable to see what will likely be obvious to you—how these developmental influences effect present day events.

How do you recognize these connections? A good way is to watch for signs in the person's language. Hearing "all or nothing" words and phrases—like *good* and *bad,* and *always* and *never*—are signs the patient's developmental age is currently sometime before age 7. Watching the way your patient's body moves can give you similar hints—young children move quite differently from adults. And after a while, recognizing these signs becomes an intuitive part of diagnosis.

For instance, Athena (she is currently eating something), you look like you are reliving something from an earlier age.

Can anyone tell me what age she appears to be reliving?

To me, it looks like you're reliving something from about age 12—a time you were at a holiday or a family meal. Here, you've in some sense been told, either by your inner voice or by someone else, to present yourself so your family looks good.

What makes me say this?

You're eating so slowly and perfectly. Granted, you may not be aware of this because it's just such a part of who you are. But you're currently eating in front of a large group of people—all of us. Hence my saying it's likely a family event, as more people are present than would be at your usual family dinner table.

After a while, recognizing these kinds of visual and verbal patterns becomes self-evident. And obviously, there's no diagnostic meaning to the way Athena is eating—I gave this example merely to point out the kinds of things which can be seen. Okay. Linda, can you tell us your patient's first name, chronological age, and her presenting problem in her own words?

Linda: Ouch. I think I screwed up. The client's age? She's 13. And her first name is Alyssa. But the presenting problem I have is stated in the mother's words.

Steve: Okay. How about the things Alyssa said to you in her first session with you? Do you recall anything she said that sounded notable to you in that session?

Linda: Oh shit. My Alexa app just went off. [The group laughs].

Anyway, I do have the words Alyssa gave the intake person.

Steve: Did this intake person write down Alyssa's own words?

Linda: There are quotes around them—so they're definitely her own words. There are also some of the mom's words as well. The thing is, if I only give you Alyssa's words, I don't know if this will make sense to you all without first hearing what the mom initially said.

Steve: Okay Linda, pause. Group, can anyone tell me the mistake Linda just made in presenting the case?

Linda, you're not breathing. We're just here to learn. So please stay with us.

Tom: She gave too much information?

Steve: Yes, Tom. That's true. But that's not the real problem.

The real problem is, Linda wants to give us additional information. Her explanation for needing to do this? She claims, without it, we won't understand what she's saying.

The thing is, I don't want to *understand* what she's saying. Why not? Because *understanding* gives us a "preconceived notion" of what Alyssa's words mean. Schools pressure people to learn to do this as they diagnose. But doing this is just plain wrong. Why? Don't we want all the information we can get?

Actually, no, we don't. We only want what the patient says in their own words.

Why? Think about it. Believing you already understand what something means will bias what you then ask your patient. It will also put a spin on the meaning of every answer the patient gives. Then, if these things *don't* fit your preconceived notions, then you won't see them as important. And if they *do* fit your preconceived notions? Then you risk seeing them as more diagnostically significant than they are.

Linda, realize, we are not trying to *understand* the evidence. We're only looking to *gather* it. So do try to let go of having to make sure we understand it.

Rather, just give us the genuine evidence.

[Said to the group] Recall what your task here is. Each time Linda gives us data, the rest of us will be looking to ask Linda diagnostic questions. The goal? To gather enough genuine evidence from what's said for the diagnostic patterns to begin to emerge from the evidence. Okay. So now, let's begin. Linda, can you tell us what the intake person's notes say?

Linda: Okay. But I'd just like to read one sentence from the mom. Then I'll give you the client's words.

Steve [in frustration]: Linda, please don't do that. Please set aside these urges to override what I'm asking you for. And yes, I know what you were likely taught to do back in school. They taught you to do the very thing I'm asking you to not do. This said, please do your best to set these urges aside. Only then can you personally experience for yourself what happens when you do it this way.

Linda (speaking very quickly now): Okay, I'll read the . . .

Steve: Linda, slow down. I'm trying to get you to see *why* doing this is important.

Linda: Because you want the client's words, not someone else's?

Steve: Yes. But why? Let me try again. In wanting to give us the mother's words, you're putting the focus on getting us to "understand." This means you're trying to get us to assign meanings to the evidence you're about to give us *before you even give it to us.* I know you're trying to help us here. But I wish you could let this go. Why? Because in your efforts to get us to understand your client, you'll be biasing everything you tell us—along with everything we then say and think in this group.

So say a client comes in and says, "I want to work on better communication with my partner." To me, that phrase is a throwaway. Why? Because if, at this point, you try to understand what they mean by "better communication," you lose. You've yet to gather any genuine evidence. Yet already, you'll have biased your entire sense of what these people are actually there for.

Also, "better communication" is not a diagnostically discernible problem. Why not? Because there's no human on earth who couldn't benefit from better communication, including me. Worse yet, it's likely a phrase they learned from another therapist, or from a TV therapy show, or that they read in one of those bad self-help books—rather than something they're voicing in their own words.

My point here? The minute you try to *understand* what evidence means, you've stopped *collecting* evidence, because you've created a hypothesis. You'll then try to fit the evidence you do gather to what you think you already know. "Confirmation Bias" and all that rot. This will eliminate a whole lot of questions you might have asked.

Linda's Case | A 13 Year Old Girl Named Alyssa - Intake (part 1)

Steve: So Linda, could you please just read the client's own words and skip the mother's?

Linda: Okay. So "the client's own words."

> **Alyssa (her intake):** "I don't know why I'm acting like this. I'm acting dumb. I'm also on my phone, doing stuff I shouldn't be doing."

Steve: Linda (who is still beating herself up), [said softly] please stop beating yourself up. Would you please reread the first part of what your patient said?

> **Alyssa (her intake):** "I don't know why I am acting like this?"

Steve: Okay. Stop.
Can anybody tell me what they can see here?
It's already pretty revealing.
Clancey?
Clancey: The patient is blaming herself?
Steve: Oh, yes. One sentence in and already we can see that.
Well done, Clancey. Thank you.

Steve: Me? I'm putting myself in Alyssa's place. As I do, I can see how this one sentence points to a 13-year-old girl who has already struggled a lot in life. It also tells me she is someone who tries to reflect on herself and on her life. Also, when she says, "I don't know why I am acting like this," she's being self-critical. Here, she's either feeling regret or remorse or both. [Note: where Steve got these things from will be explained after the case.]

Tom: Would this be evidence for her having a You state in her Character Type?

Steve: It certainly is, Tom. Keep in mind though, it's only one piece of evidence. So we shouldn't assume anything yet. If you think you know something from a single piece of evidence, this will bias what you look for going forward. And with tipping-point based evidence, like remorse vs regret, or Character Type (Me state vs You state), you're then going to assume you already know which it is—when in truth, at this point, we have too little evidence to know.

Steve: Jesse, you had your hand up?

Jesse: Yeah. I wonder if what she said here points to that she has ***Understanding*** as her fourth Social Priority. ***Understanding*** is my fourth Social Priority. So when I'm really stressed, that's where I go. Could this be true for Alyssa? [Note: again, what these things mean will be explained after the case.]

Steve: That's an excellent question, Jesse.

Jesse: Yeah, like, "Why is this happening to me? Why am I like this?"

Steve: You're right, Jesse. And based on what we see in this sentence, it's possible, Alyssa has ***Understanding*** as her lowest Social Priority. Why? Because she's obviously suffering as she's arriving in therapy. And the first thing she says is, "I don't know why I do this." This is evidence that, when she's at her worst, she looks to understand. That's brilliant, Jesse. Really good. Anyone else?

Okay. So Linda, can you see how Jesse just did the opposite of what you've been taught to do in school? And yes, I know, when you tried to make sure we understood the evidence—before we even heard it—I know you were trying to help us. Also, I'm quite sure this was what you were required to do back in school. There, I'm sure you had to present—and analyze—cases during the presentation. They wanted you to try to logically understand what evidence meant almost before you finished hearing it.

Now consider what we're doing here, by limiting what we're proposing to things based entirely on personality and human nature. Already, we can know a lot about Alyssa, all this from a single, six-word sentence. What do we already know?

One: That it's possible Alyssa is **You first**.
Two: That by age 13, Alyssa's **already self-reflective**.
Three: That it's likely **Alyssa has already suffered a lot**.

My support for this third statement?

Thirteen-year-olds who haven't suffered a lot don't come to therapy already having had insights about themselves. By this age, people definitely have begun to question why *the world* is the way it is. But they don't usually question why *they* are the way they are.

Shelby, I'd guess you were like Alyssa by age 4 (she nods, yes). Maria, I'd bet you were likely like that by age 6 or before (she smiles).

Okay. Linda, what was Alyssa's next sentence?

Alyssa (her intake): "I'm acting dumb. I'm also on my phone, doing stuff I shouldn't be doing."

Steve: Okay, we have several things to look at here. Let's look, one at a time.

Alyssa (her intake): "I'm acting dumb."

Steve: Okay. Clancey? I've heard you say things like this about yourself. Any thoughts about this girl? She says, "I'm *acting* dumb." You'd more likely say, "I *am* dumb." But Alyssa said, "I'm *acting* dumb." What do you think about this?

Clancey: I'm not sure. It could mean a lot of things.

Steve: Yes, that's true. This said, can you offer any thoughts?

Clancey: It's hard to put into words. I know I've felt like her a lot. This makes me wonder who she surrounds herself with, and if she feels she has to impress them—or if she feels judged. I'd definitely want to know more about her social life.

Steve: That's excellent, Clancey. Notice, though, that you prefaced what you told us with, "It could mean a lot of things" and "it's hard to put into words."

These things, especially your saying, "I'm not sure," are apologies.

Then when you slowed down—and when you took your time—look what happened. The apologies went away.

Excellent, Clancey.

Shelby?

Shelby: I feel like I may be regressing. So this may be more about me than about Alyssa.

Steve: That's fine, Shelby. All we're doing at this point is throwing out possible things about this person based on what we know about personality and human nature. We're not supposed to know for sure whether these things are true yet.

Shelby: Okay. So I'm picturing a time when I lied to my mom in order to keep myself safe and she said to me, "Don't act dumb!"

Steve: So you're saying, Alyssa may literally have been startled by hearing that or a similar phrase? That's absolutely a possibility.

You may be right.

Tom?

Tom: This sentence reminds me of me where, somewhere deep down, I perceived myself as being smart. But I would act like I was dumb.

Steve: That's also interesting.

Tom: You don't say "act" dumb if you "are" dumb. I don't know. Does this make sense?

Steve: It does. You know better, but you do it anyway. David?

David: So I heard these two sentences, and what went on inside my body is a question. Obviously we need more information. But can this girl be Body first? [Note: again, what this means will be explained after the case.]

Steve: Did you hear something that would point to this?

David: So the words I latched onto were *act* and *being on the phone,* all of which I know a lot of teenagers say and do. It's still a question in my mind. But *something in my body* makes me wonder.

Steve: Okay. So similar to feeling either remorse or regret, at this point, all we can say is, we have one thing which points to her being Body first.

Okay. Linda. Would you read that sentence again.

There were two ideas in that sentence. "I act dumb" and . . .

Linda: "I act dumb," and, "I am on my phone doing stuff I shouldn't be doing."

Steve: Okay. Anyone have a comment about any of this? Sam? "Doing stuff I shouldn't be doing"? Thoughts?

Sam: Yeah. I often hear people say that phrase. "I shouldn't be doing it." It's confusing. I always need to ask a lot of questions about that. If I don't, I never know if it's coming from the inside or the outside. I can't tell if it's a personal rule or a theoretical idea. It's confusing.

Steve: Keep in mind though, this is a 13-year-old teen who's probably not going to have the defenses of a 50 year old woman. Her age gives us some clues about this.

Sam: I'm imagining someone once telling her, she shouldn't do "something."

Steve: Athena? "I am on my phone doing things I shouldn't be doing." You have two daughters who are frequently on phones doing things they shouldn't be doing. What do you think?

Athena: Yeah, I'm curious where, what Alyssa's saying here, is coming from.

It confuses me too.

Steve: Okay. Tom?

Tom: Well, she's 13. I mean, at what age would she normally start rebelling?

Steve: Normally, the change from seeing "your parents being *heroes*" to "your parents being *stupid*" occurs between ages 11 and 13.

Tom: So should we put this at the same spot on both the chronological and developmental timelines?

Steve: Definitely. Why?

For one thing, because this is obviously being reported currently.

For another, because what she's saying is obviously age appropriate. So it also tells us things about Alyssa's current developmental age as well.

In effect, we can see several things here.

"I act dumb," may indicate that she's been told, "You know better. Why did you do that?" As for that next sentence, thoughts?

Alyssa (her intake): "I'm also on my phone, doing stuff I shouldn't be doing."

Steve: Here, she's not saying, "I stay up late on the phone." She's saying, "I do things I shouldn't be doing." This statement makes me really curious.

What kinds of things is Alyssa doing?

Linda, are you beginning to see how—by limiting what we look at to "a patient's actual words," that we can learn much more—all this without ever having met the person? For instance, none of what Alyssa reports so far has happened to her in school. And while we don't know what it all means yet, it begs more questions.

We've also not been biased by the mother's ideas as to why Alyssa should be there. Hence my having asked you to not tell us this. My point? Small amounts of the patient's original words can reveal a lot. But for this to happen, we can't complicate these words by adding in the mother's—or a therapist's—take on these things.

Doing this also gives us hundreds of starting points from which to diagnostically formulate more questions. This can make the hand-off from intake to treatment far more focused. Jesse, you had your hand up.

Jesse: Yeah. It just sounds like there is a lot of blame going on in Alyssa's house.

Steve: Okay. Where are you getting that from? Where's your evidence?

Jesse: From her saying, "I act dumb." She sounds like she's blaming herself.

Steve: Okay. Yes. I can hear that. But why say, "blame in that house?" Are you assuming Alyssa's parents are blaming her, rather than it's her being hard on herself?

Jesse: Yeah. I can see both things are possible. But I'm still wondering.

Steve: Realize Jesse, no genuine evidence has surfaced so far for where this blame is coming from. Yet you just inferred her parents are blaming her. This is why I so often say, "Please, don't infer. Try to limit what you say to what you see."

You could say, "I hear blame in the way she speaks. I wonder where this is coming from." Voiced as a question, this would be fine. But voiced as a hypothesis?

As I've said, doing this will bias everything you do going forward.

Jesse: Yeah. Okay. I can see that.

Steve: Jesse, can you feel the difference between wondering if there's blame in the house, in effect, blaming the parents—versus that Alyssa is blaming herself?

Jesse: This tells us we need more evidence before we can know?

Steve: Yes. And by not reading into what Alyssa's said, there's no extra stuff. This limits what we can claim we know to what was actually said. So yes, we can ask patients all sorts of questions. But we should base our questions, and limit them to, those which come directly from genuine (actually observed) evidence.

Realize, this is the key to getting an accurate picture for who your patients are. You limit your diagnostic evidence to what patients literally say. You then try to never complicate this evidence by reinterpreting or misrepresenting what's been said.

Linda, are there more sentences there?

Linda: Yeah. There was something after that. I didn't want to give it away. But when she said, "I'm on my phone doing stuff I shouldn't be doing," she was referring to speaking to an older guy. She said . . .

> **Alyssa (her intake):** "I was speaking to an older guy. I lied about my age and made up stories."

Tom: I need to hear that again. Linda, could you repeat it?
Linda: Should I read what she said from the beginning?
Steve: No. From the part where she says she was on her phone, please.

> **Alyssa (her intake):** "I'm also on my phone, doing stuff I shouldn't be doing."

Linda: Here, she's referring to that she's "speaking to an older guy." Then she says . . .

> **Alyssa (her intake):** "I lied about my age and made up stories."

Steve: Hmm, anyone? Who has thoughts about what this tells us? Maria, you're likely going to catch your daughters doing this someday. (Maria's twin daughters are currently turning three).

Maria: You know, this sounds like what I was like as a teen.

Steve: Oh, yeah, definitely [the group laughs].

Maria: But in my case, I don't think I ever revealed these things—even when I got caught. She's actually admitting what she did.

Steve: What would you do? Would you lie, then stick to the lie?

Maria: Yeah. There are lies I told as a teenager that even now, I don't know if my parents know.

Steve: So you were a "bad" girl [more laughter].

Maria: Yeah, I guess I was. Even my AOL messenger name. I forget what it was. But it was something like, "bad ass chick."

Steve: And that was probably accurate back then [laughter].

Maria: It's interesting that she's actually admitting to the things she's doing.

Steve: Why is this interesting?

Maria: Mainly because I so wasn't like that. I wasn't honest, even when I could have been. I'm curious about whether, when she said those things, if her mother was with her at that intake. That would be very different.

Steve: Yes. That's true. But keep in mind, we need to limit our evidence to things Alyssa literally said. Also keep in mind that some of the things she said are likely to be phrases she heard other people say *about* her, perhaps even things that were said *to* her. Why mention this? These ways of saying things sound like things adults often say to teens. So based on the words she's using and the way they're phrased, it sounds like someone must have said those words to her many times. This makes me question whether they're coming from her alone. At the same time, she is the one saying these words. So they are still genuine evidence.

Tom?

Tom: It seems kind of important that she's telling the truth that she's lying—if that makes sense. Something about her "telling the truth about lying." As of now, we don't actually know what she's referring to. But I feel like her doing that makes me trust her a little more.

Steve: Excellent. What else? Anybody? Thoughts? Shelby?

Shelby: I'm wondering what made her make these confessions. Was she suffering when she said these things? My reason for asking this? Her first sentence about "not knowing why she's like this." This said, I can't tell if she admitted these things because her mother pressured her to confess—or if she felt pained by keeping these things secret.

Steve: Those questions would be good to ask her in a therapy session. But in a case presentation—with no chance to actually ask the patient? These questions could bias what we look for. Better that we limit our thoughts and questions to things coming directly from what was said. At the same time, I don't want to inhibit any of you by saying this. You're doing great, all of you. But before sharing your thoughts about this case, please do take a minute to ask yourself where your questions are coming from. What evidence are you basing your question on?

For instance, one of you mentioned Alyssa may be "You first." Was that you, Tom? Yes? Okay. In that case, Tom had evidence. Alyssa's not just "reflecting" on herself. She's acknowledging she's done things that aren't right. Linda, what was it she said about talking to an older—what did she say—a boy or a man?

Linda: A guy. An older guy.

Steve: Okay. We know she lied about her age. She actually said that. But she also said she lied about other things.

Linda: She made up stories—and there's more after that.

Steve: Okay. But Linda, for now please hold off on telling us those other things.

First, did anyone notice anything unusual about the sentence Linda just gave us? It references more than one idea. Please realize, when this happens—when a sentence contains more than one idea—it's best to explore each idea, one at a time.

What happens when you don't? This is like trying to look at any two or more things simultaneously. The more you try to do this, the more blurry these things become. The same thing applies to intake sentences which contain more than one idea. It's best to consider each idea by itself, and only then, look at combinations.

With Alyssa, we don't yet know what she was doing on her phone—let alone what things she was referring to when she said, "doing things I shouldn't be doing."

Linda: This sounds like she was blaming herself again.

Steve: That's true, Linda. But if you'd told us everything Alyssa said right from the start, we wouldn't have realized a lot of what we've discovered about her.

Why not? Because we'd probably have tried to address all those things at once. But those things aren't everything. She's done other things as well. It's also likely the things she did mention aren't the first things she's done wrong. They're probably just the things which finally led her mother to force her into therapy.

Clancey: It also seems to me, Alyssa often goes against her own sense of what's right for her. This makes me wonder how often Alyssa gets peer pressured into doing things.

Steve: Your evidence for this question, Clancey? For instance, is it the way she speaks?

Clancey: Mm-hmm, right. Totally. Yeah.

Steve: Can anybody else sense the pressure Clancey is referring to in the way Alyssa speaks? Does she sound pressured to you? My thoughts? No one's going to self-disclose so honestly without feeling pressured. She's actually acknowledging how she acts dumb and that she doesn't know why she does things.

She's also saying she does things on her phone she shouldn't be doing.

All three of these things point to that she's likely You first. Or at least, that she has a You state in her Character Type. For instance, she could have a You second state. She could be a Three upside down. But we've no evidence that Alyssa has a Me state yet. So we can't know for sure. Okay, Linda, would you read the next piece.

Linda: Mm. So after that, Alyssa said she made up stories. Mm. And that this led to CPS (Child Protective Services) coming to her house last year.

Steve: Stop. CPS came to the house last year! Okay. That's huge.

Clearly, we do not know why CPS was called at this point. And Linda, rather than explaining this to us by adding more information to what we've just heard, please consider what you would think here were you to only look at the information you've already given us.

What things can we say based only on the evidence we have? We can say . . .

[1] That CPS came to Alyssa's house [Child Protective Services].
[2] That Alyssa was 12 at the time.
[3] That CPS coming to a kid's house is normally a traumatic event.

Whenever CPS goes to someone's house, everyone in the house will feel anxious. Certainly this is true if someone's being abused—but it's true even when no abuse is going on. Thoughts anyone, before Linda goes on? Very well. Linda, will you read the next piece.

Linda: Mm, okay. Alyssa said . . .

> **Alyssa (her intake):** "CPS came to the house last year. I was talking with friends and we got into a fight. We stopped being friends. I was trying to get their attention."

Steve: Okay. Thoughts? Clancey, you look like your wheels are spinning.

Clancey: Yeah. I'm wondering if her parents were actually abusing her or not—or if she was merely trying to get attention.

Steve: Mm. I'm more curious about what she's referring to—why CPS was called. What kind of abuse was reported? Keep in mind, at this point all I'm doing is wondering about these things. Still, CPS doesn't normally go to a house unless they have evidence that some serious abuse is going on.

Clancey: Yeah, yeah.

Steve: In truth, in almost every state I know about, CPS tends to *underreact* to calls, rather than *overreact*. Linda, would you please read what Alyssa said again.

Linda: Mm. Okay.

> **Alyssa (her intake):** "CPS came to the house last year. I was talking with friends and we got into a fight. We stopped being friends. I was trying to get their attention."

Steve: Any thoughts about how she was "trying to get their attention?" I could sense something immediately. Did any of you?

Sam: Yes. I don't like how that sounds—it sounds like she's blaming herself. Also, I can't sense if what she said is true or not—whether she's actually done anything wrong. Personally, I don't buy it.

Steve: Do her words sound like the language a 13-year-old girl would use?

Sam: No. In fact, most of what she said here sounds like answers which were fed to her—things she's just repeating. Her entire explanation as to why CPS was called feels like she's parroting someone else's words.

Steve: I agree. Much of what she's said so far sounds like things her parents may have said to her. "You act dumb." "You do things you shouldn't do."

Okay. Anyone else have any thoughts?

BTW Linda, you're doing a good job. Are you taking that in? Also, are you realizing how much easier it is to get to know someone if you limit the evidence you look at to one idea at a time? For instance, are you seeing how doing this is already paying benefits with Alyssa's case?

Linda: It just opens up to so many things that you could dig into later with patients, things which would ordinarily get overlooked because the therapist assumed they understood what the patient's words meant.

Steve: Yes, Linda, that's exactly what I've been trying to point out. Unfortunately, schools pressure therapists into thinking they need to be able to understand—and *logically* explain—what evidence means *on the fly*. All this before they've even seen all the evidence. Worse yet, doing this ensures they'll gather most of the evidence having already made assumptions as to what it means.

After that, because they're under pressure, they'll look for evidence which supports these assumptions—in part, so their supervisors don't catch them doing something that sounds stupid, or is incorrect, or is something which may hurt the patient, or whatever.

Did Alyssa say anything else?

Linda: She mentioned, in a school email, that her parents were abusing her. This is what led to CPS being called and sent to her house. But she also said it wasn't true—that her parents weren't abusing her. And there's more.

Steve: Are these words Alyssa's own words, or are they what the intake person recorded?

Linda: They're Alyssa's quoted words. And there are more quoted words here.

Steve: Okay. Can you read the next piece?

Linda: Okay.

> **Alyssa (her intake):** "The website I was on was called, ***Emerald Chat***. It's a site where you get matched with someone by talking to random people. And there's an app—LMK. You get put in a call with multiple people and you're matched with random people. And in the big chat, I lied about my age. I was sending nudes and was naked in some of the videos."

Steve: Am I right that this happened last year, when Alyssa was 12 years old? I'm wondering if this was the real reason CPS got called. Thoughts, anyone?

Linda, I know Alyssa's intake implies they were called because of something which happened between Alyssa and her friends. But there's a much more obvious pattern which those words reveal. And actually, given the evidence we have at this point, I see two patterns that are really obvious.

What does Alyssa saying "she posted nudes, online, at 12 years old" say about who she is? I'm not asking what it implies about *why* she did this. I'm asking what it says about who she is as a person. Sam?

Sam: This may be way off base. But I'm thinking of a client I had once who was sexually abused at a young age. Then later, this person repeated this kind of thing with another person in a way that very much resembled the original event. So for me, this raises a question. I'm wondering if something took place with her previously that involved photographs or something of that nature?

Steve: Good question, Sam. And realize, *how* you're stating this is absolutely the right way to state it. *"I've heard of something like this before. So I'm wondering if this is what's going on here."*

Okay, Maria. I know this is a bit personal. But I'm curious. Did you ever post nudes at 12 years old?

Maria: *Post* nudes? No. But I did *send* them to boyfriends. But post pictures on a website with a group of strangers? At 12 years old? No way.

Even now, I feel afraid even just thinking about me doing that. So that's interesting . . .

Steve: Maria, realize, the idea that you felt afraid to do this at 12 was actually a good thing. You had a limit. Your parents bitched and moaned about these things and some of it stuck. Okay. You do realize that these fears will affect how you raise your daughters.

Tom? I see your hand up. Go ahead?

Tom: I once had an adolescent patient who did something similar. She was a trafficking victim. We ended up having to sort out a whole bunch of problems with her. For one thing, we had an iPad in the day room where all the kids were. She found a way to get onto this website. She was talking to all these men and was giving out the personal information of other patients. Several men ended up calling our phones. We had to block them and notify the police and stuff.

Steve: So Tom, like in any Grand Rounds group, what you just shared is stuff which can help us to think of questions about this case. But a word of caution. Rather than assume this is the case with Alyssa, let it simply create more questions in you.

For instance, is this kind of thing possible in Alyssa's case? Obviously, we can't know yet. Certainly the thing Maria said about sending nudes to boyfriends is pretty common for girls in their teens.

But posting nudes to a group where you are randomly matched with older people?

Definitely not.

Okay. Is anyone beginning to see a big picture yet?

I'm not referring to what it all means. Rather, I'm asking if anyone sees how what Alyssa's saying here connects to the other things she's said. David?

David: This may be a bit of a stretch. But I suspect this points to a pattern. Alyssa did something *extreme* with her friends. And she did something *extreme* herself as well. Both of these things seem "extreme."

Steve: That's pretty insightful, David. Yes. And the way you're voicing this—as a question—is also well done. You acknowledge you have no specifics, but that she impulsively did some risky things with her friends.

She also impulsively did some risky things with this group of men. So you're wondering if engaging in these kinds of behaviors may be a pattern for her.

Also, this connects back to the thing Alyssa said about "not knowing why she does what she does," including things she does on her phone.

"I don't know why I do the things I do. I don't know why I act dumb."

What she was referring to here may connect to what she's reporting about posing nudes. Why say this? Because it's highly likely she used her phone to go online and meet those men.

Okay. Any other thoughts about the character of this girl? And realize, this time I am asking you to infer. Why ask you to do this, when I normally would ask you to avoid doing it. Because now, I want you to feel what it's like to have the opposite experience while gathering evidence.

Up to now—because we've gone slow, and because we've looked at the evidence one idea at a time, we've managed to collect enough genuine evidence to have asked a bunch of really good questions.

Who is this 13-year-old girl?

We're beginning to get a picture for this.

Shelby, you have your hand up?

Shelby: When I think about Alyssa, I feel a lot of fear. I don't know why. Again, it might just be something related more to me than to Alyssa.

Steve: Well I think, if you were doing the things she's doing, you would be feeling afraid.

Shelby: It's just that I had a similar situation when I was a kid, where I told my friends my parents were abusing me. Like Alyssa, the lie I told was a more extreme version of what was actually happening.

What I was afraid of back then, I still don't know. But I felt afraid all the time. So I don't know. It's possible I may just be projecting that onto her.

Steve: Shelby, that may be true. And that you're questioning how much is you projecting is excellent. Then again, you seem to be sensing a genuinely existing similarity.

Okay. Anyone else?

Athena, what does this girl sound like to you?

You have two daughters.

First of all, you'd probably be appalled if this was one of your daughters. Right? Any thoughts? Remember, I am not asking you to answer as if you are a therapist. I'm asking you to answer as a mother and a human being.

Athena: I see shades of gray and I'm wondering what makes this girl go so far down into the gray? That's what I'm asking myself.

Steve: That's good, Athena. That piggybacks onto what David was suggesting.

Athena: I mean, I've told lies. But I would never have dreamed of going that far. My daughters? I should hope they don't go there.

Steve: Right. Yeah. And as far as you know, they haven't done anything like that.

Athena: Right, right. So I'm asking myself, what pushes someone to go so far down into the gray?

Steve: That's good. David, you had your hand up?

David: Mm, first of all, this case really makes me anxious. So I'm glad it's not mine.

Steve: Anxious?

David: Yes. It seems to me that this girl is in Baby Mind a lot of the time.

Steve: Ah, excellent. Clearly, she is impulsively doing a number of risky things. And from this, we can identify two tipping-point based measures which are evidence that she is doing these things in Baby Mind.

For one thing, the "instant on, instant off" way she suddenly does things. For another, the way she seems to have no sense of how what she's doing will affect her future. Both of these things point to something missing in her: that she lacks any sense of how "what she's doing" would look like on a timeline.

This also raises questions about the things she reports doing—like sending nudes to a group of strangers and lying.

If she felt the need to lie about her age, then the people in the group were clearly older.

She wouldn't be posting nudes in a group of seven-year-olds.

Jesse? You have a comment?

Jesse: Yes. I had similar thoughts about whether she was in Baby Mind when she got in the fight with her friends. She said they got into a fight. Then she said she lost them as friends. But we don't know why that fight happened.

Steve: Wasn't that her explanation for why CPS got called—that in the conversation she had with those friends, she told them, she was being abused.

Jesse: Oh, I thought she said she lost the friends.

Steve: Jesse, realize that to understand what's going on here, we need to get a big picture view. A big picture view is one where we connect all these things in one big lump.

Linda: She did lose her friends.

Steve: But put all the things she said on a timeline.

Linda: She said she and those friends got into a fight. Then they stopped being friends. Then she wanted to get their attention. So she told her friends that her parents were abusing her.

Steve: Thank you, Linda, for that excellent recap.

Jesse: I'm wondering if Alyssa was in Baby Mind the whole time?

Steve: You know, that's probably true, Jesse. Contrary to what Shelby said then—this girl totally lacks fear—she was probably not seeing what each of these things could or would lead to.

In Maria's case, she told us she felt fearless at that age. Yet she still had some fear about going too far, exceeding limits, or something.

Alyssa seems to have no limits. None whatsoever.

Realize, I'm not assuming anything about where this lack of limits came from. Specifically, I'm not making any assumptions about Alyssa's house or her parents. I can't. I have no evidence for any of that. So I cannot know. What I can say is, Alyssa does seem to be a girl traditional therapists would say is "acting out to get attention."

At the same time, I need to keep asking myself if this is true. Is it?

To me, "acting out to get attention" is a rather empty phrase.

Of course, she's acting out. And of course, she's seeking attention. But why? Based on the evidence we've been given so far, we simply cannot know.

Is she angry at her parents—and is that anger what's pushing her to do some of these things, perhaps as a kind of a revenge thing?

Is she looking to punish her parents for something?

We simply cannot and should not assume anything at all.

We need more genuine evidence.

Then there's the idea that she told these things to an intake person, a person she just met. But she didn't then tell these things to Linda, the extremely kind woman she met next.

I've sat with a lot of teens—well over eight hundred kids—most of them in a hospital inpatient setting.

Rarely have I heard a teen offer that much information in an intake. I don't care what they got sent there for.

Alyssa is obviously coming to therapy because she's in a load of trouble.

She sent nudes to a group of strangers at 12 years old.

And CPS has been to her home. But why? Because she lied? Okay. But there's something missing in what we know about this girl.

For one thing, she seems to be acting way younger than she really is. It seems the Baby Mind thing that you mentioned, Jesse, is definitely at play here.

Also, the way Alyssa's acting shows she doesn't have much in the way of healthy limits. This makes me ask, at what age is it normal for children to not have these kinds of limits?

Normal 13-year-olds, or even 12-year-olds, do have limits—Maria is a good example. At times, she may have wanted to exceed those limits. She even did exceed them at times. But Alyssa's saying these things to an intake coordinator?

This says she is much different than Maria.

Alyssa is not Shelby either. There's also a big range between Shelby and Maria as young girls. So we can suspect something else is going on here, something behind the scenes, something that predates her at 12 years old.

How can I know? Because by age 12, she's doing these things. But she stops doing them only when she gets caught—and not because she has a normal 12-year -old's internal sense of limits.

Okay. So now, Linda, can you tell us a bit about your experiences sitting with this girl in therapy?

End of Part 1: [Ed. note: this transcript has been edited for clarity]

Evidence Gathering - Alyssa's Intake | First Thoughts

If you're wondering why I've labeled what you've just read, "part 1," it's because there is a second part to this transcript.

Why divide this transcript into two parts?

Because I want you to experience the difference between "evidence gathered in an *intake*" versus "evidence gathered in *ongoing therapy sessions.*"

Up to this point, what you've read includes only the evidence gathered during Alyssa's intake—along with the group's reactions to this evidence.

Obviously, at some point, we will need to look at part 2 of this transcript—evidence gathered from her ongoing therapy sessions.

Before we do, I first want to check-in with you to see how you've done so far.

To begin with, already, there are quite a few things to consider here. So many in fact that some readers may find the thought of having to process all this information overwhelming. If this is you, just know, I'm feeling pretty overwhelmed myself right now.

You should also know though, that having these feelings tells you something important about yourself and how you've done. These feelings tell you, you've done a good job—listening to, and getting to know—the patient in this transcript.

In truth, if you gather evidence properly, all cases will feel complex.

Human beings, and especially those seeking help, never have simple lives.

What if you don't feel overwhelmed by all this? What if you feel you can already diagnose Alyssa? Then your diagnostic style is based on the old method. Here, quickly arriving at a symptom-based diagnosis is preferable over finding ways to know and help suffering human beings. This focus—where quickly arriving at a symptom-based diagnosis is the main goal—is what I described in the first pages of this book's Introduction.

There, I quoted noted psychiatrist and author, Henri Ellenberger's, take on the differences between European and American psychiatrists. In this excerpt, Ellenberger politely expresses surprise, mild shock, and concern at how—unlike European psychiatrists—American Psychiatrists see exploring a patient's life as superfluous and a waste of time. He wrote that description back in 1955. Yet American psychiatrists still are not required to be properly trained in personality and psychotherapy. No surprise then that in the US, diagnosis has not changed much since then. It still focuses on finding brokenness.

Getting to know the patient? Not so much.

How about you? Are you curious as to whether you are practicing the old way or the new? Fortunately, determining this difference is easy. Which are you focused on—symptoms or suffering? Focusing on symptoms is the old way to diagnose. Sadly today, most diagnosticians get taught—and feel pressured—to diagnose this way. Worse yet, most diagnosticians also get pressured to begin to diagnose patients from the first moment they sit down with them. This is why, throughout this book, I've urged diagnosticians to get to know their patients, and to take their time doing this. Obviously, to do this, they must be formally trained in personality and human nature—and most diagnosticians are not. Do recall, however, that I've previously acknowledged the few American psychiatrists who post-graduation do acquire this training. If this is you, I applaud you for your dedication and professional persistence. No coincidence, I personally prefer to work with these folks.

To be honest, I cannot stomach working with clinicians who treat patients like broken machines. If you are reading this, then I suspect you feel similarly.

What if you have a good heart, but do still feel pressured to practice the old way of diagnosing? In a moment, I'm going to ask you to test yourself for this.

How?

Based on what you read in part 1 of Alyssa's transcript, I'm going to ask you to propose a working diagnosis for her.

Know you'll need to reference some version of the current diagnostic manual in order to make this diagnosis. Must this be an actual, current diagnostic manual? Not really. Online? Google? Any of these versions of that book will do.

When you're done doing this, I'd then like you to imagine, you need to prove to an insurance company that this diagnosis is valid.

To do this, you'll need to support your diagnosis with evidence drawn only from the intake coordinator's written words. No inferences here, please. Use only what you read in part 1 of Alyssa's transcript.

What if you don't feel you know enough yet?

Please try to do these things anyway.

What if you aren't a licensed professional but rather, an interested grandma, young mom, and such? Even here, I'm going to ask you to try doing this just the same. Experiencing for yourself how diagnoses are made will pay benefits for the entire rest of your life. At the very least, you'll learn to ask good questions about any diagnosis you or your loved ones are given.

Now before you begin, I first need to address a few things—things which may have confused some readers. For one thing, why have I not referenced any diagrams during this transcript? After all, I've repeatedly said, diagnosis should be rooted in drawings, not in words. Why not? Because these Grand Rounds groups represent what amount to first looks at the person and the case. Our focus here is on getting better at seeing the person *as they arrive*—rather than focusing on a diagnosis. Only then do we consider making drawings which amount to diagnostic notes of this gathered evidence. And if we later find evidence which does not fit, or contradicts, what's in these drawings? As I've said, to be a proper diagnosis, no evidence can or should be overlooked. Not a single thing. Thus the patterns in these drawings must, without exception, account for all of the evidence gathered ***to date***.

What about when they don't?

Know this can and often does happen.

When it does, these drawings must be revised to include, and make sense of, all the evidence you've gathered. As for my point for having you do all this, the transcript gave you a taste for the way we gather evidence in these Grand Rounds groups—and being forced to come up with a diagnosis, the old way. Only then will the path to a diagnosis which is allowed to emerge naturally make sense to you.

Okay, it's time. Set a timer for five minutes. Now think back on what you can recall from part 1 of Alyssa's transcript. Please don't reread the transcript. Base your diagnosis only on what you recall. And yes, what I'm asking you to do here will be hard. This said, please use only the evidence you can recall. Then make your diagnosis based solely on this evidence.

Okay. Ready? Start your timer.

Now begin.

My Apologies For What I've Just Put You Through: The Old Way

Clearly, what I've just had you do goes against my advice as far as how to properly arrive at a diagnosis. That advice, to "let the diagnosis emerge from the evidence *all on its own*," can be the most difficult part of learning the new way of diagnosing. I liken that old way to how high school guidance counselors must ask high school juniors to decide on what they want to do in life—in a single half hour sitting. How can a high school guidance counselor, let alone a high school junior—or a diagnostician, be expected to make a decision like that? I don't know.

Realize, the exercise I just had you do really is this difficult. Yet it's exactly what diagnosticians are presently expected to do, every time they diagnose. They're expected to manufacture a diagnosis—and to create all the requisite inferences to support this diagnosis—without ever getting a chance to personally know their patients. Why are they expected to do this? Because in our world, poorly trained insurance company clerks—and profit based managers—often have more influence on patient care than the opinions of licensed, practicing therapists.

In truth, insurance companies routinely deny patients care despite licensed professionals having determined this care is needed. I personally know this to be true and have been forced many times to do "sham case reviews." I cannot count the times I've had to argue for care which I am licensed to say is necessary, but which clerks tell me is unnecessary. I'm sure many of you will have experienced this as well.

Now let me ask you. What diagnosis did you give Alyssa? Did you manage to limit your evidence for this diagnosis to what was in her transcript? Or did you do what most diagnosticians get pressured to do? Did you expand on this evidence, by inferring things not present in the transcript? If you did, please don't blame yourself, certainly, not in this case. After all, it was me who just asked you to do this.

ooooo

What about me? Based on the transcript so far, could I have diagnosed Alyssa? If I was using the 5th edition TR of the Dumb Stupid Manual—and if I was allowed to infer things—in theory, I could have. Just know, if you actually gave Alyssa a diagnosis, then you cannot have let the diagnosis emerge naturally from the evidence. Rather, the only way you could have arrived at this diagnosis is by having made logical inferences as to who Alyssa is and what this evidence means.

The thing is, often, this is exactly how much evidence you're expected to base your diagnoses on. So if you'd taken my advice to heart, when I asked you to diagnose Alyssa, you would have told me, "Sorry, Steve. I can't. I don't have enough evidence to make a diagnosis."

Does this feel like I've tricked you? Do you feel angry at me? Then please know this. If you did just do this exercise, then you've likely gained something which will pay huge benefits when you get to read part 2 of Alyssa's transcript.

Why did I ask you to do something I clearly see as wrong?

Because doing this written exercise will have created a baseline measurement for how much of the "old diagnostic method" is still ingrained in you.

It will also show you how not getting to know Alyssa has prevented you from knowing this suffering girl.

Do you think I'm wrong? Did you feel you already knew enough to be able to help Alyssa get the help she needs?

This last question is critical.

Obviously, we'd agree that getting her this help is the main point for giving a diagnosis.

So if you do disagree, it's likely we're only disagreeing about one thing here—how to arrive at this diagnosis. If so, then let me ask you this.

You just heard the story of an extremely troubled teenaged girl.

This girl has a name. She has an age and a presenting problem.

Now based on part 1 of this transcript AND without having reread it—would you be willing to bet, the diagnosis you just gave her could or would change this girl's life?

If you answered "yes," then without a doubt, you used the old diagnostic "method" to arrive at your diagnosis. That "method" is what this book's title refers to when I ask, "Did You Know Your Diagnosis Is Bullshit?"

That word does not refer to you. I'm not saying you are bullshit. I'm sure you have a good mind, and heart, and mean well. But that diagnosis you just gave Alyssa?

Not so much.

ooooo

As for my question as to whether you limited your evidence to the intake coordinator's words from part 1 of Alyssa's transcript—if you answered "yes," then what genuine evidence did you use to support your diagnosis? Did you feel you had enough evidence to feel confident, your diagnosis could and would change her life? Did any of this evidence fit onto any of the Diagnostic Bingo Cards? How about this? Could you chart any of her experiences on a Four States of Change event diagram? Could you profile her personality using even one of the tipping-point based measures in this book?

Be honest now. Did any of the things I just mentioned matter to you? More important, do you think I care if they did or not at this point? My answer may surprise you. At this point, none of these things should have mattered to you. All that should have mattered is that a thirteen-year-old girl named Alyssa is out there, somewhere, suffering.

Why? Because in the end, ***all that really matters is whether you've connected to the suffering human being.*** And the diagnosis? Doesn't this matter? On your best days? Yes. A good diagnosis may help a patient to get proper help. A very good diagnosis will often guarantee this. But a good diagnosis is based on the person, not just on their suffering. And getting to know a person takes time.

Now before we turn to part 2 of Alyssa's transcript, please take a few minutes to review the things Linda told us that the intake coordinator quoted, in part 1.

Alyssa (her intake): "I don't know why I'm acting like this. I'm acting dumb. And I'm also on my phone, doing stuff I shouldn't be doing."

Alyssa (her intake): "I was speaking to an older guy. I lied about my age and made up stories."

Alyssa (her intake): "CPS came to the house last year. I was talking with friends and we got into a fight. We stopped being friends. I was trying to get their attention."

Alyssa (her intake): "The website I was on was called, ***Emerald Chat***. It's a site where you get matched with someone by talking to random people. And there's an app—LMK. You get put in a call with multiple people and you're matched with random people. And in the big chat, I lied about my age. I was sending nudes and was naked in some of the videos."

Linda's Case | A 13-Year-Old Girl Named Alyssa - Linda (part 2)

Steve: So now, Linda, can you tell us a bit about your experiences sitting with this girl in therapy?

Linda: You know, there's a lot I could say. But I'm going to try to be concise and brief. To begin with, when I think about her, she's a really sweet girl.

Steve: Every kid who sits with you will feel sweet to you, Linda. You see the good in every person you sit with.

I'm not saying Alyssa's not a sweet girl. But keep in mind, you're a very kind, very warm woman. And any kid who sits with you is going to seem like a sweet kid, because you're going to be sweet with them.

Realize, what I've just said to you is really important. It points to how patients pick up on who you are and that this leads them to reflect this attitude back to you. For instance, there's no sweetness in what you told us Alyssa told the intake person.

Linda: Mm. Okay. What else can I say?

She's in eighth grade now. Also, I started seeing her last summer.

In sixth grade, she got suspended ten times for fighting. She was being bullied. In seventh grade, seven times. So she got suspended 17 times in two school years, and it seems she will impulsively try to kick any boy's or girl's ass.

Steve: Pause. Pause. She got bullied? Pause. So okay. That's really important to add to our big picture.

I've been asking myself why Alyssa is so angry.

I've been asking myself this because she's doing things that would piss off any parents. And Maria was rebellious and angry, and she pissed off her parents regularly. But doing these things for years and she got suspended 17 times in school for fighting . . .

Linda: Yeah. But you should know, she told me her parents had encouraged her to defend herself, and that if someone started with her, she should fight back.

Steve: Get the heck out of here.

Linda: She let me read texts on her phone from her father.

Steve: Okay. Let that go for now.

She told you she was bullied?

Linda: Yeah.

Steve: Do you know how old she was when the bullying started?

Linda: Mm. I'm going to say sixth grade—when she got suspended 10 different times for fighting—because people were bullying her.

Steve: At 11 years old?

Linda: It would have begun before that.

In sixth grade, she was self-harming.

Then there was suicidal ideation last year.

Also, she lives in a house with her mother.

Her father is her father. But her older sister and brother each have different fathers. So in all, there are three different fathers.

In addition, her mother sees another therapist in my office. That therapist shared with me that the mother has sexual abuse in her story. I asked Alyssa if she was being physically abused—is this why you fight so much?

I also asked Alyssa if she had been sexually abused.

She denied ever being physically or sexually abused.

Steve: Linda, when Alyssa's answered these questions, can you recall what her face or body looked like? How did she react to these questions?

Linda: She just spit out a quick, "no."

Steve: Mm.

Linda: She does have a 22 year old brother who no longer lives with them. She told me he's schizophrenic and that he left the home when she was four.

Also, supposedly, Alyssa has been diagnosed with ADHD. She's been taking meds for it.

Steve: Linda, did you just notice Sam's reaction? Look at Sam's face right now.

When you said those things about Alyssa's schizophrenic brother and that he moved out of the house when she was four, Sam reacted.

Also, look at Tom's face. Right?

And look at Maria's face. And David's nodding head.

Can you see something happening here? Holy shit.

So at this point, we need to put all this stuff onto Alyssa's chronological and developmental timelines; her Schizophrenic brother who is nine years older than her, who leaves the home when Alyssa is four. Is that right? Alyssa's brother is nine years older than she is?

Linda: Right now she's 13.

Steve: So when he left the house, he was 13?

Linda: Wait. I'm sorry. Alyssa's brother is 28 now and her older sister is 22.

Steve: Okay. So Alyssa's brother is 28 now and Alyssa is 13. So Alyssa was 4 and her brother was 15 when he left the house.

Fifteen would be prime time for Alyssa's brother to be curious about sex. I don't know. But Alyssa's mother reports having been sexually abused. I wonder why she is only just now seeking treatment?

It's highly likely that Alyssa's mother has in some way influenced Alyssa because of what happened to her. This same thing happened to me. I always wondered if my mother was sexually abused. Then later in life, my father told me she got molested when she was 15. She was raped when she worked as a nanny, upstate. I didn't know that until I was in my late 40s. But do you think it's a coincidence that I was sexually molested in childhood by multiple people?

How does this kind of thing happen in families?

I have no idea.

I just know this stuff often repeats in families in the strangest ways.

I'm not saying it always happens, that it's automatic. It's not. But Alyssa was 12 years old and was sending nudes to significantly older males?

This makes me wonder if her doing that was in part why CPS came to her house. Clearly, if so, then that visit would have been required. Any adult looking at those nude pictures of a 12-year-old girl would have been committing a serious offense. Holy shit.

Admittedly, Alyssa would likely not see her doing this through the lens we're seeing it through right now. But the adults around her? That's got to be there somewhere, even if only vaguely.

The brother was schizophrenic.

Schizophrenia in males doesn't usually occur until they are 18 or 19. Am I right, Tom? (Tom is a Nurse Practitioners).

Tom: I've seen it as early as age 16.

Steve: As early as age 16. Okay. But generally, isn't this something which surfaces in the person at around age 19, 20, or 21?

Sam, what do you know about this?

Sam: Mm. I got confused about one thing.

Linda, the brother is 28 years old now, right? And you say, he left the house how long ago?

Linda: Mm . . . Alyssa is 13 now. And the brother left the home 9 years ago. This means Alyssa's brother left the home right around when Alyssa turned 4.

Steve: Nine years ago means he was 19 at the time. This makes me wonder if the brother left the house *because he got diagnosed with schizophrenia.*

Linda: Alyssa told me she is not allowed to see him. But she does it anyway. Recall the texts I previously mentioned from her father. He doesn't like it that she sneaks and meets with her brother.

Steve: Is it possible the schizophrenic brother molested Alyssa when she was four? Obviously, we should not assume this happened. However, we do have enough evidence to be asking this question.

Why would the family disown Alyssa's brother? What did he do that was so bad?

[Steve realizes the group is running short on time].

Linda, before we go, what else can you tell us about this case?

Linda: The family claims Alyssa's been diagnosed with ADHD—and that she's on Ritalin. No surprise they said she doesn't take her meds consistently.

They also said Alyssa doesn't have a lot of friends.

Steve: A girl who beats everybody up? That makes sense.

Linda: Yeah. She's also had a bad reputation in school for some time now. But this year, since she started coming to me over the summer, she's gotten in trouble only once.

Steve: So the violent incidents were reduced from 10 in sixth grade and 7 in seventh grade to 1 this year.

Linda: Yes.

Steve: So Linda, the next time you feel like you're a shitty therapist, I'm going to say to you, "Linda, 17 to 1." [the group laughs]

Linda: Right now, I realize there's still a lot of digging I need to do.

I intuitively sense she's holding back a lot. She's also still way too impulsive. A boy at school said, "Can I have your number? I want to give it to my friend." She assumed the boy was referring to a local boy in school. But it turns out it was his friend who lives in another state.

Next thing you know, she's dating this boy's friend. I'm like, "He's a complete stranger. What do you mean you're dating a guy in another state that you've never met before?" Then she came in the following week and told me, she broke up with him when she left my office—right after we finished the session.

What is that thing when they tell you to watch out that your clients do everything you tell them to do and whatever?

Steve: Being too compliant?

Linda: Yes. And I'm trying to show her how to do things for herself, and not because I tell her to do them.

Steve: Yes. But Linda, think about what I said to you about why she's sweet in your office. 17 times she's suspended for being angry? That's not a "nice" girl. Probably not normally sweet. Yet she's sweet with you. So you're …

Linda: She's sweet with me. But she's smashing people's heads into lockers.

Steve: So she's a "sweet, locker head-basher." Okay. I get it. [laughter].

All right. Thank you, Linda. Thank you everyone. That was well done.

Linda: Bye guys.

Steve: Thank you. Wow, what a case.

[Ed note: again, this transcript has been edited for clarity]

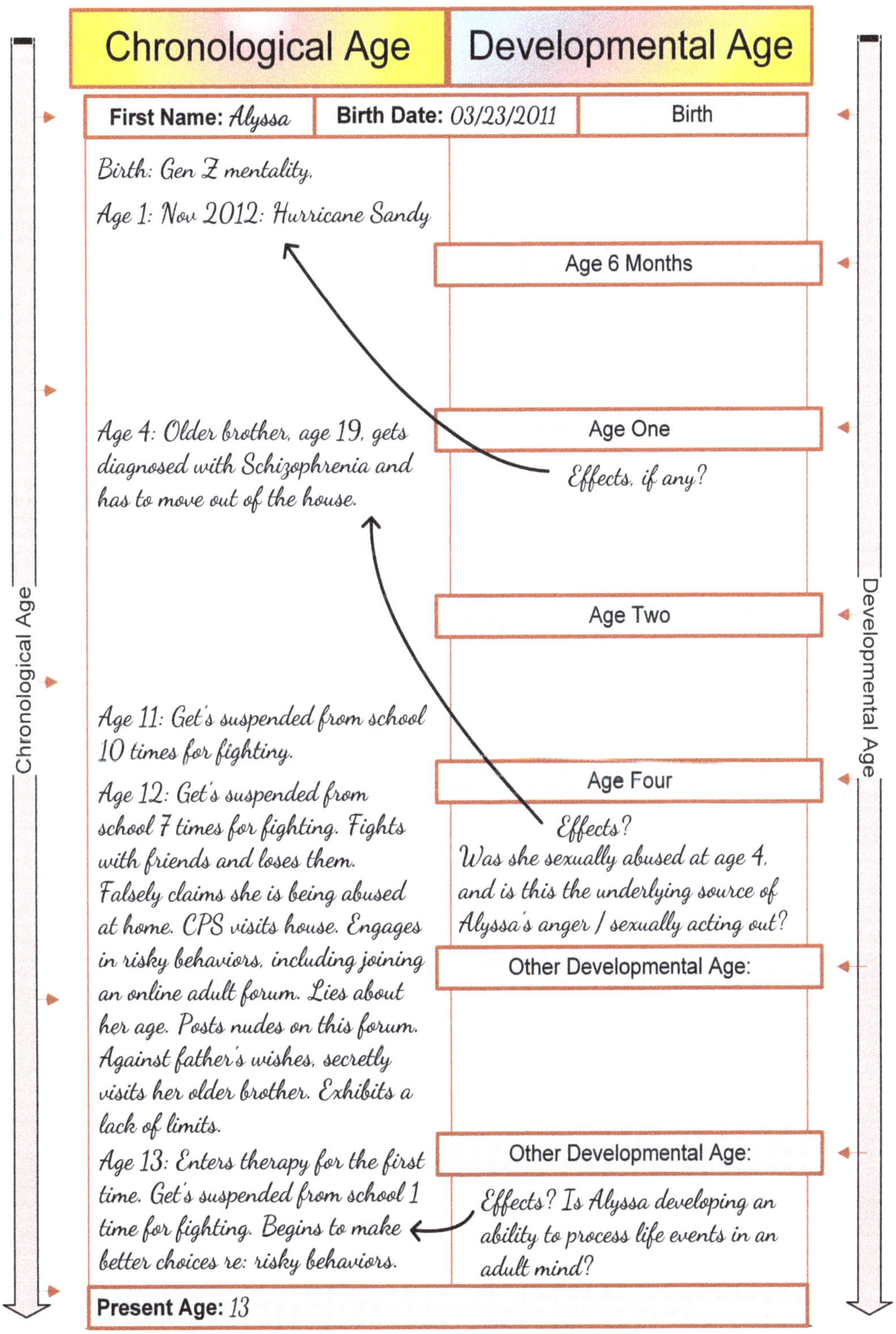
Chronological Age
Developmental Age
First Name: Alyssa
Birth Date: 03/23/2011
Birth
Birth: Gen Z mentality.
Age 1: Nov 2012: Hurricane Sandy
Age 6 Months
Age 4: Older brother, age 19, gets diagnosed with Schizophrenia and has to move out of the house.
Age One
Effects, if any?
Age Two
Age 11: Get's suspended from school 10 times for fighting.
Age Four
Age 12: Get's suspended from school 7 times for fighting. Fights with friends and loses them. Falsely claims she is being abused at home. CPS visits house. Engages in risky behaviors, including joining an online adult forum. Lies about her age. Posts nudes on this forum. Against father's wishes, secretly visits her older brother. Exhibits a lack of limits.
Effects?
Was she sexually abused at age 4, and is this the underlying source of Alyssa's anger / sexually acting out?
Other Developmental Age:
Age 13: Enters therapy for the first time. Get's suspended from school 1 time for fighting. Begins to make better choices re: risky behaviors.
Other Developmental Age:
Effects? Is Alyssa developing an ability to process life events in an adult mind?
Present Age: 13
Chronological Age
Developmental Age

Evidence Gathered in Therapy Sessions | Do You Know Alyssa?

Prior to part 1 of Alyssa's case transcript, I asked you to imagine you were sitting in on this Grand Rounds group with us.

Now I'm going to ask you to imagine that you did this, and that our group has just finished.

Did you leave this group having learned any new skills—or having identified some old ones you'd like to learn more about?

Whatever the case, can you now tell me who Alyssa is as a person?

Who is she? What are your thoughts? Does Alyssa remind you of anyone you know? Is she in any way like you? Do you think you could help her?

If you realized anything at all about who she is, then you'll have answered these last few questions with a "yes."

If not? Then please forgive my bluntness—but you've got some work to do.

Now go back over the diagnosis you gave Alyssa and especially, the evidence you previously used to support it. Did anything you read in part 2 alter who you thought Alyssa was? Do you feel the need to revise your diagnosis? Did you add any evidence to support your doing this? What overall impressions did you come away with? Most important, do you feel you know more about who Alyssa is?

I did.

I also, like many in my group, came away wishing it could be me that could be the one to help her.

Did you?

Symptoms vs Personality | Which Kind of Evidence Matters More?

Based on the many times I've already advised you to focus on personality, I'm betting what I've just had you do may have confused some of you. Isn't the point of a diagnosis to find a useful description for the patient's symptoms? Obviously, this is true. If so, then symptoms must matter. So where do they come in?

In a moment, I'm going to offer you my short list of the kinds of evidence I look for right from the start. Why? Because you cannot properly understand symptoms without first knowing the person—and this list is about the person. Said in other words, ***a diagnosis*** is ***a description of the suffering being experienced by a person***. So this person IS the *context* for these symptoms and not the other way around.

My point here?

There are ways to gather genuine diagnostic evidence, while not losing sight of the suffering human being you are trying to help. One tool I use is the thing I referred to a moment ago, something I call, my "short list." Everything on this list refers to aspects of personality and human nature. Taken together, these things create a "diagnostic baseline," a backstory for the patient's symptoms.

This then is where my diagnoses begin. I do my best to fill the upper half of the diagnostic funnel with the things on this list—while at the same time, noting—but not interpreting—the patient's symptoms.

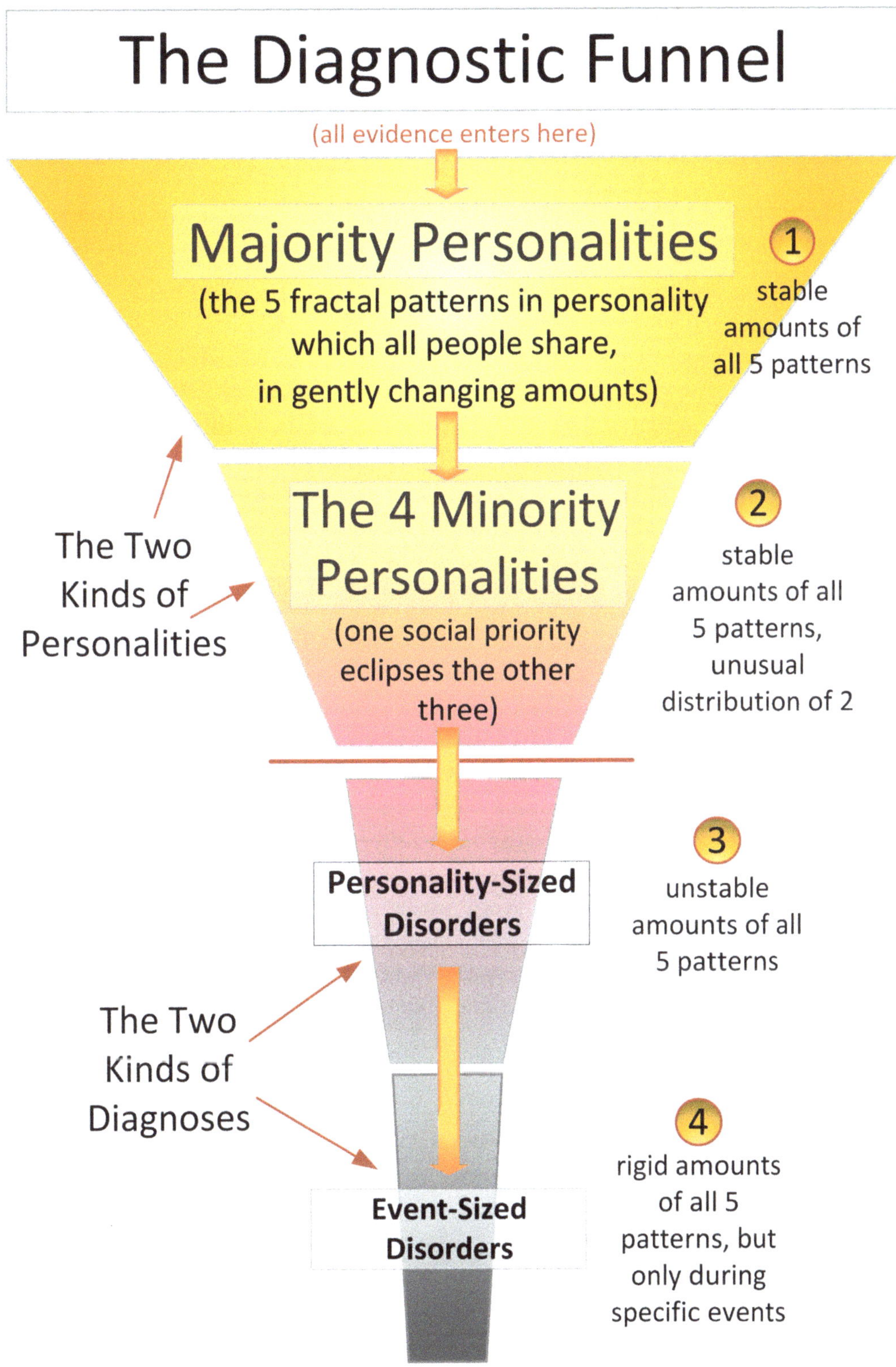
The Diagnostic Funnel
(all evidence enters here)
Majority Personalities
(the 5 fractal patterns in personality which all people share, in gently changing amounts)
1
stable amounts of all 5 patterns
The 4 Minority Personalities
(one social priority eclipses the other three)
2
stable amounts of all 5 patterns, unusual distribution of 2
The Two Kinds of Personalities
Personality-Sized Disorders
3
unstable amounts of all 5 patterns
The Two Kinds of Diagnoses
Event-Sized Disorders
4
rigid amounts of all 5 patterns, but only during specific events

My Short List of Diagnostic Baseline Elements

All diagnoses should begin with these three pieces of information.

[1] The Patient's First Name
[2] The Patient's Present Age
[3] The Presenting Problem Stated In The Patient's Own Words

Then—***while*** slowly processing the presenting problem, ***one idea at a time***—look to learn as much as you can about the following baseline personality identifiers.

[4] Language preference (either "fussy" or "fuzzy"; **Personality**)
[5] Mental acuity (Mind Body preference; **Personality**)
[6] Physical dexterity (Mind Body preference; **Personality**)
[7] Tendency to place blame on others or self (Character Type; **Personality**)
[8] Default urge-categorizing (Social Priorities; **Personality**)
[9] Strategies when life is hard (Lowest Social Priority; **Personality**)
[10] Biases for and against each of the four types of **Information.**
[11] Ability to process life sequentially (child/adult; default sense of **Time**)
[12] Event onsets/endings (abrupt or gradual; how the person processes **Time**)

If the second part of this list sounds daunting, please, don't fret. I've addressed these things—at least briefly—in previous chapters, in this book. I've also elaborated on these aspects of personality, and the mind, in several previously published books. Please feel free to go back and review them as often as you need to.

Keep in mind though, if you truly wish to learn these things, then like learning who your patients are, this will take time. What you shouldn't do is waste time trying to memorize these things—let alone use them to logically determine diagnoses. Why not? Because memorizing destroys learning—and logic is the heart and soul of making inferences. And making inferences is the most common way diagnosticians get lost during the diagnostic discovery process.

To see why I'm saying this, simply juxtapose the following two words—***Inference*** and ***Evidence***. Now contrast and compare these two words.

Inferences are pseudo-evidence. They take effort to arise in the mind. So ***Inferences*** function similarly to how it would feel to "live in the Matrix," where everything feels like you're doing well—but these feelings are fake.

Evidence, on the other hand, arises in the mind *naturally*, effortlessly, as you gradually and gracefully notice things in life. So with ***Evidence,*** you feel like you're living in "the literal, functional, natural world," where you're walking on solid—but always changing, living "mental" ground.

Now let's turn to yet another important point—the idea that patients can need more than one diagnosis. This raises yet another diagnostic skill you'll need to develop. Current diagnostic criteria for diagnoses often overlap so badly that they often make it difficult to tell them apart.

How then do you determine a patient's ***primary diagnosis***?

This skill is what we are about to explore. The key word here? The "***differential.***"

Finally, please know, the stuff we're about to look at is theoretically dense. So feel free to skip it—*for now*— if it's too hard. Do keep in mind though that determining a patient's primary diagnosis is a necessary diagnostic skill. So please, do at least try.

Diagnosis & Treatment | Beginning the Differential Assessment

Everything in patients' minds will in some way affect everything they claim is happening to them. This is true, even when they can't see it happening. To properly diagnose patients then, diagnosticians must determine the primary diagnostic focus. By this I mean, what "the biggest lump in the snake" is at the present time.

Then too, the mere fact that you're evaluating a patient can cause his or her reporting to vary quite a bit. For instance, some patients fear "getting a diagnosis," thinking this will force them to do, or face things, they don't want to deal with. Other patients may worry you will not take their suffering seriously, if they don't offer enough evidence. In the first case, patients may try to "be on good behavior," omitting serious concerns during the evaluation. In the second, patients may distort or exaggerate their symptoms and presenting problems—in an effort to make sure you don't overlook their needs.

Yet other patients may present as being seriously mentally ill. Yet they may actually just be extremely stressed. Here you'll need to sort through what may seem to be lies, distortions, or outright nonsense. Regardless, in all these cases, you must treat what patients tell you as genuine evidence—no matter how strange it sounds. Evidence for what? For what's currently true to them. This, after all, is what you're diagnosing—the patient's own sense of their current state. But this then raises many questions. This brings us to what I call, "The Overarching Clinical Concern."

The Overarching Clinical Concern: How Is Stress Affecting Patient Reporting?

Accounting for the effect of stress on patient reporting is the overarching clinical concern. You should not proceed without first assessing for this. This includes not only mental illness, but also situational stress. So the question here is …

Is the patient reporting accurately or not, based on their presenting state?

Realize, assessing for this—and all diagnostic differentials—*never ends*. Each time you acquire new evidence, you must first assess—and record— this evidence as seen through the lens of the patient's *current* life state. Do keep this in mind then as not doing this risks contaminating the entire diagnostic process. Your diagnosis should above all accurately reflect and address the patient's truth.

Significant stress can cloud these, and your, diagnostic reflections.

The 1st Differential: Sort Evidence to Determine Features of Personality

Now we come to a biggie. It's basically a summary of what's just been said.

All diagnostic evaluations should begin with getting to know the patient as a person.

Know this holds true even when you've seen a patient many times.

The Diagnostic Funnel

(1) The 1st Differential

Determine Personality

(look for evidence for the 5 fractal patterns in personality which all people share)

Personality rarely changes. But presentation often does.

Realize too, each time you add evidence into the uppermost portion of the diagnostic funnel, patient personality is the first thing you must assess for. Here the main thing you're looking to do is to identify measurable features of this patient's personality—each of which will further frame, point to, indicate, and support or contradict previous assessments.

What you should not try to do, at any point, is to try to process a patient's suffering separately from their personality. Why?

Because separating symptoms from personality is the core deficit present in most traditional diagnostic evaluations.

Admittedly, determining personality in suffering people can be quite difficult.

This is why it's normally best to assess for features of personality only when people are in normal states of mind. Diagnosticians rarely have this luxury.

Either way, to arrive at an accurate diagnosis, you must first create the patient's diagnostic baseline. This baseline amounts to a best estimate of what this patient is like in normal times. So not doing this risks mistaking things like cultural differences for diagnostically significant features.

Finally, please realize, these baseline assessments must be ongoing.

New evidence can and should cause you to reconsider even the surest of baseline assessments.

Why is this so important?

Because a patient's personality will always affect how their symptoms present.

This means, it's simply not possible to properly diagnose without accounting for personality.

The point here is simple.

All symptoms must be seen in the context of personality.

No exceptions.

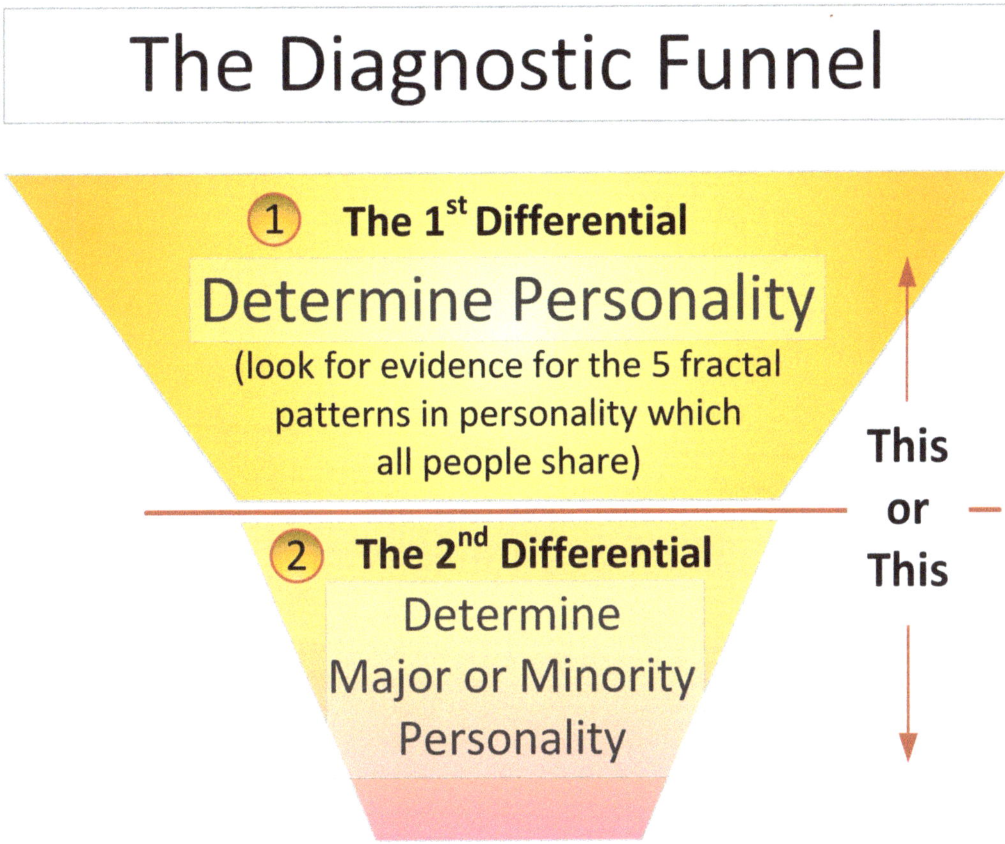

The 2nd Differential: Determine Major vs Minor Personality

At some point, sufficient features of the patient's personality will have emerged for the second differential to come into play. At this point, you'll need to begin to look for features which indicate, the person may have a **Minority Personality.**

Realize I've described the specifics of making these determinations in detail, in earlier chapters, in this book. Here again, learning when, where, and how to use these tipping-point based measures can take time. So please be patient with yourself.

Keep in mind too, that learning how to make these assessments is critical—as patients with Minority Personalities and patients with Majority Personalities process life events very differently.

Also—previous diagnostic manuals have treated these four Minority Personalities as diagnosable conditions.

They are not. Difference isn't brokenness. Period. End of story.

This said, learning to speak with—and assess the evidence you gather from patients with Minority Personalities requires special skills and experience.

What can help here is to imagine these patients were raised in a foreign country, where English is a second language. How would this affect your questions to these patients, as well as your sense of what they say?

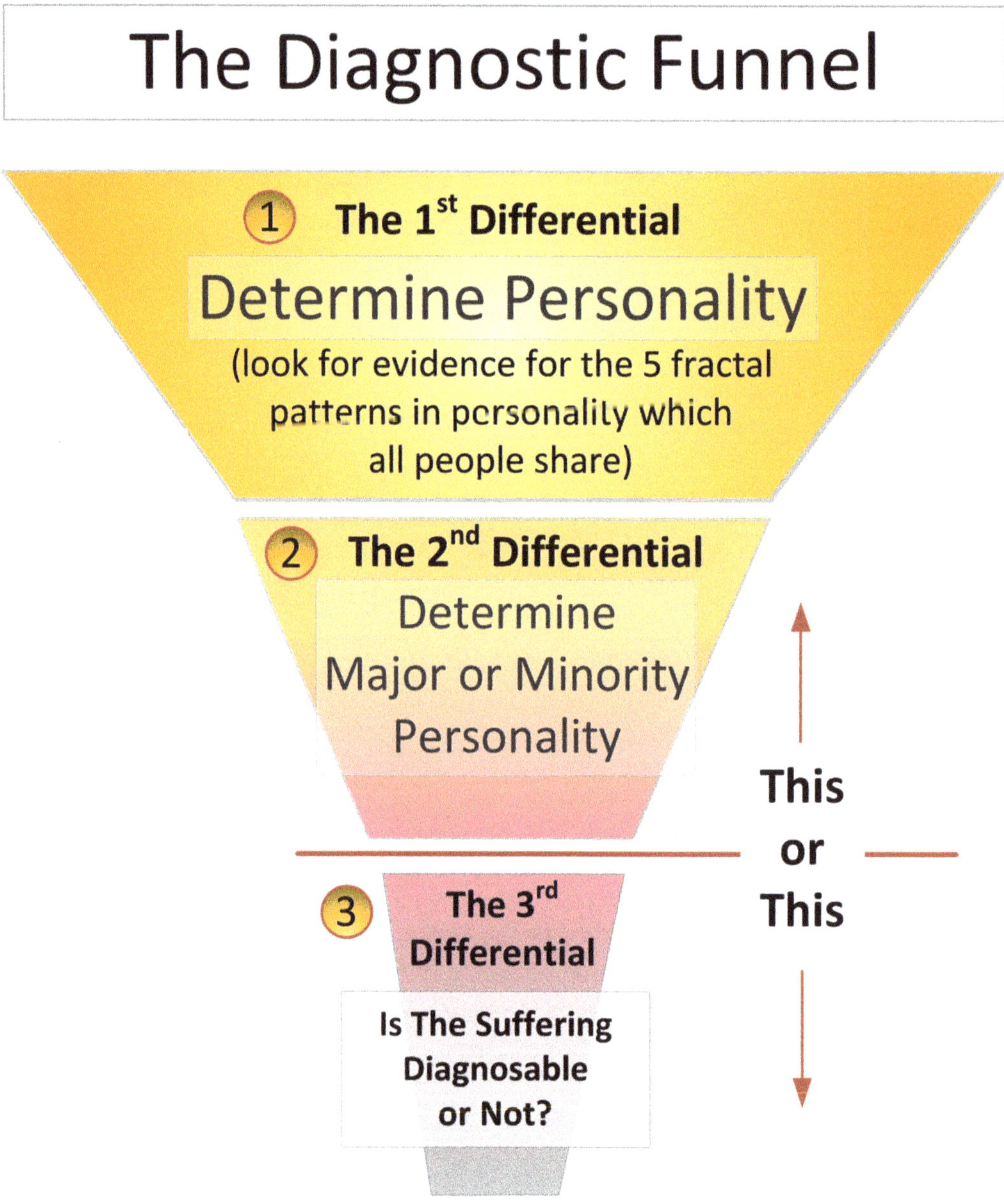

Know I've written extensively, in previous books, about how people with Majority differ from people with Minority Personalities. I've also posted many articles about this on online sites, such as Quora.com. Of particular importance is the idea that while all English speakers use the same sorts of dictionaries, at the same time, there are five ways people can assign meanings to these words.

In the first, which I call, "*fuzzy*" usage, people assign word meanings fluidly, *based on context*. This is the way folks with Majority Personalities use words. For people with Minority Personalities though, context often doesn't matter. So word meanings are often more rigid, pattern-based, and literal. I call this, "*fussy*" usage.

An example of this difference? Phrases like, "how are you?" For people with Majority Personalities, being asked "how are you?" is—most times—a greeting. However on rare occasions, they can also hear it as a personal question, depending on the context. Whereas people with the AS Minority Personality, most times, interpret this phrase as a literal request for a description of what they are currently doing. And people with the OCD Minority Personality hear the phrase, "how are you?" as a request for all currently relevant, small, organizational details.

Can you see it? Same English words. Different meanings. These changes all rest on how the patient does or does not employ context to assign meanings to language. Here again, the point is the same. Before you can diagnose, you must first account for the patient's personality. Now that we have, we come to the 3rd Differential.

The 3rd Differential: Diagnosable or Not?

In the 3rd Differential, you'll be looking to separate evidence which points to ordinary human suffering from that which points to a diagnosable condition. Obviously, this step also requires significant experience and skill. Keep in mind, though, that at this point, you are not trying to determine ***which*** diagnosis to give. Rather, you're merely trying to rule out evidence which does not refer to diagnosable suffering, the stuff which refers to normal, human suffering.

The point this time? That the overall goal of the Diagnostic Funnel is to narrow down what you will—and will not—use as evidence for a diagnosis. Some evidence will remain in the upper half of the Diagnostic funnel. Some will not.

Evidence you sort into the upper half of the funnel refers to aspects of personality—things which exist within normal human-nature ranges. These things do not indicate diagnosable problems. So they can, for now, be set aside.

Evidence you do not sort into the upper half of the Diagnostic Funnel then automatically gets sorted into the lower half of the funnel—where it becomes the focus of the work. Realize, by doing this, you will accomplish two important things.

First, the evidence which remains in the upper half of the funnel enables you to create the patient's diagnostic baseline—a picture of what this patient's normal life context looks like.

Second, as I just said, by creating this baseline, you separate evidence which refers to *context* from evidence which points to *diagnosable symptoms and signs*.

Current diagnostic methods rarely separate these two things and only do this in extreme, life situations. Yet to not create this diagnostic baseline means you effectively treat all suffering patients as if there is a single standard human being.

Said in other words, if you fail to account for your patients' personalities, in effect, you treat all patients as if their differences do not matter. This amounts to ignoring the humanity in your patients, by treating them as if they are all the same.

Doing this then this leaves you with no way to discern between the patient's normal responses to difficult life situations—and their diagnosable, over or under reactions, regressions, and such. In effect, their humanity is gone and forgotten and they become lab rats, one and all.

My point for repeating these ideas ad nauseam? To insure I sufficiently annoy you, so that they become unforgettable. Here there are two main points. One.

Evidence which remains in the upper half of the funnel is the stuff that describes and defines the patient's norms (the diagnostic baseline).

This means, there is no way to accurately know which evidence should go into the lower, diagnosable half, without first determining these norms.

Even here, it's possible you may gather new evidence which alters what you've previously believed to be the patient's baseline. And if your patient's personality baseline changes, then the diagnostic implications of the evidence gathered must change as well.

Realize too, the more you learn to recognize and identify your patients' baseline personality identifiers, the more you'll be able to zero in on the diagnosable data—and the more accurate your diagnoses will become. Why? Because you'll be limiting the evidence you use to diagnose to what is clinically relevant.

This alone will reduce the chances you'll mistake one diagnosis for another.

Also, do keep in mind, there will be times where evidence may appear to point to a specific diagnosis—only to later turn out to be the result of unusual, but otherwise ordinary, life circumstances. This makes this 3rd Differential extremely important. Suffering can come from diagnosable conditions. But it can also come from unusual, but otherwise normal, circumstances. Thus, the second point.

Is the evidence you see diagnosable or not?

Now take a few moments to consider what you've accomplished so far.

At this point, you will have divided the evidence into what you will—and will not—be looking at, during your attempts to find a diagnosis. At the same time, you will NOT have begun to decide on which diagnosis this will be. You will only have decided on which evidence you will use to make this decision. This brings us to the fourth and final step in the diagnostic process.

Know this step is so complex, it requires a second, four part funnel.

The goal of this second funnel? To break the fourth and final level of the Diagnostic Funnel into a hierarchy of four separate, smaller, sub-steps.

Complexity broken down becomes relevant data.

Only then can something as complex as human suffering begin to make sense.

The 4th Differential: Creating the Diagnostic Hierarchy

Clearly, what you see on the opposite page—in the fourth and final level of the funnel—is a variation of the previous larger, "Diagnostic Funnel." You've already used the first three levels of that funnel to separate ***evidence which is diagnosable*** (signs and symptoms) from ***evidence which is not*** (personality). Now you'll use this second, four-step, "hierarchical" funnel ***to resolve differences between overlapping constellations of symptoms which occur within the diagnosable evidence.***

The end result is something I call the patient's, "Diagnostic Hierarchy."

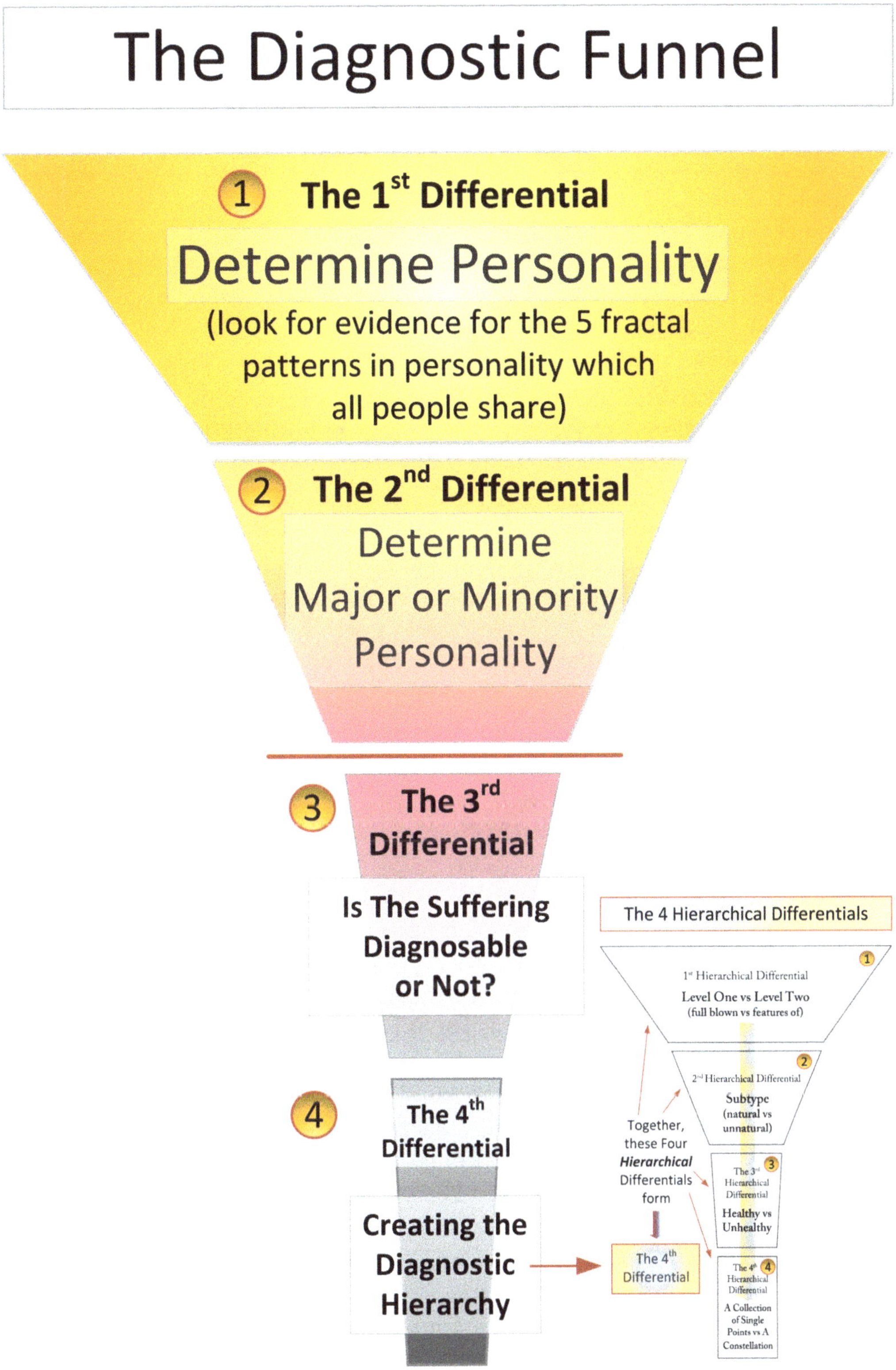
The Diagnostic Funnel
1 The 1st Differential
Determine Personality
(look for evidence for the 5 fractal patterns in personality which all people share)
2 The 2nd Differential
Determine Major or Minority Personality
3 The 3rd Differential
Is The Suffering Diagnosable or Not?
4 The 4th Differential
Creating the Diagnostic Hierarchy
The 4 Hierarchical Differentials
1 1st Hierarchical Differential
Level One vs Level Two
(full blown vs features of)
2 2nd Hierarchical Differential
Subtype
(natural vs unnatural)
3 The 3rd Hierarchical Differential
Healthy vs Unhealthy
4 The 4th Hierarchical Differential
A Collection of Single Points vs A Constellation
Together, these Four Hierarchical Differentials form
The 4th Differential

The good news is, once you've learned how to use this second four-level hierarchy, you'll be able to resolve conflicts between any and all similar diagnoses. Know this will remain true even when the diagnoses in existing manuals get updated or deleted.

Unlike the prior diagnostic manuals then—where hundreds of poorly defined differentials can disappear, reappear, or change—once you learn to use this hierarchy of four differentials, you'll be able use it for the rest of your career.

Now if you've been using the Diagnostic Funnel, then this is the point where you'll begin to look for the patient's 4 Hierarchical Differentials. What does doing this look like? This is what we'll turn to next. Here we'll briefly touch on a few examples which can often confuse diagnosticians.

First example? The differential between Bipolar and Bipolar features.

Do you feel you already know enough about this Personality-sized Disorder? In truth, you may. If so, I applaud you. Acquiring and using this knowledge takes quite a bit of experience.

Let me ask you this though. Can you teach what you know to others, and do this in ways which allow them to do it as well as you?

Most people can't do this. Again, you may. If so, bravo. You're quite skilled. Either way though, what I'm about to show you can raise even the most experienced diagnostician's skills a notch or two—always a good thing.

In any case, I promise, the simple hierarchy I'm about to expose you to can definitely add a thing or two, or four, to what you know.

1st Hierarchical Differential | Level One vs Level Two

The first thing you'll need to address is called, the *1st Hierarchical Differential.* In this step, you'll differentiate between a serious diagnosis and similar, but less severe, conditions.

For example, say you're looking to distinguish between a Personality-sized Disorder (in the case, Bipolar) and a similar, less serious cluster of Event-sized Disorders. Here, to get diagnosed with Bipolar (or any other Personality-sized Disorder), the patient *must* either be a Character Type One—or be living as if they are, such as when the person has an active Substance Use Disorder.

According to the present book, to be diagnosed with Bipolar Disorder, the person must be a Character Type One—and also, his or her primary symptoms must be the clinically necessary symptoms for this diagnosis. Only when both conditions (Character Type and symptoms) are met does the person's diagnosis fall into the category, Personality-sized Disorders | Level One.

And if the person's symptoms do look like the clinically necessary symptoms, but he or she is not a Character Type One? Then this person's diagnosis falls into the category, Personality-sized Disorders | Level Two.

Realize, this distinction differs quite a bit from what the current diagnostic manual states. For one thing, the current diagnostic manual completely ignores

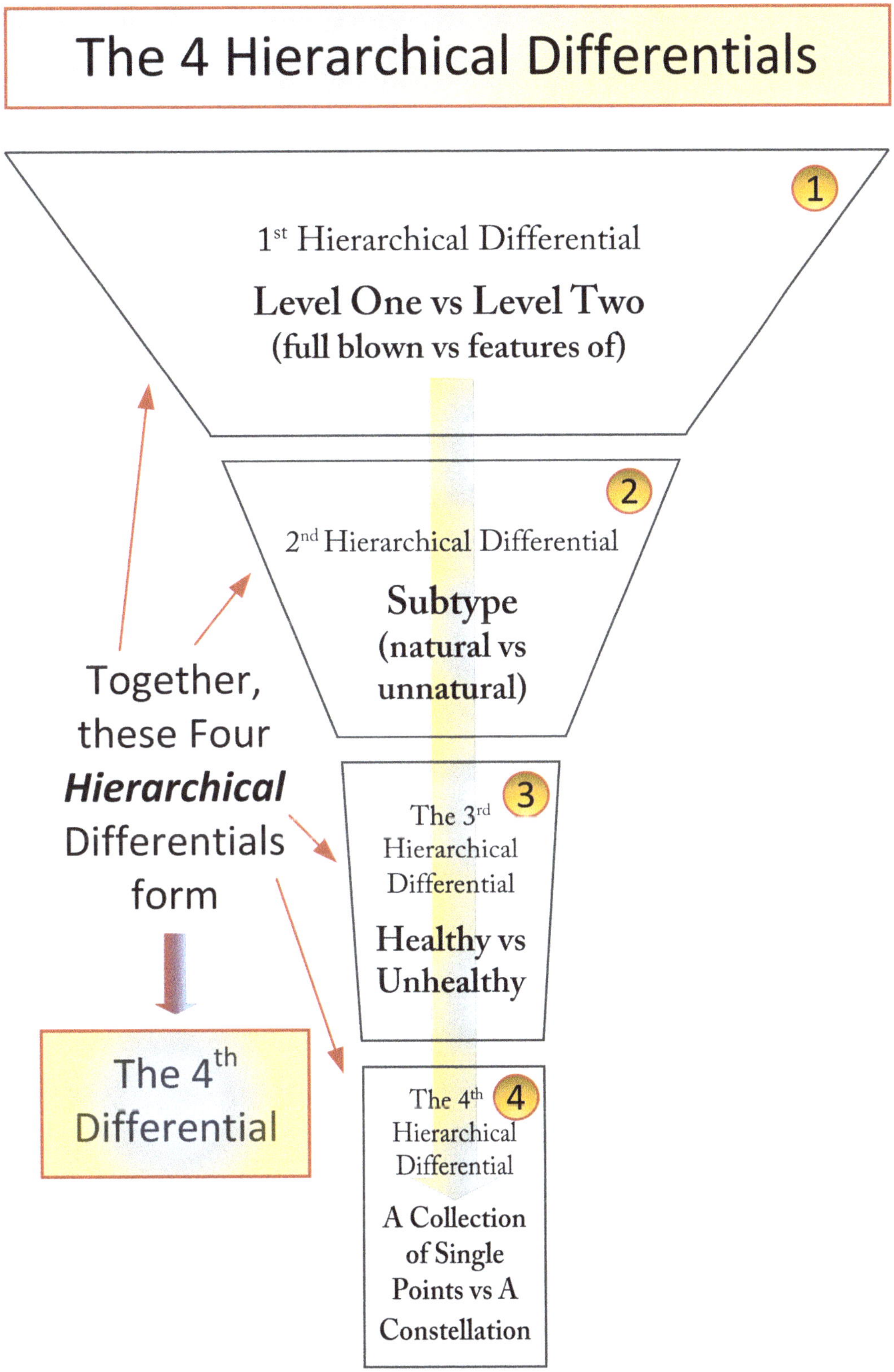
The 4 Hierarchical Differentials
1
1st Hierarchical Differential
Level One vs Level Two
(full blown vs features of)
2
2nd Hierarchical Differential
Subtype
(natural vs
unnatural)
3
The 3rd
Hierarchical
Differential
Healthy vs
Unhealthy
4
The 4th
Hierarchical
Differential
A Collection
of Single
Points vs A
Constellation
Together,
these Four
Hierarchical
Differentials
form
The 4th
Differential

personality as a factor when diagnosing. This first step in the Hierarchical Differential is meant to take this into account.

It also then clarifies and redefines treatment objectives between two levels—Levels One and Two.

The difference between these two levels?

That despite two patients presenting with identical symptoms, a patient whose Character Type is One is a completely different case from say a patient whose Character Type is Two.

I've personally sat with a number of patients who display these two Hierarchical Levels. Possible therapeutic outcomes here change dramatically. And this distinction lies entirely in a feature of personality.

In this case, Level One refers to patients whose Character Type is One.

Level Two then refers to patients with the other three Character Types.

In both cases, the level of severity, symptom-wise, is the same.

In every case, treatment requires hospitalization.

Realize, this difference is far more than a mere observational distinction.

Of the five truly measurable personality traits, Character Type, more than any other, predicts and determines the potential gains a client will make in treatment.

This means the Level One | Level Two qualifier differentiates between the categories of, goals of, and strategies used during treatment.

In Level One cases, therapists can expect—and should try to help clients to focus on—making significant ***temporary*** improvements in their abilities to create order in their lives.

In Level Two cases, therapists can expect—and should try to help clients to make—significant ***permanent*** improvements in their abilities to create order in their lives.

Realize, this differential accounts for the differences between patients who require medication for life and those who can eventually live normal lives without it. But even for those whose symptoms require medication for life, patients with Character Type One will at best be able to live normally for only brief periods, if that. Whereas patients with one of the other three Character Types, with medication, once stable, will live what amount to fairly normal lives.

I have a close friend who was like this.

He was once hospitalized for Bipolar for an entire year.

During this time, he lost everything—a beautiful home, a professional career, a teaching professorship. Yet once he was stable, he regained much, including the ability to have healthy interpersonal relationships.

Sadly, patients with Character Type One will never be able to achieve such a thing.

The takeaway here?

That all Personality-sized Disorders, both Level One and Level Two, are comprised of two principle parts.

One. The primary constellation of symptoms which meet those necessary to clinically give the diagnosis. This is what Level One and Level Two have in common; the thread of similarity.

Two. To be given a Level One Dx, the person must be a Character Type One. Otherwise the Dx is Level Two.

Here, Bipolar 1 would be a Personality-sized Disorder | Level One. And a Bipolar II would be a Personality-sized Disorder | Level Two.

Finally, keep in mind how we define "disorder" in this book.

In this book, "**disorder**" is defined as "***a clinically significant lack of order in the person's life.***" And "**clinical significance**" is defined as "***a notable inability to bring order into everyday life activities.***"

2nd Hierarchical Differential | Natural vs Unnatural Subtype

In the *2nd Hierarchical Differential,* you add the "subtype qualifier." This time, the therapist differentiates between two types of suffering—the type which gets seen as ***normal suffering*** and the type stemming from more serious conditions.

This differential gets determined by a simple test. Does the disorder present in the person's life match this person's life circumstances?

If yes, then this diagnosis is a *Natural Subtype.*

If no, then this diagnosis is an *Unnatural Subtype.*

Can you see which type the friend I told you about a moment ago has?

People in both subtypes suffer badly. But he now suffers from things which can be explained by his life.

What he no longer suffers from is a constant inability to maintain normal healthy relationships.

What he still suffers with is the need to constantly be vigilant regarding taking his medications.

3rd Hierarchical Differential | Healthy vs Unhealthy

A further diagnostic distinction can now be made, based on the next pair of subtypes—the differential between *Healthy* and *Unhealthy Suffering.*

Here *Healthy Suffering* is defined as suffering wherein the person's urges and behaviors tend to blend and combine towards order. Whereas with *Unhealthy Suffering,* a significant amount of the person's urges and behaviors diverge towards disorder.

Obviously, for the *Healthy/Unhealthy* differential to be useful, it must account for all situations—both those which are *Natural* and those that are *Unnatural.* This raises an important point—the idea that all four hierarchical steps affect and interact with the other three. Thus in order to diagnose, the visual diagnostic constellation must address and include all four hierarchical differentials. More important, this visual constellation (the way the parts fit together) cannot be seen as four separate qualities. Why not?

Because a diagnosis can emerge only when you've acquired a fully baked "visual constellation."

This criterion is similar to not being able to know what a cake will taste like until all the ingredients are baked. The visual constellation for a patient's diagnosis emerges only after a fully baked version of all four Differentials appears. This fully baked version is one which creates a personal picture of the patient's life. And to be personal, this must be a picture you yourself can picture in your mind.

4th Hierarchical Differential | Single Points vs A Constellation

This idea—that therapists must visually constellate their observations in order to diagnose—now brings us to the very nature of disorder and to the 4th Hierarchal Step.

In what way?

In truth, this IS what the 4th Hierarchical Differential differentiates between.

It allows you to further differentiate between the suffering which does, and does not, apply to a single, specific diagnosis.

Obviously, to do this, you must have resolved the 3rd Differential.

Either the evidence is a ***Collection of Single Points*** or it is a ***Diagnostic Constellation***.

For example, take the case we looked at in the Grand Rounds group, the case of Alyssa. Consider how differently you would have diagnosed her had you not heard the information about her older brother.

Him moving out.

The father wanting Alyssa to not see him.

How these things coincided with the onset of Alyssa's problems.

Each of these things in some way reframed the entire case. In doing so, it created a likely constellation—a direction to be explored during therapy.

This direction is the single most important reason for giving a diagnosis.

Finally, as an aside to all this, I want to mention what one of my colleagues, Jesse, said when he first learned about this Four-Step Hierarchy. He wrote the following in an email to me.

I include it here as Jesse has so clearly pointed out the benefits of using even the first step in this hierarchy.

> *"Damn that distinction between Level One and Level Two is incredibly calming. Knowing your limits with a client and understanding what to shoot for—**temporary** change in Level One, and **permanent** change in Level Two. I'm thinking of how many times I've killed myself for not being able to move a Level One client or person in my life in a permanent way. In the past, not knowing this limit made me question myself, my worth as a person, and my worth as a therapist in so many ways."*

A Nine-Month Journey To A Provisional Diagnosis

How does it feel to diagnose like this?

To me, it feels solid.

You feel confident you're doing your best for your patient.

You feel surprised at how well your diagnosis fits the evidence.

Moreover, the longer you diagnose like this, the more confident you become.

You also feel surprised by how you sense the diagnosis was there, hidden in the evidence, all along.

At this point in the process, it is a good idea to double-check your work. Unlike previous advice against using logic, this is a good time to use logic. Please do keep in mind though that doing this earlier in the process can derail your diagnostic efforts. Thus use logic only where logic is suited best—as part of a good "end game," to make sure you haven't missed anything.

Realize too, in some cases, even arriving at a provisional ("working") diagnosis can take a long time. Some evidence can be so confusing and convoluted that you may wish you'd never accepted a patient. This brings to mind a case I had some years back which took an extremely long time to diagnose.

The patient—who was 12 at the time—was the daughter of an already existing patient. The mother had had no babysitter on her appointment days. So she'd bring her daughter to therapy with her. And yes, if you already see something, you're right on track.

A 12-year-old girl needed a babysitter?

The mother thought she did.

Often the girl, whom we'll call Lisa, would wait outside in my waiting room. But on occasions, the mother would ask her daughter if she'd like to come in with her. Sometimes the girl would nod, "Yes." Each time she did, she'd sit on the same love seat with her mother—always silent, shy, withdrawn, and unresponsive.

Being as the majority of my experience as a therapist had, back then, been spent helping teenagers, I'd seen this kind of thing before. So at first, I saw nothing notable. But over time, I acquired plenty of clear visual evidence that Lisa was regressing in those times. For instance, the first time she came in with her mom, she, at age twelve, laid on my couch with her head on her mother's legs.

Notably, this seemed to be normal to them both—almost unconscious.

Add to this that the few times I tried to speak to Lisa, she would wordlessly look up at her mother—in effect, cuing her mother to answer for her. At which point, her mother would tell me "what her daughter was thinking."

Now, to be honest, it would take far too long to tell you all the things I learned over the next year—each of which caused me to revise my assessment of this girl. More important, I knew for a good part of that year that I could give her a number of diagnoses. All of these diagnoses could have fit the criteria. None of them accounted for all the evidence. Moreover, not once during this time did I feel I knew what was troubling this girl.

Ultimately, her close to complete silences led me to give her a provisional diagnosis of Selective Mutism. The thing is, on a few occasions, she spoke like this diagnosis didn't exist. Why give her this diagnosis then? Because she needed something to qualify her for assistance in school.

As of today, based on more than a year of observations, clearly, she has the formerly Asperger's variety of Autism Spectrum Disorder (level 2). The regressions? Event-sized Disorders not directly correlated to her AS Minority Personality. More important, proper diagnosis has resulted in notable improvements between this mother and daughter. To be continued, for sure.

One Final Reminder: The Goal Here—Let The Diagnosis Emerge Naturally

As I begin to think about how to close this chapter, I recall reading something Plato wrote. The following two quotes come from the same paragraph in his Seventh Letter, pg. 344.

> "For both must be learnt together; and together also must be learnt, by complete and long continued study, as I said at the beginning, the true and the false about all that has real being."

> "After much effort, as names, definitions, sights, and other data of sense are brought into contact and friction one with another, in the course of scrutiny and kindly testing by men who proceed by question and answer without ill will, ***with a sudden flash there shines forth understanding about every problem***, and an intelligence whose efforts reach the furthest limits of human powers."

To me, these two quotes summarize much of what I have been trying to teach you throughout this book.

The first quote?

It refers to what you do in Part One.

You employ tipping-point based definitions.

Why?

Because to know something, you must know both what it is and what it is not. Moreover, together, these things must account for all possible patterns.

And the second quote?

Part Two—that you must continuously be pre-learning, until, ***"with a sudden flash, there shines forth understanding about"*** the diagnosis.

Makes you realize, Plato was a pretty smart dude.

Realize, you too can be this smart.

In the epilogue which follows, you'll find a few of the things I've discovered during the writing of this book. Can you find the places in this book which led me to these discoveries? Hopefully, you can.

In any event, see you in a bit, in the epilogue.

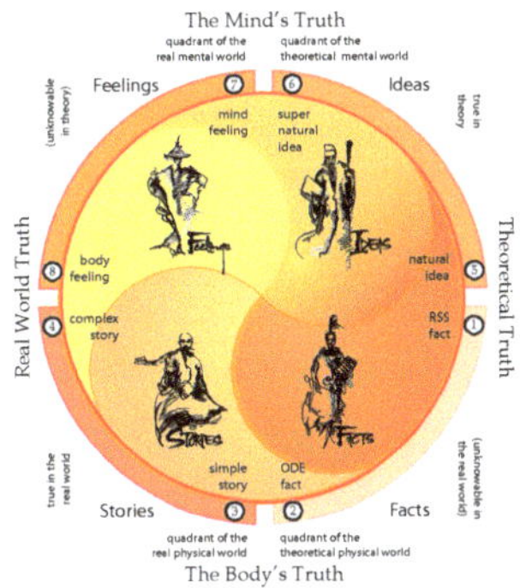

Epilogue

Questions & Comments
(what have I learned . . . ?)

Diagnosis | What Have I Learned From Writing This Book?

So what have I learned that I didn't know when I began to write this book?

My first thoughts? A whole shitload of stuff, much more than I expected to learn when I first attempted to write this book, five years ago.

Back then, I wrote for some ten months. Then I quit. Why? Because I realized, I simply didn't know enough yet about the nature of diagnosis.

I then tried—and failed—three more times, before I began the present effort.

In each of those previous times, I found, I still did not know enough yet.

Please take this in. I tried—and failed—to write this book, four other times.

Of course, this begs the question, what makes me think I know enough now?

My thoughts? I still don't know enough. But I realized, I will never know enough to write this book—not completely anyway. Neither will my colleagues, you, or anyone else ever know enough.

Why write this book then? Because I realized something during this, my fifth attempt. I realized—with my life partner, Hanna's, help—that much of what we do in life involves "diagnosis."

Meaning what? When you take your car to your mechanic, he tells you he's going to diagnose the problem. Same with your computer tech, your plumber, your "lawn doctor," and on and on.

What in the hell am I saying?

That the diagnostic principles I've offered you in this book apply to far more than mental health conditions. Rather, they apply to any and all situations which, in some way, involve human suffering. And that's most of life.

Have I just confused you? Think about it. We "diagnose" everything which involves suffering. This not only includes the suffering we experience when our minds struggle. It also includes the suffering we experience when our tools and technology malfunction. It should come as no surprise then that the way we diagnosis our stuff must have a lot in common with the way we diagnose ourselves. After all, we fashion most of our stuff in the likeness and image of our minds.

Ok. What else have I learned from writing this book?

Here's my short list. Nothing comprehensive. Just a (hopefully) brief list.

My Diagnostic Takeaways | A Short List

First and foremost is the significance of the tipping-point between ***Genuine Evidence*** vs ***Inferred Evidence***. Especially surprising is the degree to which all people infer. Most human beings do this constantly, all day long, hundreds of times a day. I had no idea and only discovered this later on in the writing of this book.

It seems, then, that inferring is the default mental state of most humans. Wow—what a waste of our brain power. We truly live in "the matrix"; a fake world of our own making and design.

An example of this fake world?

Imagine your water heater has malfunctioned.

Imagine you then call your repair person and during your call to him, he tells you what you "likely" need.

Obviously, he's inferred what you need.

He hasn't even visited your home, let alone looked at your water heater.

Now imagine that he's already told you that you likely need a new water heater. Imagine what you would have been feeling at the time. No hot water! Shit! So you infer he's right and decide to do this. But what if later, you find that all you actually needed (based on ***Genuine Evidence***) was a $5.00 part? What would you think then? Would you infer he was a shithead? A con man? A "dumb-as-a-stump," brain-dead moron? Worse yet, that you should have known?

Do you realize how many inferences are at play in this simple story? This example shows how quickly inferences can layer on top of one another. In truth, if all of this did happen to you, I'd bet the inferences would fly, fast and furious. For instance, many people would likely infer this repair person deliberately sold you something you didn't need. [Did you notice, I just inferred what many people would feel?]

Some kinder souls would infer he was simply overworked (his wife just had a baby?). Or they'd get mad and infer he was just plain stupid.

On and on and on the inferences would come. After all, the story involves suffering. The thing is, he wouldn't have been the only person who inferred when making this decision.

Given you hadn't seen it necessary to get a second estimate, you'd have inferred as well. Then again, the thought of "no hot water" can do that to people.

Now let me ask you. Do you think you rarely—if ever, infer things? Or if you do, then only in those urgent kinds of situations? If so, then try going through a single day without once inferring. Could you do it? Try. Or let me make it easier on you. What if I say you're allowed twenty inferences a day—but not one more.

Do you think you can manage to do this? A hint. If you can, then you have a superpower. Then again, to do this, you'd first need to learn to see yourself inferring *in real time*. Most people tell me, learning to see inferences—in real time—is really difficult. And we have yet to address the definition problem.

Are you sure you know what I mean by this word? You may. Then again, my current estimate of most people's ***Inferred*** to ***Genuine Evidence*** ratio is something like 95% / 5%. A whole lotta shakin' going on here.

How about a few hints as to what I mean by this word. For instance, do you know which situations people are most likely to infer in? The most common? Those times when you're faced with having a sticky conversation—a conversation which may lead to a fight, or to a rejection, or worse.

Getting fired. Getting left. Arguing until 3 AM. In times like these, people use inferences to try to plan what to say. In effect, they're mentally playing out what may happen so as to avoid the suffering.

Have you ever realized that when you do this, that your brain experiences these imaginary scenes as if they have actually happened?

Please take a minute to take this in. Know this claim has been scientifically studied and proven many times. Brain scans based on people picturing things estimate, we experience something like 90% of the real thing. In truth, the more skilled you are at these mental role plays (and the higher your IQ), the more likely you'll suffer like this in life.

Ironically, the inferences therapists make during sessions are the source of most of what they themselves struggle with during sessions. After all, most schools pressure talk therapists to make inferences about all manner of things in sessions. Despite the good motives behind these suggestions, these therapists suffer nonetheless. As do their clients when these therapists suggest "better inferences" and mistake these inferences for better mental health (CBT anyone?).

Ironically, therapist or not, these good intentions create a world of confusion and stress for everyone involved. This stress then multiplies when other people then infer hidden meanings in the inference which has just been said. Think I'm wrong? Then try my suggestion. Try going a single day without prefacing a conversation with mental attempts to tailor this conversation so it won't go badly.

Finally, know a good way to learn to see inferences in real time is by keeping a stroke count for just one day, each stroke marking one inference.

The takeaways here? I see quite a few. Here is but a short list.

A Few of My Takeaways

- Inferences are the source of 95% of all human suffering. Maybe more.
- All inferences are attempts to "predict the future and in doing so, avoid future suffering."
- This makes seeing inferences rather easy. Just notice when you are trying to predict the future. All inferences—even those which accurately draw on the past—are attempts to predict the future.
- The most egregious inferences? Hypotheses. All hypotheses are *attempts to predict the future.* Know this is true even when these predictions are done by the most talented and well-intentioned scientists.
- Indeed, based on this idea alone, we can say the reverse is true as well—*that all inferences are hypotheses.*
- Then there's the idea that most people believe in "cause and effect." The philosopher, David Hume, proved this wrong over five hundred years ago. In effect, he said, we can never actually see "cause and effect." We can only infer that it has happened based on the sequences in which things occur.
- Take a moment to take this in. All claims of cause and effect are inferences, based on seeing repetitions. This is why scientists design all lab-based experiments so they remove all but one or two variables. By doing this, they artificially up the odds their inferences will come true. But in real world situations where there are infinite variables? A whole lot of iffyness remains.
- Think what I just said is a whole lot of bullshit? Then consider medicine. The pills you take—are they guaranteed to change you in some exact way? Are they even guaranteed to work? Ever seen a guarantee on a pill label? And how much do inferences "that they will work" affect what we claim to feel?
- No surprise then that with all this guessing going on, that scientists so rarely make breakthroughs. And yes, when they do, these breakthroughs often benefit us greatly. But think of how much this success rate would go up were scientists to limit what they worked with to ***Genuine Evidence***. Then again, doing that would require gross admissions of how much their inference-based methods have caused them to fail. I "predict" this is not likely to happen anytime soon. I'm not sure it will ever happen.
- Next comes one of my most surprising realizations—***the idea that diagnoses can either be based on*** **"things that have already happened"** ***or on*** **"things diagnosticians predict may or will happen."**
- This gives us the critical tipping-point based measure needed to discern between genuine diagnoses and inferred diagnoses. Genuine diagnoses are based entirely on things which have already happened, even if only a moment ago. Whereas inferred diagnoses are based at least in part on things which may or may not occur in the future.
- This brings us to what I see as the biggest diagnostic takeaway of all. The entire point for giving diagnoses is to prevent past suffering from recurring.

Yet it seems, most diagnostic evidence comes from inferring the future. Ironically, gaining an accurate picture of the past and present IS the only way to guarantee the diagnosis you give today will be effective down the road. Why? Because the source of the vast majority of human suffering is "living in the future," as opposed to "living in the present." Meditators have known this forever. Diagnosticians? Not so much.

- My final takeaway? That to give your patients the best chance at having a better future, you must restrict the evidence you use to diagnose things which have already happened. At the same time, you must do your best to not contaminate this ***Genuine Evidence***, by inferring how this diagnosis will turn out. You are not Madame Zola, the Asbury Park boardwalk fortune teller. Unless you are. In which case, you have no business diagnosing. A genuine diagnosis refers only to the present moment's views of the past. Period. No exceptions.

My Most Surprising Personal Takeaway: *Compatibility*

Of all the things writing this book has led me to discover, the one I personally value the most has implications far beyond diagnosis. This realization has to do with how we diagnosticians do and do not connect to those we're looking to help.

In a word, I'm referring to "compatibility." How compatible are we with our patients? And is there anything we can do to up the chances we are compatible?

Where should we start? Let's start where I always begin, with how I define the word, "compatibility."

I define **compatibility** as ***"the degree to which two people are being themselves with each other."***

Obviously, defining compatibility this way can have no real meaning until and unless I also define the phrase "being themselves" as well.

How then do I define "being themselves?"

When two people ***ARE being themselves,*** these two people are together, exchanging ***Genuine Evidence***.

Conversely, when two people are ***NOT being themselves***, these two people are together, exchanging Inferences.

Can this single idea be what's been missing from our understanding of how relationships work? I am claiming, it is. In fact, I am claiming, this is the main source of suffering in all of our relationships.

I only wish I'd known this back in 2011, when my book on personality was first published (***Unraveling Human Nature***, 2011). In this book, I'd originally planned to discuss what I call "The Four Primary Motives" in human nature.

What I did write—and publish in that book— was a chapter on the first three motives. I then wrote a chapter on the fourth motive, but decided to omit it, as it seemed to stray too far from the book's main points.

So what is The Fourth Motive in human nature?

To predict the future and in doing so, prevent future suffering.

Now, thirteen years later, I see why I felt that chapter didn't fit. Were it written correctly, the chapter would have stated, and focused on, what I've been saying about inferring things. For instance, I would have said, "Making inferences IS the main mechanism with which human beings try to satisfy the Fourth Motive." I would also have then added that there are two main things these inferences do.

Better late than never. Here they are.

One—We Almost Exclusively Infer About Avoiding Bad Things

Similar to newspapers and news commentators, inferences almost always focus on bad news. The human mind pays fleetingly little, if any, attention to good news. And yes, newspapers and news commentators do occasionally focus a bit on ***Genuine Evidence***. But more often, they focus on inferring the terrible things which they claim may or will likely happen.

Extending this a bit further, some say we live in the "a-factual age." Translation. Most of what we get fed as facts are either taken out of context or altered to create false beliefs. Here, the "a" refers to the Latin prefix for *not* or *without*. For example, the "a" in the word, "amnesia," means *not* able to remember things. So the "a" in a-factual refers to something people claim is a fact, but which is supported by little to no ***Genuine Evidence***. So it's not a fact. It's bullshit.

Two—The Mind Treats Inferences As Facts; as Something That Has Happened

Once the mind infers something, the mind then treats this thing as something that has already happened. And technically, this is true. It did happen—but it only happened in the person's mind. Despite this statement being obviously accurate, the mind sees little difference between ***Genuine Evidence*** (things which have already happened) and ***Inferred Evidence*** (things which we imagine may happen in the future).

Why?

The Fourth Motive.

We so feel the need to predict the future, in order to prevent future suffering.

Now come back to where we began a moment ago, with my definition for compatibility. **Compatibility** is ***"the degree to which two people are being themselves with each other."*** And when two people ***ARE being themselves***, these two people are together, exchanging ***Genuine Evidence***.

My claim here? That making inferences means people are not being themselves. This renders one or both of these two people incompatible with the other.

A Few Places To Look When Trying To Find Inferences

- When you **Rehearse For What May Be Difficult Conversations.**
- When you **Hear A Word You Don't Know And Try To Guess The Meaning.**
- Anytime you use **Statistics.** Statistics is 100% inference and is an example of the "gambler's fallacy."

- Whenever you **Resent Someone** (all resentments are based on inferences).
- Anytime you **Trust a Clothing Size Label** (all clothing size labels are based on statistical inferences about size).
- Whenever you **Blame Someone** (all blame is based on inferences about cause and effect).
- Whenever you **Punish Someone** (all punishment is based on inferences).
- Whenever you **Do Damage Control** (restrain yourself). All damage control stems from inferences about the future.
- Whenever you are sure "**Plans Are Not Going To Work Out**."
- Inferring in general about **What Body Sensations Mean About Your Health**. For example, when you feel sure a headache means you have a brain tumor.
- Whenever you try to predict how you **Will Feel In The Future**. For instance, if I marry so and so, I will live happily ever after.
- Whenever you think you know how a new relationship, job, or situation **Will Turn Out**.

Using Context Independence to Determine Minority Personalities

Like all writers of technical books, there is always more to say. That's because, by writing a book, you learn to see the incompleteness in the things you thought you knew. My work on Minority Personalities is currently more than two decades old. Yet the implications of this idea may extend far beyond my lifetime.

I personally pray they will.

As for what I've discovered about them during the writing of this book, there are quite a few things. Diagnostically, the most significant is this.

To begin with, as I've said in this book, there are four Minority Personalities. I've written about this idea for years. Here, each Minority Personality has its own bias towards what is, and is not, considered useful ***context***.

What this means is that, because each Minority Personality has a single Social Priority which eclipses the other three, people with Minority Personalities limit the context for their life events to things which fit this one priority.

- For the AS type, the context is limited to Meaning and Understanding.
- For the OCD type, the context is limited to Neatness and Organization.
- For the KA type, the context is limited to Comfort and Sensation.
- For the ADD type, the context is limited to Social Freedom.

What I realized only after reaching this point in my writing is how this bias can be used during diagnosis—specifically, to discern between Majority and Minority personalities. For people with Majority Personalities, all four Social Priorities can be considered. For people with a Minority Personality however, people limit the context of life events to one of the four classes of context—and this bias then blinds them to all the rest. In effect, the rest just get ignored.

What does this have to do with diagnosis? More important, how can knowing these four things help diagnosticians to identify each of these four Minority Personalities? At this point, I must apologize. I've no space to properly describe this to you. What I will offer is yet another hopefully brief story.

The following story outlines how I've begun to use this realization in therapy sessions. This case involves a middle-aged man we will call Harold. Harold has the OCD Minority Personality. Like me, Harold's son, Benjamin, has the AS Minority Personality. Do you see it yet? Both of these people have a different Minority Personality. So they cannot understand what the other is saying. Why? Because each one creates the context for life events from a different kind of data.

This story involves how I recently taught them to speak to each other, this after years of being unable to understand what the other said. To begin with, these two men are both engineers by profession. Harold is a civil engineer and works for a major transportation agency. Benjamin is a nuclear engineer and works for a major company as well.

People with Minority Personalities often chose STEM based technical careers. These careers are usually highly technical but focus less on interpersonal relationships. Here, people's actual choices get based largely on whichever Social Priority remains visible. Harold and Benjamin were no exceptions.

Harold's visible priority is Neatness and Organization. So organizing details is his forte, and this causes him to struggle with interpersonal relationships. Whereas Benjamin's visible priority is Meaning and Understanding. So his forte is rapidly understanding critical situations. Except when they involve interpersonal relationships.

In Harold's case, his bias has repeatedly led to him getting in trouble—mainly for taking too long to deliver reports. OCD at its finest. He cannot turn in work without creating and organizing every single detail. Nothing can be left out, no matter how insignificant or small. So most of what he does gets delivered late.

Benjamin, on the other hand, has been falsely accused, at work, of inappropriate behaviors towards others. I know him well. None of these accusations have a shred of merit. The thing is, most of his understanding of human relationships is context independent. So he's frequently quiet and awkward, especially with female coworkers, leading them to at times misunderstand his motives.

The point here? To see it, first set aside any thoughts as to their workplace difficulties. Our focus here will be on teaching them to be able to talk to each other. I recently spent about six weeks introducing Harold to the idea that each Minority Personality uses a different context for conversations. This amounts to picking and using words differently.

Those with OCD—and most people whose first Social Priority is Neatness, see conversations as a time to offer the other person copious amounts of details.

Those with AS—and most people whose first Social Priority is Understanding, see conversations as a time to offer the other person copious amounts of "subheads."

Subheads?

To see what I mean, take a moment to look at the subhead on this page.

Can you see how I offer the reader both kinds of data?

And over the years, I've learned that most people never read the subheads. People with AS cannot do this. They need subheads in order to organize the words which come next. In effect, these subheads function like book-page street signs. They each create a "Meaning and Understanding-based" context for the section that follows.

This then allows AS minds to organize what they then begin to read. They literally know what mental neighborhood they're in. The point?

When Harold talked to his son, he would never offer subheads. All he'd offer was endless details, all of which only further confused his son.

In a way, all these details would be like puzzle pieces falling onto Benjamin's mental floor. And the more Benjamin would get lost, the more details Harold would offer him. Meanwhile, Benjamin would be begging Harold to give him a subhead (a mental road sign) to guide him. But this only resulted in Harold giving Benjamin even more details.

Harold's context for everything he says and does gets created from just the details. So he mistakenly thought Benjamin wasn't understanding him because he hadn't given Benjamin enough details. Benjamin creates the context for what he hears from the gist of what's being said. But when he asked his father for this gist, all he got was more details.

Now, only weeks later, they've had several good conversations, all because I taught them to see their contextual biases. Diagnosticians can watch for this and use what they see in many ways. Look for a high proportion of straight lines of ideas in conversations. Possibly AS. Look for the absence of straight lines of ideas and the presence of endlessly meandering details. Here, it's possible the person has OCD.

What Do We Do With The Existing Diagnostic Manual?

A question I've not addressed anywhere in this book is, "What do we do with the existing diagnostic manual?" Obviously, for our clients to be reimbursed—and until someone creates a more adequate dictionary of symptoms (this person won't be me), we will all need to continue to use that "manual."

So what good is this book, if that one is the authority?

That other book is merely an overstuffed collection of cold-hearted dictionary style definitions.

In no way does it offer any guidance as to how to actually use it, let alone offer proper definitions.

This book, on the other hand, is an actual manual.

It's a how-to guide to diagnosing with kindness—a guide to treating suffering people with the empathy and compassion they deserve.

For now, then, these two books must be used together.

To do this, you'll need to be familiar with the diagnoses in that other book.

At the same time, when that other book refers to words like "depression" or "mania," you'll use the visual definitions in this book. Then, and only then, you will use this book to guide you through the evidence gathering process, including that you let the diagnosis emerge from this evidence naturally.

Hopefully, in this way, we will all learn to better offer suffering people kindness. This includes using the drawings in this book to teach suffering people what their diagnosis means.

Closing Comments And Thoughts on Future Books

As some may have noticed, this is the fifth book in this series. The first book, which documents the flow of Information in the mind, was released in 2010. That book is now almost 15 years old. Yet despite this time passing, nothing in the present book contradicts what's in that first book. Indeed, were you to read all five books in order, you'd find, each book merely refines and adds detail to the previous books.

Why mention this?

Because books based on conventional science tend to age poorly. As new discoveries are made, previous "discoveries" must get "revised," usually by adding ad hoc corrections. These five books, however, are based on a new scientific method which guarantees nothing ever needs to change—or be revised. Hence my saying nothing in this book contradicts what's in the previous four books.

My point?

I expect many readers will claim this book isn't based on actual science. Please do try to hold off on making these judgements until you can study this new method for yourself. How? By reading the third book—The Science of Discovery. In it, I've thoroughly documented this new method in ways which hopefully will address any concerns. Please try to avoid **skimming** through any of my books, including that one. At best, all you'll come away with is a terrible feeling that none of it makes sense.

These books make sense only if you put in the time to actually read them.

What's coming next? God willing, I'll get to finish my planned next book. My friend and coauthor of book 4, Sam, has been encouraging me to write this book for years. No title exists yet. It may be another in the lineage of the "what you've been told is bullshit" line. Or not.

The subject? ***Everything You Thought You Knew About* Love *Is* ….**

Think about it.

Everything in the present book also applies to every part of every human relationship. Correctly defining our struggles is but one part of connecting to each other. I'd like to think that I'll leave the planet having made a lasting difference in people's lives. And what better way than to up the bar for what is surely our most important asset—love.

And with that said, I wish you all well.

Until the next book,

Steven